Nanocarriers-Based Antimicrobial Drug Delivery

Nanocarriers-Based Antimicrobial Drug Delivery

Guest Editor

Anisha D'Souza

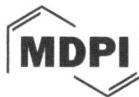

Basel • Beijing • Wuhan • Barcelona • Belgrade • Novi Sad • Cluj • Manchester

Guest Editor
Anisha D'Souza
Otolaryngology–Massachusetts
Eye and Ear Infirmary
Harvard Medical School
Boston
United States

Editorial Office
MDPI AG
Grosspeteranlage 5
4052 Basel, Switzerland

This is a reprint of the Special Issue, published open access by the journal *Antibiotics* (ISSN 2079-6382), freely accessible at: www.mdpi.com/journal/antibiotics/special_issues/UZ724F964Q.

For citation purposes, cite each article independently as indicated on the article page online and using the guide below:

Lastname, A.A.; Lastname, B.B. Article Title. *Journal Name* **Year**, *Volume Number*, Page Range.

ISBN 978-3-7258-2874-6 (Hbk)
ISBN 978-3-7258-2873-9 (PDF)
https://doi.org/10.3390/books978-3-7258-2873-9

© 2024 by the authors. Articles in this book are Open Access and distributed under the Creative Commons Attribution (CC BY) license. The book as a whole is distributed by MDPI under the terms and conditions of the Creative Commons Attribution-NonCommercial-NoDerivs (CC BY-NC-ND) license (https://creativecommons.org/licenses/by-nc-nd/4.0/).

Contents

Preface . . . . **vii**

Ariane Boudier, Nour Mammari, Emmanuel Lamouroux and Raphaël E. Duval
Inorganic Nanoparticles: Tools to Emphasize the Janus Face of Amphotericin B
Reprinted from: *Antibiotics* **2023**, *12*, 1543, https://doi.org/10.3390/antibiotics12101543 . . . . . **1**

John Jackson and Claudia Helena Dietrich
Synergistic Antibacterial Effects of Gallate Containing Compounds with Silver Nanoparticles in Gallate Crossed Linked PVA Hydrogel Films
Reprinted from: *Antibiotics* **2024**, *13*, 312, https://doi.org/10.3390/antibiotics13040312 . . . . . . **22**

Sinazo Z. Z. Cobongela, Maya M. Makatini, Bambesiwe May, Zikhona Njengele-Tetyana, Mokae F. Bambo and Nicole R. S. Sibuyi
Antibacterial Activity and Cytotoxicity Screening of Acyldepsipeptide-1 Analogues Conjugated to Silver/Indium/Sulphide Quantum Dots
Reprinted from: *Antibiotics* **2024**, *13*, 183, https://doi.org/10.3390/antibiotics13020183 . . . . . . **37**

Jolanta Flieger, Sylwia Pasieczna-Patkowska, Natalia Żuk, Rafał Panek, Izabela Korona-Głowniak and Katarzyna Suśniak et al.
Characteristics and Antimicrobial Activities of Iron Oxide Nanoparticles Obtained via Mixed-Mode Chemical/Biogenic Synthesis Using Spent Hop (*Humulus lupulus* L.) Extracts
Reprinted from: *Antibiotics* **2024**, *13*, 111, https://doi.org/10.3390/antibiotics13020111 . . . . . . **50**

Ance Bārzdiņa, Aiva Plotniece, Arkadij Sobolev, Karlis Pajuste, Dace Bandere and Agnese Brangule
From Polymeric Nanoformulations to Polyphenols—Strategies for Enhancing the Efficacy and Drug Delivery of Gentamicin
Reprinted from: *Antibiotics* **2024**, *13*, 305, https://doi.org/10.3390/antibiotics13040305 . . . . . . **69**

Luana Dutra de Carvalho, Bernardo Urbanetto Peres, Ya Shen, Markus Haapasalo, Hazuki Maezono and Adriana P. Manso et al.
Chlorhexidine-Containing Electrospun Polymeric Nanofibers for Dental Applications: An *In Vitro* Study
Reprinted from: *Antibiotics* **2023**, *12*, 1414, https://doi.org/10.3390/antibiotics12091414 . . . . . **94**

Muhammed Awad, Timothy J. Barnes and Clive A. Prestidge
Lyophilized Lipid Liquid Crystalline Nanoparticles as an Antimicrobial Delivery System
Reprinted from: *Antibiotics* **2023**, *12*, 1405, https://doi.org/10.3390/antibiotics12091405 . . . . . **106**

Olivia Lili Zhang, John Yun Niu, Iris Xiaoxue Yin, Ollie Yiru Yu, May Lei Mei and Chun Hung Chu
Antibacterial Properties of the Antimicrobial Peptide Gallic Acid-Polyphemusin I (GAPI)
Reprinted from: *Antibiotics* **2023**, *12*, 1350, https://doi.org/10.3390/antibiotics12091350 . . . . . **117**

Khadeejeh AL-Smadi, Vania Rodrigues Leite-Silva, Newton Andreo Filho, Patricia Santos Lopes and Yousuf Mohammed
Innovative Approaches for Maintaining and Enhancing Skin Health and Managing Skin Diseases through Microbiome-Targeted Strategies
Reprinted from: *Antibiotics* **2023**, *12*, 1698, https://doi.org/10.3390/antibiotics12121698 . . . . . **129**

Ali M. Nasr, Noha M. Badawi, Yasmine H. Tartor, Nader M. Sobhy and Shady A. Swidan
Development, Optimization, and In Vitro/In Vivo Evaluation of Azelaic Acid Transethosomal
Gel for Antidermatophyte Activity
Reprinted from: *Antibiotics* **2023**, *12*, 707, https://doi.org/10.3390/antibiotics12040707 . . . . . . **147**

Preface

Fighting microbial infections has become increasingly difficult due to the rapid emergence of multi-drug resistance. Infectious diseases caused by microorganisms can range from acute, short-term illnesses to chronic and long-lasting conditions. Intracellular pathogens, such as those responsible for brucellosis, salmonellosis, and tuberculosis, target the body's initial defense mechanisms—macrophages and other non-professional phagocytes—where they continue to survive and multiply. In contrast, extracellular pathogens, which cause conditions like pneumonia, osteomyelitis, and scarlet fever, employ virulent strategies to evade immune defenses and reproduce outside host cells.

Nanocarriers—ranging from polymer- and lipid-based systems, liposomes, micelles, metal-based carriers, silica nanoparticles, fullerenes, dendrimers, zeolites, and quantum dots to hydrogels and composites—have been investigated for their antimicrobial properties in various infections, including those associated with biofilms. However, the selection of appropriate nanocarriers for targeting intracellular versus extracellular pathogens requires careful design and innovation. These carriers must be tailored to enhance specific microbial targeting, overcome drug resistance, minimize toxicity, and disrupt biofilms while also expanding their potential for theranostic applications and use in cosmeceuticals.

This reprint delves into the various polymeric and inorganic nanocarrier formulations developed to enhance the effectiveness of drugs such as gentamicin and amphotericin. It also explores novel strategies for managing skin health through microbiome-targeted therapies. Additionally, this reprint presents original research regarding improving the antimicrobial activity of drug conjugates, nanoparticle-based formulations, and nanosized materials for a range of applications, from dental care to skincare.

We are pleased to present this reprint to the scientific community and anticipate that it will foster continued advancements and innovations in the field of nanotechnology application for microbial infection management. We sincerely thank all the contributors for their valuable expertise, dedication, and commitment to furthering this critical area of research. Their contributions have been instrumental in making this reprint possible, and we are confident that it will serve as an essential reference for future studies and applications in the field.

Anisha D'Souza
Guest Editor

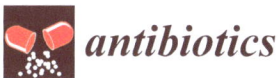

Review

Inorganic Nanoparticles: Tools to Emphasize the Janus Face of Amphotericin B

Ariane Boudier [1,*], Nour Mammari [2], Emmanuel Lamouroux [2] and Raphaël E. Duval [2,3,*]

1. Université de Lorraine, CITHEFOR, F-54000 Nancy, France
2. Université de Lorraine, CNRS, L²CM, F-54000 Nancy, France; nour.mammari@univ-lorraine.fr (N.M.); emmanuel.lamouroux@univ-lorraine.fr (E.L.)
3. ABC Platform®, F-54505 Vandœuvre-lès-Nancy, France
* Correspondence: ariane.boudier@univ-lorraine.fr (A.B.); raphael.duval@univ-lorraine.fr (R.E.D.)

Abstract: Amphotericin B is the oldest antifungal molecule which is still currently widely used in clinical practice, in particular for the treatment of invasive diseases, even though it is not devoid of side effects (particularly nephrotoxicity). Recently, its redox properties (i.e., both prooxidant and antioxidant) have been highlighted in the literature as mechanisms involved in both its activity and its toxicity. Interestingly, similar properties can be described for inorganic nanoparticles. In the first part of the present review, the redox properties of Amphotericin B and inorganic nanoparticles are discussed. Then, in the second part, inorganic nanoparticles as carriers of the drug are described. A special emphasis is given to their combined redox properties acting either as a prooxidant or as an antioxidant and their connection to the activity against pathogens (i.e., fungi, parasites, and yeasts) and to their toxicity. In a majority of the published studies, inorganic nanoparticles carrying Amphotericin B are described as having a synergistic activity directly related to the rupture of the redox homeostasis of the pathogen. Due to the unique properties of inorganic nanoparticles (e.g., magnetism, intrinsic anti-infectious properties, stimuli-triggered responses, etc.), these nanomaterials may represent a new generation of medicine that can synergistically enhance the antimicrobial properties of Amphotericin B.

Keywords: redox properties; oxidative stress; Amphotericin B; antimicrobial; inorganic nanomaterials

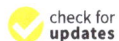

Citation: Boudier, A.; Mammari, N.; Lamouroux, E.; Duval, R.E. Inorganic Nanoparticles: Tools to Emphasize the Janus Face of Amphotericin B. *Antibiotics* **2023**, *12*, 1543. https://doi.org/10.3390/antibiotics12101543

Academic Editor: Anisha D'Souza

Received: 25 September 2023
Revised: 11 October 2023
Accepted: 13 October 2023
Published: 15 October 2023

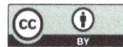

Copyright: © 2023 by the authors. Licensee MDPI, Basel, Switzerland. This article is an open access article distributed under the terms and conditions of the Creative Commons Attribution (CC BY) license (https://creativecommons.org/licenses/by/4.0/).

1. Introduction

Amphotericin B (AmB) is the leading compound of the polyene macrolide family, so named because of the numerous conjugated double bonds in a large macrolactone ring (Figure 1). Its structure also contains a polyol domain and a deoxysugar mycosamine group.

AmB is an old molecule as it was first discovered and extracted in the 1950s in Venezuela from *Streptomyces nodosus* [1,2]. The molecule rapidly reached the market after the FDA approved it in 1958 [2]. AmB is considered to have a broad spectrum of activity not only on fungi (i.e., filamentous, molds, yeasts, etc.) but also on parasites (e.g., Leishmania). Thus, AmB is efficient against different fungal genera/species: *Candida* spp., *Aspergillus* spp., *Histoplasma capsulatum*, *Coccidioides immitis*, *Blastomyces dermatitidis*, *Rhodotorula* spp., *Cryptococcus neoformans*, *Sporothrix schenkii*, *Fusarium* spp., *Cladosporium* spp., *Scytalidium* spp., and Zygomycetes. Conversely, the genera/species *Candida lusitaniae*, *Candida auris*, *Trichosporon* spp., *Geotrichum* spp., *Scedosporium* spp., *Fusarium* spp., and *Aspergillus terreus* are resistant or less sensitive to this molecule [3,4]. It should be noted that resistance to polyenes still remains rare (i.e., compared to resistance to other antifungal drugs, such as azoles). Furthermore, although several mechanisms of resistance to polyenes have been described in the literature, the main mechanism of resistance remains associated with a modification in the sterol composition at the level of the cell membrane or even a depletion of ergosterol, attributable to gene-level mutations involved in its biosynthesis [5,6]. Noteworthily, it is more and more common to find conflicting data regarding the activity of AmB against different fungal species/strains in the literature [4].

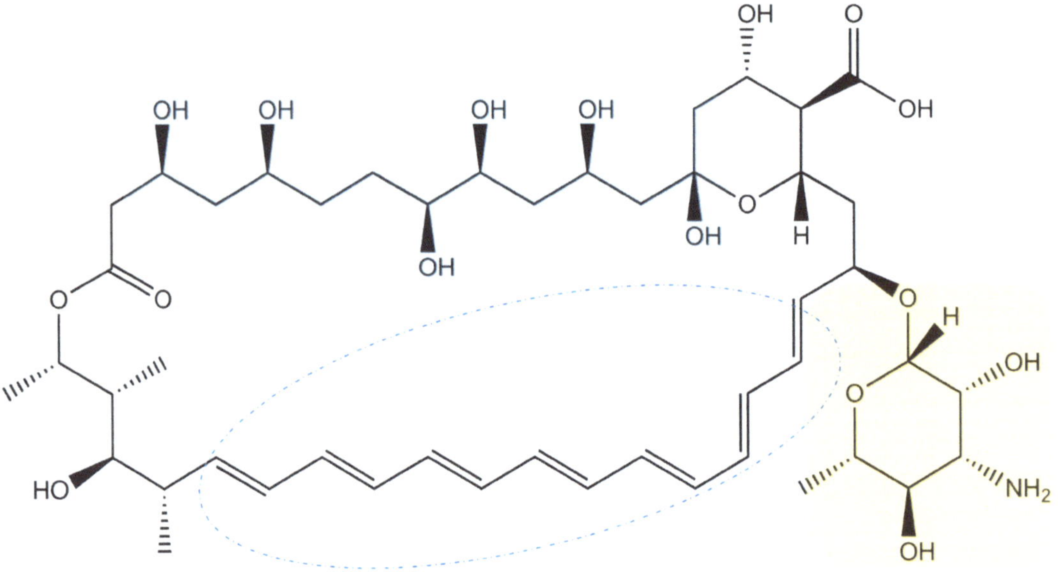

Figure 1. Molecular structure of AmB. Blue zone: polyol domain, yellow zone: deoxysugar mycosamine group.

The affinity of AmB for the ergosterol of the membranes of microorganisms gives it its selective microbial activity. This selectivity is only slightly higher compared to that of cholesterol from mammalian cell membranes, making its therapeutic efficacy very narrow [4–6]. Considering the structure of the compound, studies demonstrated that the dimers forming AmB are toxic for eukaryotic cells. While the polyaggregated forms present reduced resistance for host cells, they retain antiparasitic activity at the same time [7]. AmB is mainly used in monotherapy, rarely as first-line, except for in the management of serious systemic fungal infections. AmB can also be used in combination with other antifungals such as flucytosine or fluconazole depending on particular clinical situations [8]. However, treatment with AmB is not devoid of side effects, which occur in 25 to 90% of patients [3,9]. The reported symptoms range from infusion-related reactions up to anaphylaxis, which can be prevented by drugs (e.g., corticoids, antihistamines, analgesics, etc.). Another serious side effect is a significant risk of nephrotoxicity which limits its use [10]. The formulation of AmB is an important topic of research with the aim to develop forms which improve its therapeutic effect and lead to less nephrotoxicity [11,12]. All the formulations are based on lipidic compounds mixed with AmB due to the amphiphilic nature of the antifungal. The lipid formulations of AmB which have been developed are either AmB in a colloidal dispersion, or AmB in a lipid complex or liposomal AmB. Thus, these three formulations differ in their lipid composition and therefore in their physical and pharmacokinetic characteristics, their efficacy, and their tolerance to efficacy [13]. Evidence has been shown that self-assembled mixed micelles containing AmB based on a combination of lecithin with polymers have reduced in vitro cytotoxicity and improved AmB solubility results with increased parenteral and oral bioavailability in rats compared to Fungizone® [14]. Moreover, the oral administration of AmB encapsulated in nanoparticles (N-palmitoyl-N-methyl-N,N-dimethyl-N,N,N-trimethyl-6-O-glycol chitosan) has also showed high efficacy in mouse models of candidiasis, aspergillosis or visceral leishmaniasis compared to AmBisome® administered parenterally [15]. Data have highlighted that using the lipid-based formulation of AmB is more expensive than conventional micellar deoxycholate AmB, which is why its use is limited in clinical practice [3,4]. This evidence has been discussed in numerous bibliographic reviews presenting the various formulations of AmB. Table S1 summarizes and compares the main content of these studies, and these will not be emphasized in the present paper. The development of an orally active formulation of AmB capable of reducing the systemic drug toxicity, avoiding infusion-related adverse events, improving patient compliance, and reducing the costs associated with the intravenous administration of commercial formulations of AmB is an urgent requirement. Up until now, in contrast to lipid formulations, no inorganic nanoparticles, as an agent to carry AmB, have been brought to clinical trials. However, they have unique specific properties (such as magnetic, optical, redox, etc.) that can be added to those of AmB or beneficially influence those of AmB synergistically. Moreover, there are many reports of the pre-clinical development of such objects as carriers of AmB or for the development other anti-infectious strategies [16]. Inorganic nanoparticles are structured with a well-organized core made of metal or carbon atoms surrounded by an organic corona (i.e., inorganic/organic core–shell particles). The core can bring, depending on the material it is made with, magnetic or optical properties, while the corona can be functionalized by drugs (e.g., AmB) or other molecules. They represent ideal tools for the targeting and the recognition of the site of action (antibody, aptamer, substrate for an enzyme, ligand for a receptor) [17]. They can be combined with other properties (i.e., interact with radiation) to succeed in the development of nano-objects dedicated for both therapy and diagnostics (i.e., theranostic) [17,18]. These nanoparticles often exhibit redox properties. This is very interesting since it has now also been described that AmB is characterized by both oxidant and reductive activities, usually known as a Janus face. Indeed, Janus was a Roman god depicted with two faces; one looking ahead, the other behind.

In this review, in the first step, the similarities between inorganic nanoparticles and AmB will be emphasized according to their redox character. In the second step, the different strategies to synthesize inorganic nanoparticles as AmB carriers will be discussed. A specific emphasis will be given to the capacity of inorganic nanoparticles to enhance either the prooxidant or the antioxidant effects of AmB. An explanation of the involved mechanisms and the synergistic anti-infectious effects will be described, which represents the originality of the present review.

2. Similarities in Redox Behaviors between Amphotericin B and Inorganic Nanoparticles

2.1. Redox Properties of Amphotericin B

2.1.1. The Janus Face of Amphotericin B

AmB possesses a double role, either as a prooxidant or, in some publications, as an antioxidant. The main mechanisms for this are illustrated in Figure 2. This redox role is implied in the mechanism of anti-infectious action, as well as other (such as polyene-sterol: ergosterol) interactions leading to membrane destabilization with pore formation and/or surface adsorption and/or the formation of sterol aggregates (or "sponges") outside the cell membrane causing the loss of ions and the accumulation of reactive oxygen species (ROS) [5,19,20].

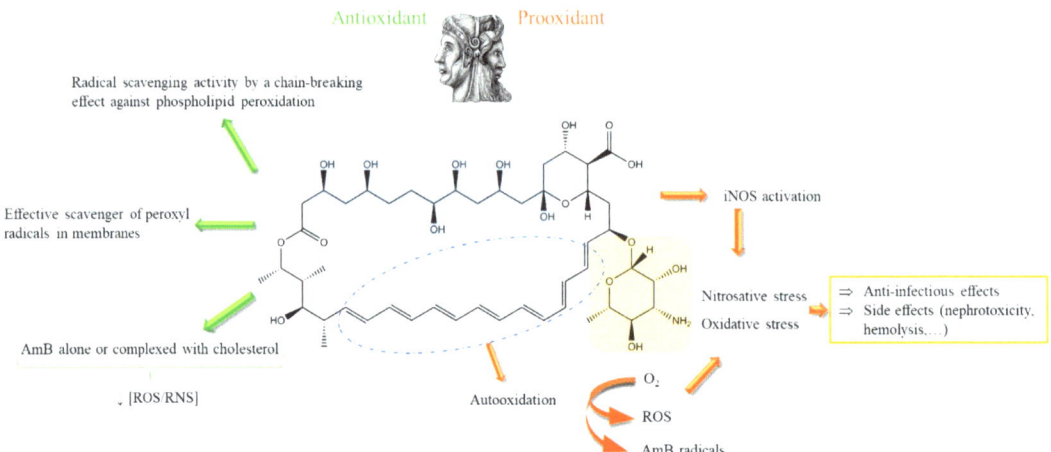

Figure 2. Janus face of AmB: prooxidant and antioxidant effects described in [5,21–23]. ROS: reactive oxygen species; RNS: reactive nitrogen species; iNOS: inducible nitric oxide synthase.

The prooxidant effect of AmB is quite significantly described in the literature. It leads to both oxidative and nitrosative stresses through the expression of stress genes, including an increase in the inducible form of nitric oxide synthase, the generation of ROS and reactive nitrogen species (RNS), respectively, and the production of proinflammatory cytokines [5,20,21]. Radicals originating from AmB itself were also identified using electron-spin resonance (ESR) spectroscopy [24]. Oxidative and nitrosative stresses damage the plasma membrane, the intracellular proteins, the mitochondria activity, and the nucleic acids [5]. AmB has been shown to have the ability to trigger a common dependent cell death pathway through oxidative damage in fungi such as *Candida albicans*, *Saccharomyces cerevisiae* or *Cryptococcus gattii* via the production of ROS in a tricarboxylic acid cycle and respiratory chain-dependent manner impacting, consequently, the inhibition of its DNA repair systems [20,25–27].

It is worth underlining that the antioxidant property of AmB is less described in the literature. The antioxidant effect may originate from the polyol part of the molecule [21]. It was evidenced in vitro [22] and was also highlighted in rat aortic smooth muscle cells [23]. This dual behavior has already been described for other molecules such as retinol [28], ascorbic acid [29] or Trolox [30]. As a function of the imposed conditions, a conversion from one property of AmB to the other (i.e., pro- to anti-oxidant and vice versa) may occur. The questions of how important the antioxidant phenomenon is, or how the equilibrium between the prooxidant and antioxidant properties of AmB is balanced, for the activity and/or toxicity of AmB, remain unsolved. These issues are extremely difficult to address due to the intimate interdependence of this phenomenon.

2.1.2. Amphotericin B Activity, Resistance, and Toxicity, and Its Possible Modulation

The impact of both oxidative and nitrosative stresses are well-described for AmB activity in fungi (i.e., filamentous, molds, yeasts, etc.) and parasites [5,26,31], as well as for AmB-resistant pathogens [5,31–33]. These elements were deeply reviewed by Carolus and coll. recently [5]. One less-studied aspect in the literature is the impact of oxidative and nitrosative stresses on AmB-induced toxicity. These stresses are identified as actors in the induced side effects of AmB in clinical settings, on kidney and liver [34–37]. Its dose-dependent toxicity is caused by ROS (and maybe also by RNS, even if this is usually less studied) and the oxidized forms of AmB.

Because of the consequences implied by oxidative and nitrosative stresses on AmB activity, resistance, and toxicity, the modulation of redox status by the co-administration of other oxidants or antioxidants with AmB has been considered by researchers with the aim of the enhancement of its anti-infectious property and/or limitations of its toxicity [5]. A great variety of components were shown to enhance AmB activity when co-administered with redox-potent molecules. For example, Kim and coll. showed that thymol enhances AmB activity on *Candida albicans* and *Candida krusei* [38]. They also demonstrated that dihydroxybenzaldehydes promote AmB activity against *C. albicans*, *C. krusei*, *C. tropicalis*, and *Cryptococcus neoformans* [39]. One can also mention the effect of butylated hydroxyanisole, *n*-propylgallate, or nordihydroguaiaretic acid on *C. albicans* and *C. parapsilosis* [40], and ascorbic acid on *Aspergillus terreus* [41]. The four involved mechanisms were (i) the co-disruption of the redox signaling on the response capacity of pathogens [39], (ii) the targeting of at least one common cellular component in the antioxidant system of the organism [39], (iii) a prolonged duration of AmB activity via a stabilizing effect probably preventing its auto-oxidation and stabilizing the polyene moiety of the molecule [39,40], and (iv) a synergistic prooxidant effect, increasing the concentration of ROS, lowering the minimal inhibitory concentration (MIC) and restoring the sensitive phenotype of a AmB-resistant strain [41].

On the contrary, well-known antioxidants failed to induce any anti-infectious activity. *N*-acetylcysteine (a precursor of glutathione) improved the survival of *A. fumigatus* in the presence of AmB [42]. This molecule also showed a protective effect against ROS induced by AmB in *Aspergillus terreus* [41]. Similarly, the addition of reduced glutathione or cysteine revived the endospores of *Coccidioides immitis* previously treated with AmB by modulating the redox potential of the medium [43]. In parallel, cysteine stopped the AmB-mediated growth inhibition of *C. albicans* [44].

Several redox-balancing agents were also tested to counterbalance the toxicity induced by AmB. For example, pre-treatment with diosmin hesperidin in Wistar rats followed by AmB administration showed an antioxidant protective effect on the kidneys [36]. In another study, the co-administration of vitamins A and E with AmB attenuated the side effect of the antifungal on the kidneys and liver of Wistar rats. The combination of both vitamins was more efficient than each vitamin alone [37]. Another antioxidant, caffeic acid phenethyl ester, showed an effectiveness as an adjuvant agent for AmB nephrotoxicity in rat models [34].

In addition, the mechanisms of AmB resistance of certain clinical isolates such as the *Candida haemulonii* species complex (*C. haemulonii*, *C. duobushaemulonii*, *C. haemulonii* var. *vulnera*) have been explored. Consequently, studies on the molecular composition of the wall in this group of fungi revealed that the vast majority of the membrane sterols were intermediates of the ergosterol pathway, and not ergosterol itself, highlighting the absence of an AmB target and thus explaining (at least in part) the resistance phenotype [45]. These results were supported by the fact that the deletion of the genes encoding ergosterol (*ERG11* and *ERG3* genes; encoding lanosterol 14-demethylase and C-5-sterin desaturase, respectively) affect the resistance of *C. lusitaniae* and of *Saccharomyces cerevisiae* strains [46–48]. Thus, a decrease in sterol (i.e., ergosterol) content causes a decrease in the membrane permeability to the compound [45]. The majority of studies have shown that AmB induces the formation of ROS as described above; however, this phenomenon was slightly observed in the strains of the *C. haemulonii* species complex. Evidence has determined that these fungal strains have undergone an alteration of the respiratory chain: poor growth in unfermented carbon sources, low oxygen consumption, and an alteration of mitochondrial membrane potential. These data explain the resistance presented in this multi-resistant fungal complex with respect to AmB [45].

2.2. Redox Properties of Inorganic Nanoparticles

There are important similarities between the behaviors of AmB and inorganic nanoparticles as they are both characterized by prooxidant and antioxidant properties. Inorganic nanoparticles behave as redox-potent agents using an important variety of mechanisms which are depicted in Figure 3. For a detailed view of this chemistry, the reader is referred to the following reviews [48–53].

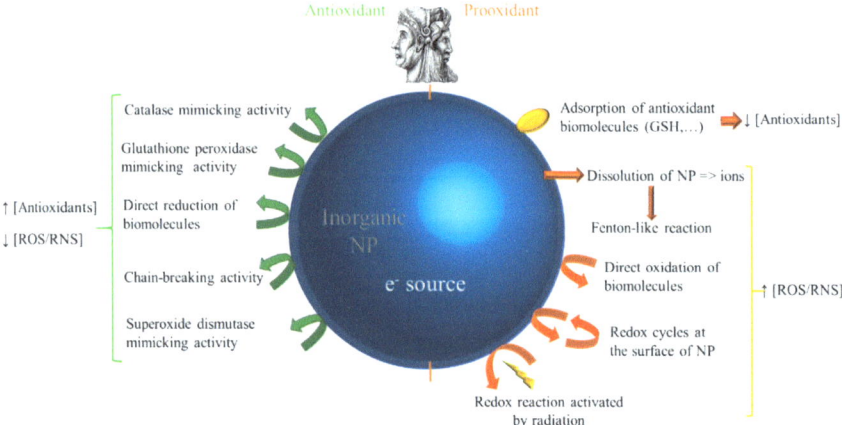

Figure 3. Summary of the main mechanisms conferring antioxidant or prooxidant properties to inorganic nanoparticles. ROS: reactive oxygen species; RNS: reactive nitrogen species; GSH: reduced glutathione; NP: nanoparticle.

Nanoparticles interfere with the redox homeostasis of a medium via different pathways: either directly, e.g., by providing electrons for the direct self-conversion of an antioxidant to a prooxidant molecule and vice versa [54], or indirectly, e.g., by the nanoparticle degradation via dissolution [55] or upon radiation [56].

The redox properties of nanoparticles are highly dependent on the type of material that they are made of (e.g., carbon, metal, metallic oxide, etc.) [48,50], the process by which they were prepared [56], the shape and their isotropy/anisotropy [57], their capping in terms of type/force of interaction, and the nature of the capped molecule [58,59]. The redox potential of nanoparticles or their oxidative potential (prooxidant character) remains difficult to assess because of the low concentrations of, for example, synthesized nanoparticles, possible interference with the analytical method, and the relevance of the incubation medium [48,49]. In parallel to what was explained as the case for AmB, the redox properties of inorganic nanoparticles are involved in their related activity in cells and in their induced toxicity, even if this last point is a matter of debate in the literature [49]. The possible biological impact of this double-faced redox property is observed on the cell wall and membrane, on the proteins, and on the nucleic acids [60]. The overall response of the organism is either a regulation of redox homeostasis via redox signaling or stress that can lead to necrosis, apoptosis, autophagy, etc. [49]. This prooxidant effect has been used as a bacterial-killing agent, which is now being explored for further use in antimicrobial medicine for the treatment of infections due to multi-resistant bacteria [60]. Various studies have been able to highlight the antibacterial activity of silver nanoparticles (AgNPs) [61–63]. These metallic nanoparticles promote the induction of ROS leading to structural and metabolic damage which ultimately leads to an antibacterial effect [64]. Of note, an extensive review about the oxidative-stress-mediated antimicrobial properties of metal-based nanoparticles has been recently published [60].

Some inorganic nanoparticles are functionalized by redox-potent molecules in order to obtain synergy in their antioxidant activity. These tools are sometimes named "nanoantioxidants" [65]. Many types of nanoparticles have been functionalized with different antioxidants. The main results were a prolonged release of the antioxidant, an improved biocompatibility, and a targeted delivery of the antioxidants with superior antioxidant profiles [65].

3. Inorganic Nanoparticles Carrying Amphotericin B

3.1. The State-of-the-Art of Lipidic Formulations of Amphotericin B on the Market or under Clinical Trials

Due to its chemical structure, AmB is lipophilic, completely insoluble in water, sparingly soluble in alcohol, and highly soluble in dimethylformamide or dimethylsulfoxide [66]. Even though the molecule presents two groups (carboxylic acid and primary amine) associated with ionization constants (pKa), the molecule is globally neutral at physiological pH as it is both positively and negatively charged. AmB is characterized by poor oral permeability, besides a degradation occurring in the stomach. AmB is presented in its classical formulation as micelles of sodium deoxycholate. These parameters may explain why researchers focus on its formulation in so many works. The nanoparticle formulations based on liposomes or lipids increase the therapeutic index of the molecule, decreasing its toxicity, especially nephrotoxicity, while retaining the same efficacy [67–69]. Indeed, lipid formulations of AmB limit nephrotoxicity, but tubule cells remain still vulnerable to some forms of superimposed injury [70]. In 2020, Hnik and coll. tested a single dose of an oral formulation based on liposomal amphotericin (iCo-019) on healthy people. The objective of this study was to develop a molecule that is easy to administer, stable, and non-toxic while maintaining effective pharmacological activity. The data of the randomized controlled trial has demonstrated that the single dose of iCo-019 demonstrated a good tolerance of the molecule and a reduction in its toxicity [71]. More precisely, an overview of the formulations on the market or under clinical trial is presented in Table 1.

These formulations present an innovation, particularly in limiting nephrotoxicity, which explains why they are reserved to treat people suffering from kidney diseases. The products under clinical trial clearly open new opportunities in terms of administration routes. However, from a redox point of view, they do not present any of these properties.

3.2. Inorganic Nanoparticles as Modulator of AmB Redox Properties

3.2.1. Strategies to Functionalize Inorganic Nanoparticles with Amphotericin B

Numerous nanoparticles were synthesized and functionalized to obtain particles carrying AmB. Table 2 presents an overview of the published works.

Table 1. Formulations of AmB on the market or under clinical trial (clinicaltrials.gov (accessed on 15 September 2023).

AmB Formulation (Examples)	Administration Route	Market Level/Clinical Trial	Cost (in USD) *	Reference and/or Clinicaltrials.gov Number
Micelles of sodium deoxycholate (Fungizone®)	Intravenous	Registered in 1966 (FDA)	96	
Unilamellar liposomes (AmBisome®)	Intravenous	Registered in 1997 (FDA)	1646	
Ribbon-like lipid complexes (Ablecet®)	Intravenous	Registered in 1995 (FDA)	840	
Disc-shaped liposome (Amphocil® or Amphotec®)	Intravenous	Registered in 1996 (FDA)	448	
Liposomal Amphotericin B	Intravenous	Clinical trial	-	NCT03529617 NCT05108545 NCT02025491 NCT05814432 NCT01122771 NCT00003938 NCT02283905
Amphotericin-B	Intravenous	Clinical trial	-	NCT00001017 NCT00002277
Amphotericin B Lipid Complex	Intravenous	Clinical trial	-	NCT00002019 NCT03196921
Encochleated Amphotericin B	Oral	Clinical trial	-	NCT05541107
Liposomal Amphotericin B gel 0.4%	Topical	Clinical trial	-	NCT02656797
Lipo-AB® (Amphotericin B) liposome	Intravenous	Clinical trial	-	NCT03511820 NCT02320604 NCT00628719
Liposomal Amphotericin B (AmBisome®)	Intravenous	Clinical trial	-	NCT00418951 NCT00936910 NCT00362544
Liposomal Amphotericin B Amphotericin B deoxycholate Liposomal Amphotericin B (AmBisome®)	Single infusion	Clinical trial	-	NCT00628719
Liposomal Amphotericin B	Intravenous	Clinical trial	-	NCT00467883
Amphotericin B Lipid emulsion (Amphomul®) Liposomal Amphotericin B	Single infusion	Clinical trial	-	NCT00876824
Cochleated nanoparticles	Oral	Clinical trial	-	NCT02629419 [72]
Amphotericin B Cream 3%	Topical	Clinical trial	-	NCT01845727

Table 1. *Cont.*

AmB Formulation (Examples)	Administration Route	Market Level/Clinical Trial	Cost (in USD) *	Reference and/or Clinicaltrials.gov Number
Nebulized liposomes (AmBisome®)	Pulmonary	Clinical trial	-	NCT00177710 NCT00263315 NCT04502381
		Clinical trial	-	NCT00263315 NCT02273661 NCT04267497
		Clinical trial	-	NCT00177684
Nebulized lipid complexes (Abelcet®)	Pulmonary	Clinical trial	-	NCT00235651 NCT04225195
Nebulized AmB deoxycholate	Intravenous	Clinical trial	-	NCT01857479
Nebulized Amphotericin B lipid complex	Pulmonary	Clinical trial	-	NCT01615809
Liposomal AmB	Intrathecal	Clinical trial	-	NCT02686853
Liposomal AmB	Oral	Clinical trial	-	NCT04059770

* per day for a 70 kg patient with the upper-limit dose.

Table 2. Results obtained from inorganic nanoparticles as AmB carriers.

Type of Nanoparticle	Core (dc) and Hydrodynamic (Dh) Diameter	Targeted Microorganism	Main Conclusion	References
Ag	dc = 10 nm to 15–20 nm (TEM) Dh = 8–15 nm to 15–25 nm (DLS)	*Leishmania tropica*	Synergic effect of nanoparticles and AmB Prooxidant effect	[73]
	Dh = 10–90 nm (AFM)	*Naegleria fowleri*	Synergic effect of nanoparticles and AmB Prooxidant effect	[74]
	dc = 8–15 nm (TEM) Dh = 10–17 nm (DLS)	*C. albicans* *C. tropicalis* *Malassezia furfur*	Synergic effect of nanoparticles and AmB Prooxidant effect	[75]
	dc = 12.7 nm (SEM)	*C. albicans* *Trichophyton erinacei*	Synergic effect of nanoparticles and AmB Prooxidant effect	[76]
	dc = 10–18 nm (TEM)	*C. albicans*	Synergic effect of nanoparticles and AmB even on biofilms Prooxidant effect	[77]

Table 2. *Cont.*

Type of Nanoparticle	Core (dc) and Hydrodynamic (Dh) Diameter	Targeted Microorganism	Main Conclusion	References
	dc = 7–15 nm (TEM); Dh = 11–17 nm (DLS)	C. albicans A. niger Fusarium culmorum	Synergic effect of nanoparticles and AmB No redox property studied	[78]
	Dh = 170 nm (DLS)	P. aeruginosa C. albicans	Effect on bacteria and on fungi No redox property studied	[79]
Ag	Dh = 30 nm (DLS)	Resistant clinical isolates C. glabrata C. albicans C. tropicalis	Effect on fungi No redox property studied	[80]
Ag	Dh = 18–60 nm (DLS)	C. krusei C. parapsilosis C. glabrata C. neoformans C. gattii, C. albicans	Effect on fungi No redox property studied	[81]
Pd@Ag nanosheets	Hexagonal shape; dc = 11 nm, 30 nm, 80 nm, and 120 nm (TEM) with Ag/Pd ratio = 6 (ICP-MS)	C. glabrata C. krusei C. tropicalis C. parapsilosis A. fumigatus Rhizopus oryzae	Synergistic fungicidal effect with AmB. More susceptibility for Cryptococcus spp. and C. glabrata whereas R. oryzae was insensitive Prooxidant effect	[82]
	dc = 50–200 nm (AFM)	Ancathamoeba castellanii	Increased bioactivity No redox property studied	[83]
Au	Dh = 50 nm (DLS)	C. albicans	Slightly more effective than bare AgNP Prooxidant effect	[84]
	Estimated absolute crystallite size = 40 and 78 nm (XRD)	C. albicans (2 strains) C. glabrata C. geochares C. saitoana	Synergic effect of nanoparticles and AmB Antioxidant effect	[85]
	Dh = 10–15 nm (DLS)	Resistant clinical isolates C. glabrata	Effect on fungi No redox property studied	[80]

Table 2. Cont.

Type of Nanoparticle	Core (dc) and Hydrodynamic (Dh) Diameter	Targeted Microorganism	Main Conclusion	References
Carbon	dc = 38.5 ± 10.6 nm (TEM)	Aspergillus niger, A. flavus, A. fumigatus, A. terreus	Effect on fungi. No redox property studied	[86]
	Graphene–carbon nanotubes composite	Leishmania donovani	Synergic effect of nanoparticles and AmB. No redox property studied	[87]
	Ammonium functionalized multi- and single-walled carbon nanotubes dc = 140–500 to 1500–4000 nm (TEM)	C. parapsilosis, C. albicans, C. neoformans	Increase effect of nanoparticles and AmB. No redox property studied	[88]
	Ammonium functionalized multi- and single-walled carbon nanotubes dc = 140–500 × 1500–4000 nm (TEM)	C. neoformans and acapsular mutants, Rhodotorula rubra, S. cerevisiae, Pichia etchellsii, C. albicans, C. parapsilosis	Activity even against AmB-resistant strains. Redox mechanisms hypothesized	[89]
	Functionalized carbon nanotubes dc = 40–70 nm × 2–8 μm (TEM)	L. donovani	Superiority over AmB in terms of toxicity and efficacy. No redox property studied	[90]
Ca₃(PO₄)₂	Dh = 112–165 nm (DLS)	L. donovani	More efficient to treat intracellular leishmania. No redox property studied	[91]
	dc = 13 nm (TEM)	Candida spp., C. glabrata, C. albicans	Synergic effect of nanoparticles and AmB even on biofilm. Prooxidant effect	[92]
Fe	Dh = 184 nm (DLS)	A. castellanii	Synergic effect on trophozoites and on cysts. No redox property studied	[93]
	dc = 10 nm (TEM) Dh = 15 nm (DLS)	L. donovani	Synergic effect of nanoparticles and AmB. No redox property studied	[94]
	dc = 6–7 nm (TEM) Dh = 85 nm (DLS)	P. brasiliensis	Similar activity. No redox property studied	[95]
	Sub-micronic particles (SEM)	C. albicans, C. glabrata, C. geochares, C. saitoana	Synergic effect of nanoparticles and AmB. Antioxidant effect	[85]

Table 2. *Cont.*

Type of Nanoparticle	Core (dc) and Hydrodynamic (Dh) Diameter	Targeted Microorganism	Main Conclusion	References
	Dh = 193–218 nm (DLS)	*A. castellanii*	Synergic effect of nanoparticles and AmB No redox property studied	[96]
	Dh = 30–40 nm (DLS)	*C. albicans* *C. glabrata* *C. krusei* *C. parapsilosis* *C. tropicalis*	time-dependent cellular uptake in *C. albicans* and *C. glabrata* clinical isolates, and improved efficacy over conventional AmB No redox property studied	[97]
Silica	Mesoporous included in a resin dc = 85 nm (TEM)	*C. albicans* *Streptococcus oralis*	Long-term effect of nanoparticles and AmB No redox property studied	[98]
ZnO	Doped with Fe or Mn or Co or Cu Not indicated	*C. neoformans* *Trichophyton mentagrophytes*	Synergic effect of nanoparticles and AmB mostly when doped Prooxidant effect	[99]
	dc = 10–30 nm (SEM)	*C. albicans* *C. tropicalis* *C. krusei* *C. parapsilosis* *C. lusitaniae*	Effect on fungi No redox property studied	[100]
Se	Dh = 105–209 nm (DLS)	Resistant clinical isolates *C. glabrata* *C. albicans* *C. tropicalis*	Effect on fungi No redox property studied	[80]
TiO$_2$	dc = 10–25 nm (SEM)	*C. krusei* *C. parapsilosis* *C. lusitaniae*	Effect on fungi No redox property studied	[100]

The nanoparticles were made of a metal or metallic oxide (e.g., silver, gold, iron, and zinc), or they were based on carbon (with carbon quantum dots, graphene, nanotubes) or on calcium phosphate, or on layered double hydroxides, or on silica, or even based on core–shell particles (Pd@Ag nanoparticles) [75,83,100,101]. The synthesis of nanoparticles was realized mainly via the bottom-up approach (using building blocks that further organize in nanoparticles upon a trigger, e.g., reduction, irradiation, etc.). A majority of researchers used chemical processes, while some research described the production of nanoparticles (Ag, Au and iron oxide) via different methods: phytosynthesis using extracts of *Isatis tinctoria*, *Maytenus royleanus* [75], *Cucumis melo L var makuwa*, *Prunus persica* L. [85], using Chinese cabbage or maize silky hair [102]; or using a green synthesis by *Punica granatum* [103]; or by biosynthesis using *Acidophilic Acinetobacter P. columellifera* subsp. *Pallida* [76]; or 14 *Acinetobacter* spp. isolates [77]. In addition, two studies used AmB to directly reduce the Ag^+ into Ag^0 or Au^{3+} into Au^0 with success, highlighting the antioxidant character of AmB [78,83]. The strategies used to obtain nanoparticles carrying AmB are illustrated in Figure 4.

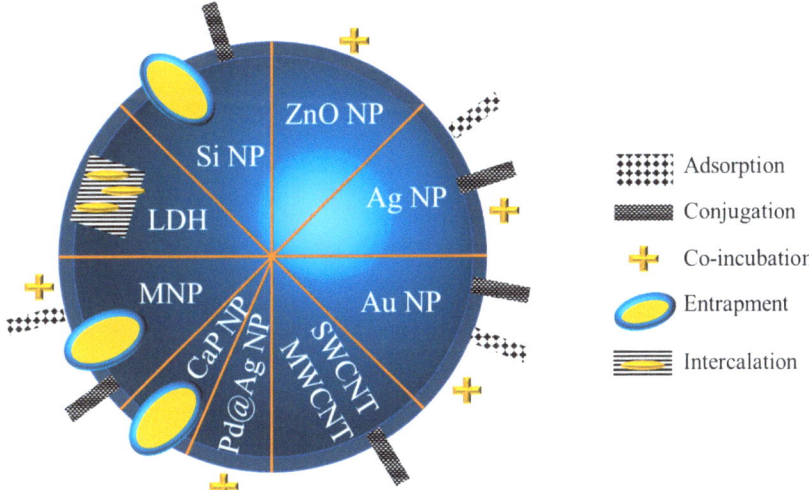

Figure 4. Different strategies employed to carry AmB. NP: nanoparticles; LDH: layered double hydroxide; MNP: magnetic nanoparticles; CaPNP: calcium phosphate nanoparticles; SWCNT: single-walled carbon nanotubes; MWCNT: multi-walled carbon nanotubes.

Common strategies were developed to carry the drug: they rely on adsorption, i.e., a weak interaction between the silver core and mycosamine group or polyol group [78,104] or between the nanoparticle and AmB; or conjugation, realized by a strong interaction, e.g., covalence with the use of a spacer [84,88]; or entrapment or intercalation between layers [105] within the nanoparticle and the simple co-incubation of nanoparticles and AmB.

In some studies, the authors took advantage of the unique properties of the inorganic nanoparticles, besides their capacity to modulate the redox signaling of the organisms (see Sections 3.2.2 and 3.2.3). For example, Ahmad and coll. demonstrated an increase in the activity of their silver nanoparticles carrying AmB upon UV irradiation [73]. AgNP are particularly studied because they have also been known for years for their anti-infectious activity as explained above. In another study, carbon quantum dots were functionalized by AmB and used as a new method for the specific detection of *C. albicans* for diagnostic purposes [106]. Iron oxide nanoparticles are also interesting due to their response to a magnetic field that can induce the generation of controlled non-invasive heat and efficient drug delivery at the selected site [85]. Various designs of iron oxide nanoparticles

(34–40 nm) coated with bovine serum albumin and targeted with AmB (AmB-IONP), were formulated via a layer-by-layer approach, and tested for their antifungal activity. These compounds showed improved antifungal activity efficacy against *C. albicans* and *C. glabrata* clinical isolates [97]. There are numerous works developed in that sense (Table 2).

3.2.2. Inorganic Nanoparticles as Synergic Prooxidants

Among the published articles, a lot of studies highlight the combined or synergistic redox properties of nanoparticles carrying AmB. Only a few papers concentrated on their activity against pathogens without exploring the involved redox mechanisms. The proposed redox mechanisms are represented in Figure 5. One can easily understand that oxidative stress can be generated by nanoparticles and/or AmB and then self-sustained. It is very difficult to determine the first actor due to the tight interconnectivity of the mechanisms.

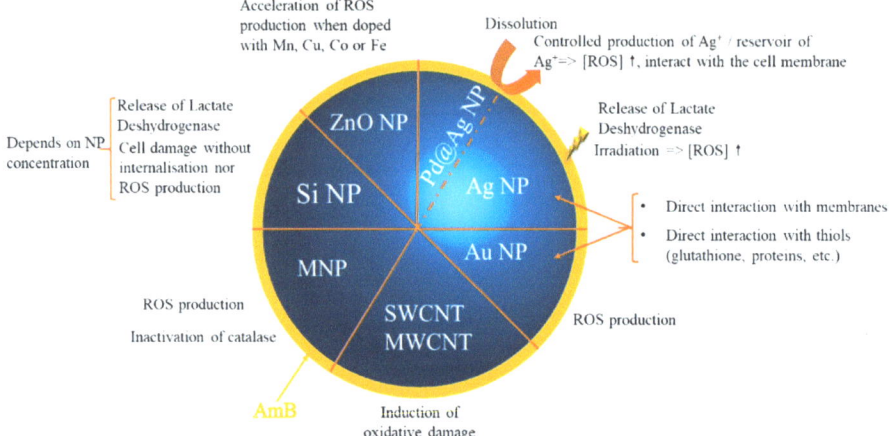

Figure 5. Main mechanisms implied in the prooxidative effect of nanoparticles carrying AmB at the origin of the described synergistic activity. NP: nanoparticles; MNP: magnetic nanoparticles; SWCNT: single-walled carbon nanotubes; MWCNT: multi-walled carbon nanotubes; ROS: reactive oxygen species.

A synergistic effect was almost always highlighted when an oxidative stress was either demonstrated or hypothesized. The effect is therefore superior to the one induced by nanoparticles or AmB alone. Recently, the same phenomenon was observed with AmB and gentamicin-loaded nanosheets/nanoneedles-based boron nitride films [107]. These films exerted an anti-infectious activity against *Neurospora crassa* and antibiotic-resistant *E. coli*. Another study using molecules other than AmB also showed the synergic effect of nanoparticles carrying antibiotics explained by oxidative stress, for example, silver nanoparticles combined with ampicillin, chloramphenicol, and kanamycin [108] or with neomycin or gentamicin [109]. However, besides their redox properties, nanoparticles possess other advantages, since they can pass through physiological barriers and penetrate more easily into pathogens due to their small size [77,110]. After entering into the cells, the nanoparticles disrupt the membrane integrity which creates a passage for drugs across the cell membrane, improving their action at the target site. This was shown for silver nanoparticles [77]. Amphotericin B-silver hybrid nanoparticles (AmB-Ag) have been reported to be a highly effective form of this antibiotic to combat fungi. In a study analyzing the interaction of AmB-Ag with *C. albicans* cells using molecular spectroscopy and imaging techniques, the antifungal activity of the nanocomplex system of the disintegration of the cell membrane was demonstrated, which occurs within a few minutes of treatment. This activity increases considerably when the treatment is in the form of hybrid silver nanoparticles. Experimental results show that AmB-Ag can effectively cross the cell wall barrier and deliver antibiotic molecules to cell membranes, thus activating oxidative stress [111].

Nevertheless, this prooxidant effect was sometimes the origin of a toxicity [112]. Researchers have demonstrated that the toxicity of silica nanoparticles carrying AmB was more important than that of the unloaded silica nanoparticles on human fibroblasts and on human endothelial cells. Moreover, the same authors have demonstrated that amphotericin B-functionalized SiO_2 NPs with an average size of 5 and 80 nm have antifungal activity against several strains of *Candida* species [113]. This effectiveness was also demonstrated when SiO_2 NPs were immobilized using amphotericin B in the case of dental resins [114]. In another study, AmB macrocyclic polyene was used as a reducing agent and stabilizing agent during the manufacture of Ag NPs. AmB-Ag nanoparticles (with an average size of 4 nm) have an inhibitory effect on the growth of *Aspergillus niger*, *Candida albicans*, and *Fusarium culmorum*. The authors attributed the high antifungal effectiveness of AmB-Ag NPs to the synergistic effect between AmB and Ag^+ ions [78].

ZnO-PEGylated AMB (ZnO-AmB-PEG) nanoparticles demonstrated their antifungal effects on two strains of *Candida* spp. When comparing the results obtained by treatment with ZnO-AmB NPs and free AMB against *C. albicans* and *C. neoformans*, it was determined that ZnO-AmB-PEG NPs significantly reduced the growth of fungi. Additionally, the toxicity was studied using in vitro blood hemolysis, in vivo nephrotoxicity. ZnO-AmB-PEG significantly reduced leukocyte counts, creatinine, and blood urea nitrogen levels, compared to AmB. The authors suggested that ZnO-AmB-PEG could be tested and used clinically [115]. On the contrary, other works reported an absence of toxicity on the kidneys, liver, and spleen of Golden Syrian hamsters [87], Swiss mice [91] and Balb/c mice [95] as well as on red blood cells [79]. In the latter, this was explained by the association of the functionalized nanoparticles with the circulating high-density (HDL) and low-density lipoproteins (LDL). Toxicity issues related to inorganic nanoparticles are a long-running story. Among others, the physicochemical parameters of nanoparticles, the material they are made with, and their possible degradation products are key points to understand since they may explain the observed phenomenon. It remains very difficult to express general rules about this toxicity [61,116].

3.2.3. Inorganic Nanoparticles as Synergic Antioxidants

Two publications focused on the antioxidant activity of nanoparticles carrying AmB [85,102]. In both, nanoparticles (made either of magnetite iron oxide or of gold) were synthesized using plants: either the silky hair of corns or the outer leaves of Chinese cabbage or other aqueous extracts of outer oriental melon peel and peach. It is likely that the nanoparticle corona contained antioxidant biomolecules such as flavonoids and polyphenols besides the activity of the metallic core of the nanoparticles. In the two works, the authors highlighted a strong antioxidant property due to the scavenging of radicals (i.e., 1,1-diphenyl-2-picrylhydrazyl, 2,2′-azino-bis(3-ethylbenzothiazoline-6-sulphonic acid) and nitric oxide) and also a strong proteasome inhibition. It has already been described that the antioxidant activity coming from the inorganic core of nanoparticles can be enhanced when functionalized by other antioxidants such as reduced glutathione [117]. These nanoparticles, when combined with AmB, proved to have synergic activity against *Candida* spp. The level of antioxidant property was correlated to the antifungal activity.

The synergic antioxidant effect is less studied in the literature. The obtained antioxidant effect may be linked to the corona of such nanoparticles that are based on extracts of plants, which can bring an antioxidant activity by themselves. The synergistic aspect of the nanoparticle combined with AmB is not totally obvious in these examples. Other studies will certainly bring more robustness to this activity in the future.

4. Summary and Future Directions

Both AmB and inorganic nanoparticles exhibit a Janus face through their redox activities. The first generation of formulations is already on the market and is based on lipids. In this review, a second generation of nanoparticles carrying AmB was reviewed to highlight their capacity to behave as synergic prooxidants or antioxidants enhancing the redox properties of the molecule, and, as a consequence, increasing the therapeutic activity of AmB. Due to the unique properties of the inorganic nanoparticle, the pre-clinical development of objects carrying AmB will certainly be dedicated to the development of agents for theranostic (e.g., using light responsive nanoparticles) and/or for targeted delivery (e.g., using magnetic nanoparticles with the application of a magnetic field on the desired site). Indeed, one can easily imagine core corona nanoparticles (or even core multi-corona nanoparticles) combining the different advantages of their materials. For example, nanoparticles made with an iron oxide core for magnetic properties surrounded by a silver corona for their anti-infectious properties and, used for both, and their capacity to respond to UV-vis radiation to generate oxidative stress at the targeted site. The functionalization of such objects via AmB would be of great potential for precision therapy.

The future steps for such objects to reach the clinical level remain challenging: requiring proof of non-toxicity as well as non-immunogenicity (no adverse reaction, no accumulation in organs, etc.), and of their benefit vs. other therapies, provided that the industrial translation (e.g., scale-up, long-term stability) is feasible.

Supplementary Materials: The following supporting information can be downloaded at: https://www.mdpi.com/article/10.3390/antibiotics12101543/s1, Table S1. References [67,68,118–124] are cited in the supplementary materials.

Author Contributions: N.M., writing—original draft preparation; E.L., conception of figures; N.M., A.B., E.L. and R.E.D., writing—review and editing; A.B. and R.E.D., supervision. All authors have read and agreed to the published version of the manuscript.

Funding: This research received no external funding.

Institutional Review Board Statement: Not applicable.

Informed Consent Statement: Not applicable.

Data Availability Statement: Not applicable.

Conflicts of Interest: The authors declare no conflict of interest.

References

1. Nicolaou, K.C.; Chen, J.S.; Dalby, S.M. From Nature to the Laboratory and into the Clinic. *Bioorg. Med. Chem.* **2009**, *17*, 2290–2303. [CrossRef] [PubMed]
2. Volmer, A.A.; Szpilman, A.M.; Carreira, E.M. Synthesis and Biological Evaluation of Amphotericin B Derivatives. *Nat. Prod. Rep.* **2010**, *27*, 1329–1349. [CrossRef]
3. Pound, M.W.; Townsend, M.L.; Dimondi, V.; Wilson, D.; Drew, R.H. Overview of Treatment Options for Invasive Fungal Infections. *Med. Mycol.* **2011**, *49*, 561–580. [CrossRef]
4. Cavassin, F.B.; Baú-Carneiro, J.L.; Vilas-Boas, R.R.; Queiroz-Telles, F. Sixty Years of Amphotericin B: An Overview of the Main Antifungal Agent Used to Treat Invasive Fungal Infections. *Infect. Dis. Ther.* **2021**, *10*, 115–147. [CrossRef] [PubMed]
5. Carolus, H.; Pierson, S.; Lagrou, K.; Van Dijck, P. Amphotericin B and Other Polyenes-Discovery, Clinical Use, Mode of Action and Drug Resistance. *J. Fungi* **2020**, *6*, 321. [CrossRef]
6. Cowen, L.E.; Sanglard, D.; Howard, S.J.; Rogers, P.D.; Perlin, D.S. Mechanisms of Antifungal Drug Resistance. *Cold Spring Harb. Perspect. Med.* **2015**, *5*, a019752. [CrossRef]
7. Brunet, K.; Diop, C.A.B.; Chauzy, A.; Prébonnaud, N.; Marchand, S.; Rammaert, B.; Tewes, F. Improved In Vitro Anti-Mucorales Activity and Cytotoxicity of Amphotericin B with a Pegylated Surfactant. *J. Fungi* **2022**, *8*, 121. [CrossRef]
8. Pappas, P.G.; Kauffman, C.A.; Andes, D.R.; Clancy, C.J.; Marr, K.A.; Ostrosky-Zeichner, L.; Reboli, A.C.; Schuster, M.G.; Vazquez, J.A.; Walsh, T.J.; et al. Clinical Practice Guideline for the Management of Candidiasis: 2016 Update by the Infectious Diseases Society of America. *Clin. Infect. Dis. Off. Publ. Infect. Dis. Soc. Am.* **2016**, *62*, e1–e50. [CrossRef]
9. Pathak, A.; Pien, F.D.; Carvalho, L. Amphotericin B Use in a Community Hospital, with Special Emphasis on Side Effects. *Clin. Infect. Dis. Off. Publ. Infect. Dis. Soc. Am.* **1998**, *26*, 334–338. [CrossRef]
10. Gursoy, V.; Ozkalemkas, F.; Ozkocaman, V.; Serenli Yegen, Z.; Ethem Pinar, I.; Ener, B.; Akalın, H.; Kazak, E.; Ali, R.; Ersoy, A. Conventional Amphotericin B Associated Nephrotoxicity in Patients With Hematologic Malignancies. *Cureus* **2021**, *13*, e16445. [CrossRef] [PubMed]

11. Jafari, M.; Abolmaali, S.S.; Tamaddon, A.M.; Zomorodian, K.; Sarkari, B.S. Nanotechnology Approaches for Delivery and Targeting of Amphotericin B in Fungal and Parasitic Diseases. *Nanomedicine* **2021**, *16*, 857–877. [CrossRef]
12. Alakkad, A.; Stapleton, P.; Schlosser, C.; Murdan, S.; Odunze, U.; Schatzlein, A.; Uchegbu, I.F. Amphotericin B Polymer Nanoparticles Show Efficacy against Candida Species Biofilms. *Pathogens* **2022**, *11*, 73. [CrossRef]
13. Faustino, C.; Pinheiro, L. Lipid Systems for the Delivery of Amphotericin B in Antifungal Therapy. *Pharmaceutics* **2020**, *12*, 29. [CrossRef] [PubMed]
14. Chen, Y.-C.; Su, C.-Y.; Jhan, H.-J.; Ho, H.-O.; Sheu, M.-T. Physical Characterization and in Vivo Pharmacokinetic Study of Self-Assembling Amphotericin B-Loaded Lecithin-Based Mixed Polymeric Micelles. *Int. J. Nanomed.* **2015**, *10*, 7265–7274. [CrossRef]
15. Serrano, D.R.; Lalatsa, A.; Dea-Ayuela, M.A.; Bilbao-Ramos, P.E.; Garrett, N.L.; Moger, J.; Guarro, J.; Capilla, J.; Ballesteros, M.P.; Schätzlein, A.G.; et al. Oral Particle Uptake and Organ Targeting Drives the Activity of Amphotericin B Nanoparticles. *Mol. Pharm.* **2015**, *12*, 420–431. [CrossRef]
16. Wang, C.; Makvandi, P.; Zare, E.N.; Tay, F.R.; Niu, L. Advances in Antimicrobial Organic and Inorganic Nanocompounds in Biomedicine. *Adv. Ther.* **2020**, *3*, 2000024. [CrossRef]
17. Jiang, S.; Win, K.Y.; Liu, S.; Teng, C.P.; Zheng, Y.; Han, M.-Y. Surface-Functionalized Nanoparticles for Biosensing and Imaging-Guided Therapeutics. *Nanoscale* **2013**, *5*, 3127–3148. [CrossRef] [PubMed]
18. Huang, H.; Feng, W.; Chen, Y.; Shi, J. Inorganic Nanoparticles in Clinical Trials and Translations. *Nano Today* **2020**, *35*, 100972. [CrossRef]
19. Mesa-Arango, A.C.; Trevijano-Contador, N.; Román, E.; Sánchez-Fresneda, R.; Casas, C.; Herrero, E.; Argüelles, J.C.; Pla, J.; Cuenca-Estrella, M.; Zaragoza, O. The Production of Reactive Oxygen Species Is a Universal Action Mechanism of Amphotericin B against Pathogenic Yeasts and Contributes to the Fungicidal Effect of This Drug. *Antimicrob. Agents Chemother.* **2014**, *58*, 6627–6638. [CrossRef]
20. Guirao-Abad, J.P.; Sánchez-Fresneda, R.; Alburquerque, B.; Hernández, J.A.; Argüelles, J.-C. ROS Formation Is a Differential Contributory Factor to the Fungicidal Action of Amphotericin B and Micafungin in Candida Albicans. *Int. J. Med. Microbiol.* **2017**, *307*, 241–248. [CrossRef]
21. Kovacic, P.; Cooksy, A. Novel, Unifying Mechanism for Amphotericin B and Other Polyene Drugs: Electron Affinity, Radicals, Electron Transfer, Autoxidation, Toxicity, and Antifungal Action. *MedChemComm* **2012**, *3*, 274–280. [CrossRef]
22. Osaka, K.; Ritov, V.B.; Bernardo, J.F.; Branch, R.A.; Kagan, V.E. Amphotericin B Protects Cis-Parinaric Acid against Peroxyl Radical-Induced Oxidation: Amphotericin B as an Antioxidant. *Antimicrob. Agents Chemother.* **1997**, *41*, 743–747. [CrossRef]
23. Osaka, K.; Tyurina, Y.Y.; Dubey, R.K.; Tyurin, V.A.; Ritov, V.B.; Quinn, P.J.; Branch, R.A.; Kagan, V.E. Amphotericin B as an Intracellular Antioxidant: Protection against 2,2′-Azobis(2,4-Dimethylvaleronitrile)-Induced Peroxidation of Membrane Phospholipids in Rat Aortic Smooth Muscle Cells. *Biochem. Pharmacol.* **1997**, *54*, 937–945. [CrossRef]
24. Lamy-Freund, M.T.; Ferreira, V.F.; Schreier, S. Mechanism of Inactivation of the Polyene Antibiotic Amphotericin B. Evidence for Radical Formation in the Process of Autoxidation. *J. Antibiot.* **1985**, *38*, 753–757. [CrossRef]
25. Belenky, P.; Camacho, D.; Collins, J.J. Fungicidal Drugs Induce a Common Oxidative-Damage Cellular Death Pathway. *Cell Rep.* **2013**, *3*, 350–358. [CrossRef]
26. Ferreira, G.F.; de Baltazar, L.M.; Santos, J.R.A.; Monteiro, A.S.; de Fraga, L.A.O.; Resende-Stoianoff, M.A.; Santos, D.A. The Role of Oxidative and Nitrosative Bursts Caused by Azoles and Amphotericin B against the Fungal Pathogen *Cryptococcus gattii*. *J. Antimicrob. Chemother.* **2013**, *68*, 1801–1811. [CrossRef] [PubMed]
27. Andrews, F.A.; Beggs, W.H.; Sarosi, G.A. Influence of Antioxidants on the Bioactivity of Amphotericin B. *Antimicrob. Agents Chemother.* **1977**, *11*, 615–618. [CrossRef]
28. Pravkin, S.K.; Yakusheva, E.N.; Uzbekova, D.G. In Vivo Analysis of Antioxidant and Prooxidant Properties of Retinol Acetate. *Bull. Exp. Biol. Med.* **2013**, *156*, 220–223. [CrossRef] [PubMed]
29. Putchala, M.C.; Ramani, P.; Sherlin, H.J.; Premkumar, P.; Natesan, A. Ascorbic Acid and Its Pro-Oxidant Activity as a Therapy for Tumours of Oral Cavity—A Systematic Review. *Arch. Oral Biol.* **2013**, *58*, 563–574. [CrossRef]
30. Ko, K.M.; Yick, P.K.; Poon, M.K.; Ip, S.P. Prooxidant and Antioxidant Effects of Trolox on Ferric Ion-Induced Oxidation of Erythrocyte Membrane Lipids. *Mol. Cell. Biochem.* **1994**, *141*, 65–70. [CrossRef]
31. Kong, Y.; Wang, Q.; Cao, F.; Zhang, X.; Fang, Z.; Shi, P.; Wang, H.; Shen, Y.; Huang, Z. BSC2 Enhances Cell Resistance to AmB by Inhibiting Oxidative Damage in Saccharomyces Cerevisiae. *Free Radic. Res.* **2020**, *54*, 231–243. [CrossRef] [PubMed]
32. Purkait, B.; Kumar, A.; Nandi, N.; Sardar, A.H.; Das, S.; Kumar, S.; Pandey, K.; Ravidas, V.; Kumar, M.; De, T.; et al. Mechanism of Amphotericin B Resistance in Clinical Isolates of Leishmania Donovani. *Antimicrob. Agents Chemother.* **2012**, *56*, 1031–1041. [CrossRef] [PubMed]
33. Jukic, E.; Blatzer, M.; Posch, W.; Steger, M.; Binder, U.; Lass-Flörl, C.; Wilflingseder, D. Oxidative Stress Response Tips the Balance in Aspergillus Terreus Amphotericin B Resistance. *Antimicrob. Agents Chemother.* **2017**, *61*, e00670-17. [CrossRef] [PubMed]
34. Altuntaş, A.; Yılmaz, H.R.; Altuntaş, A.; Uz, E.; Demir, M.; Gökçimen, A.; Aksu, O.; Bayram, D.Ş.; Sezer, M.T. Caffeic Acid Phenethyl Ester Protects against Amphotericin B Induced Nephrotoxicity in Rat Model. *BioMed Res. Int.* **2014**, *2014*, 702981. [CrossRef] [PubMed]

35. Gola, J.; Skubis, A.; Sikora, B.; Kruszniewska-Rajs, C.; Adamska, J.; Mazurek, U.; Strzalka-Mrozik, B.; Czernel, G.; Gagos, M. Expression Profiles of Genes Related to Melatonin and Oxidative Stress in Human Renal Proximal Tubule Cells Treated with Antibiotic Amphotericin B and Its Modified Forms. *Turk. J. Biol.* **2015**, *39*, 856–864. [CrossRef]
36. Schlottfeldt, F.D.S.; Fernandes, S.M.; Martins, D.M.; Cordeiro, P.; da Fonseca, C.D.; Watanabe, M.; Vattimo, M.d.F.F. Prevention of Amphotericin B Nephrotoxicity through Use of Phytotherapeutic Medication. *Rev. Da Esc. De Enferm. Da USP* **2015**, *49*, 74–79. [CrossRef]
37. Salehzadeh, A.; Salehzadeh, A.; Maghsood, A.-H.; Heidarisasan, S.; Taheri-Azandaryan, M.; Ghafourikhosroshahi, A.; Abbasalipourkabir, R. Effects of Vitamin A and Vitamin E on Attenuation of Amphotericin B-Induced Side Effects on Kidney and Liver of Male Wistar Rats. *Environ. Sci. Pollut. Res. Int.* **2020**, *27*, 32594–32602. [CrossRef]
38. Kim, J.H.; Chan, K.L.; Faria, N.C.G.; Martins, M.d.L.; Campbell, B.C. Targeting the Oxidative Stress Response System of Fungi with Redox-Potent Chemosensitizing Agents. *Front. Microbiol.* **2012**, *3*, 88. [CrossRef]
39. Kim, J.H.; Faria, N.C.G.; Martins, M.D.L.; Chan, K.L.; Campbell, B.C. Enhancement of Antimycotic Activity of Amphotericin B by Targeting the Oxidative Stress Response of Candida and Cryptococcus with Natural Dihydroxybenzaldehydes. *Front. Microbiol.* **2012**, *3*, 261. [CrossRef]
40. Beggs, W.H.; Andrews, F.A.; Sarosi, G.A. Synergistic Action of Amphotericin B and Antioxidants against Certain Opportunistic Yeast Pathogens. *Antimicrob. Agents Chemother.* **1978**, *13*, 266–270. [CrossRef]
41. Blatzer, M.; Jukic, E.; Posch, W.; Schöpf, B.; Binder, U.; Steger, M.; Blum, G.; Hackl, H.; Gnaiger, E.; Lass-Flörl, C.; et al. Amphotericin B Resistance in Aspergillus Terreus Is Overpowered by Coapplication of Pro-Oxidants. *Antioxid. Redox Signal.* **2015**, *23*, 1424–1438. [CrossRef] [PubMed]
42. Shekhova, E.; Kniemeyer, O.; Brakhage, A.A. Induction of Mitochondrial Reactive Oxygen Species Production by Itraconazole, Terbinafine, and Amphotericin B as a Mode of Action against *Aspergillus fumigatus*. *Antimicrob. Agents Chemother.* **2017**, *61*, e00978-17. [CrossRef] [PubMed]
43. Sippel, J.E.; Levine, H.B. Annulment of Amphotericin B Inhibition of Coccidioides Immitis Endospores. Effects on Growth, Respiration and Morphogenesis. *Sabouraudia* **1969**, *7*, 159–168. [CrossRef] [PubMed]
44. Weis, M.R.; Levine, H.B. Inactivation of Amphotericin B by Reducing Agents: Influences on Growth Inhibition of Candida Albicans and Lysis of Erythrocytes. *Sabouraudia* **1972**, *10*, 132–142. [CrossRef]
45. Silva, L.N.; Oliveira, S.S.C.; Magalhães, L.B.; Andrade Neto, V.V.; Torres-Santos, E.C.; Carvalho, M.D.C.; Pereira, M.D.; Branquinha, M.H.; Santos, A.L.S. Unmasking the Amphotericin B Resistance Mechanisms in Candida Haemulonii Species Complex. *ACS Infect. Dis.* **2020**, *6*, 1273–1282. [CrossRef]
46. Young, L.Y.; Hull, C.M.; Heitman, J. Disruption of Ergosterol Biosynthesis Confers Resistance to Amphotericin B in Candida Lusitaniae. *Antimicrob. Agents Chemother.* **2003**, *47*, 2717–2724. [CrossRef]
47. Bhattacharya, S.; Esquivel, B.D.; White, T.C. Overexpression or Deletion of Ergosterol Biosynthesis Genes Alters Doubling Time, Response to Stress Agents, and Drug Susceptibility in Saccharomyces Cerevisiae. *mBio* **2018**, *9*, e01291-18. [CrossRef]
48. Tournebize, J.; Sapin-Minet, A.; Bartosz, G.; Leroy, P.; Boudier, A. Pitfalls of Assays Devoted to Evaluation of Oxidative Stress Induced by Inorganic Nanoparticles. *Talanta* **2013**, *116*, 753–763. [CrossRef]
49. Hellack, B.; Nickel, C.; Albrecht, C.; Kuhlbusch, T.A.J.; Boland, S.; Baeza-Squiban, A.; Wohlleben, W.; Schins, R.P.F. Analytical Methods to Assess the Oxidative Potential of Nanoparticles: A Review. *Environ. Sci. Nano* **2017**, *4*, 1920–1934. [CrossRef]
50. Valgimigli, L.; Baschieri, A.; Amorati, R. Antioxidant Activity of Nanomaterials. *J. Mater. Chem. B* **2018**, *6*, 2036–2051. [CrossRef]
51. Innocenzi, P.; Stagi, L. Carbon Dots as Oxidant-Antioxidant Nanomaterials, Understanding the Structure-Properties Relationship. A Critical Review. *Nano Today* **2023**, *50*, 101837. [CrossRef]
52. Samrot, A.V.; Ram Singh, S.P.; Deenadhayalan, R.; Rajesh, V.V.; Padmanaban, S.; Radhakrishnan, K. Nanoparticles, a Double-Edged Sword with Oxidant as Well as Antioxidant Properties—A Review. *Oxygen* **2022**, *2*, 591–604. [CrossRef]
53. Fifere, A.; Moleavin, I.-A.T.; Lungoci, A.-L.; Marangoci, N.L.; Pinteala, M. Inorganic Nanoparticles as Free Radical Scavengers. In *New Trends in Macromolecular and Supramolecular Chemistry for Biological Applications*; Abadie, J.M., Pinteala, M., Rotaru, A.M., Eds.; Springer International Publishing: Cham, Switzerland, 2021; pp. 295–329, ISBN 978-3-030-57456-7.
54. Gómez-Herrero, A.C.; Sánchez-Sánchez, C.; Chérioux, F.; Martínez, J.I.; Abad, J.; Floreano, L.; Verdini, A.; Cossaro, A.; Mazaleyrat, E.; Guisset, V.; et al. Copper-Assisted Oxidation of Catechols into Quinone Derivatives. *Chem. Sci.* **2020**, *12*, 2257–2267. [CrossRef]
55. Steinmetz, L.; Geers, C.; Balog, S.; Bonmarin, M.; Rodriguez-Lorenzo, L.; Taladriz-Blanco, P.; Rothen-Rutishauser, B.; Petri-Fink, A. A Comparative Study of Silver Nanoparticle Dissolution under Physiological Conditions. *Nanoscale Adv.* **2020**, *2*, 5760–5768. [CrossRef] [PubMed]
56. Hydrogen Plasma Treated Nanodiamonds Lead to an Overproduction of Hydroxyl Radicals and Solvated Electrons in Solution under Ionizing Radiation-ScienceDirect. Available online: https://www-sciencedirect-com.insb.bib.cnrs.fr/science/article/pii/S0008622320302098?via%3Dihub (accessed on 11 July 2022).
57. Pearce, A.K.; Wilks, T.R.; Arno, M.C.; O'Reilly, R.K. Synthesis and Applications of Anisotropic Nanoparticles with Precisely Defined Dimensions. *Nat. Rev. Chem.* **2021**, *5*, 21–45. [CrossRef] [PubMed]
58. Tournebize, J.; Boudier, A.; Joubert, O.; Eidi, H.; Bartosz, G.; Maincent, P.; Leroy, P.; Sapin-Minet, A. Impact of Gold Nanoparticle Coating on Redox Homeostasis. *Int. J. Pharm.* **2012**, *438*, 107–116. [CrossRef]

59. Tournebize, J.; Boudier, A.; Sapin-Minet, A.; Maincent, P.; Leroy, P.; Schneider, R. Role of Gold Nanoparticles Capping Density on Stability and Surface Reactivity to Design Drug Delivery Platforms. *ACS Appl. Mater. Interfaces* **2012**, *4*, 5790–5799. [CrossRef] [PubMed]
60. Mammari, N.; Lamouroux, E.; Boudier, A.; Duval, R.E. Current Knowledge on the Oxidative-Stress-Mediated Antimicrobial Properties of Metal-Based Nanoparticles. *Microorganisms* **2022**, *10*, 437. [CrossRef]
61. Chernousova, S.; Epple, M. Silver as Antibacterial Agent: Ion, Nanoparticle, and Metal. *Angew. Chem. Int. Ed Engl.* **2013**, *52*, 1636–1653. [CrossRef]
62. Gouyau, J.; Duval, R.E.; Boudier, A.; Lamouroux, E. Investigation of Nanoparticle Metallic Core Antibacterial Activity: Gold and Silver Nanoparticles against Escherichia Coli and Staphylococcus Aureus. *Int. J. Mol. Sci.* **2021**, *22*, 1905. [CrossRef]
63. Singh, P.; Mijakovic, I. Antibacterial Effect of Silver Nanoparticles Is Stronger If the Production Host and the Targeted Pathogen Are Closely Related. *Biomedicines* **2022**, *10*, 628. [CrossRef]
64. Abdal Dayem, A.; Hossain, M.K.; Lee, S.B.; Kim, K.; Saha, S.K.; Yang, G.-M.; Choi, H.Y.; Cho, S.-G. The Role of Reactive Oxygen Species (ROS) in the Biological Activities of Metallic Nanoparticles. *Int. J. Mol. Sci.* **2017**, *18*, E120. [CrossRef] [PubMed]
65. Khalil, I.; Yehye, W.A.; Etxeberria, A.E.; Alhadi, A.A.; Dezfooli, S.M.; Julkapli, N.B.M.; Basirun, W.J.; Seyfoddin, A. Nanoantioxidants: Recent Trends in Antioxidant Delivery Applications. *Antioxidants* **2019**, *9*, 24. [CrossRef]
66. Liu, M.; Chen, M.; Yang, Z. Design of Amphotericin B Oral Formulation for Antifungal Therapy. *Drug Deliv.* **2017**, *24*, 1–9. [CrossRef]
67. Voltan, A.R.; Quindós, G.; Alarcón, K.P.M.; Fusco-Almeida, A.M.; Mendes-Giannini, M.J.S.; Chorilli, M. Fungal Diseases: Could Nanostructured Drug Delivery Systems Be a Novel Paradigm for Therapy? *Int. J. Nanomed.* **2016**, *11*, 3715–3730. [CrossRef] [PubMed]
68. Bekersky, I.; Fielding, R.M.; Buell, D.; Lawrence, I. Lipid-Based Amphotericin B Formulations: From Animals to Man. *Pharm. Sci. Technol. Today* **1999**, *2*, 230–236. [CrossRef] [PubMed]
69. Fernández-García, R.; de Pablo, E.; Ballesteros, M.P.; Serrano, D.R. Unmet Clinical Needs in the Treatment of Systemic Fungal Infections: The Role of Amphotericin B and Drug Targeting. *Int. J. Pharm.* **2017**, *525*, 139–148. [CrossRef] [PubMed]
70. Zager, R.A. Polyene Antibiotics: Relative Degrees of in Vitro Cytotoxicity and Potential Effects on Tubule Phospholipid and Ceramide Content. *Am. J. Kidney Dis. Off. J. Natl. Kidney Found.* **2000**, *36*, 238–249. [CrossRef]
71. Hnik, P.; Wasan, E.K.; Wasan, K.M. Safety, Tolerability, and Pharmacokinetics of a Novel Oral Amphotericin B Formulation (iCo-019) Following Single-Dose Administration to Healthy Human Subjects: An Alternative Approach to Parenteral Amphotericin B Administration. *Antimicrob. Agents Chemother.* **2020**, *64*, e01450-20. [CrossRef] [PubMed]
72. Aigner, M.; Lass-Flörl, C. Encochleated Amphotericin B: Is the Oral Availability of Amphotericin B Finally Reached? *J. Fungi* **2020**, *6*, 66. [CrossRef]
73. Ahmad, A.; Wei, Y.; Syed, F.; Khan, S.; Khan, G.M.; Tahir, K.; Khan, A.U.; Raza, M.; Khan, F.U.; Yuan, Q. Isatis Tinctoria Mediated Synthesis of Amphotericin B-Bound Silver Nanoparticles with Enhanced Photoinduced Antileishmanial Activity: A Novel Green Approach. *J. Photochem. Photobiol. B* **2016**, *161*, 17–24. [CrossRef]
74. Rajendran, K.; Anwar, A.; Khan, N.A.; Siddiqui, R. Brain-Eating Amoebae: Silver Nanoparticle Conjugation Enhanced Efficacy of Anti-Amoebic Drugs against Naegleria Fowleri. *ACS Chem. Neurosci.* **2017**, *8*, 2626–2630. [CrossRef]
75. Ahmad, A.; Wei, Y.; Syed, F.; Tahir, K.; Taj, R.; Khan, A.U.; Hameed, M.U.; Yuan, Q. Amphotericin B-Conjugated Biogenic Silver Nanoparticles as an Innovative Strategy for Fungal Infections. *Microb. Pathog.* **2016**, *99*, 271–281. [CrossRef] [PubMed]
76. Wypij, M.; Czarnecka, J.; Dahm, H.; Rai, M.; Golinska, P. Silver Nanoparticles from Pilimelia Columellifera Subsp. Pallida SL19 Strain Demonstrated Antifungal Activity against Fungi Causing Superficial Mycoses. *J. Basic Microbiol.* **2017**, *57*, 793–800. [CrossRef] [PubMed]
77. Nadhe, S.B.; Singh, R.; Wadhwani, S.A.; Chopade, B.A. Acinetobacter Sp. Mediated Synthesis of AgNPs, Its Optimization, Characterization and Synergistic Antifungal Activity against C. Albicans. *J. Appl. Microbiol.* **2019**, *127*, 445–458. [CrossRef]
78. Tutaj, K.; Szlazak, R.; Szalapata, K.; Starzyk, J.; Luchowski, R.; Grudzinski, W.; Osinska-Jaroszuk, M.; Jarosz-Wilkolazka, A.; Szuster-Ciesielska, A.; Gruszecki, W.I. Amphotericin B-Silver Hybrid Nanoparticles: Synthesis, Properties and Antifungal Activity. *Nanomed. Nanotechnol. Biol. Med.* **2016**, *12*, 1095–1103. [CrossRef]
79. Leonhard, V.; Alasino, R.V.; Munoz, A.; Beltramo, D.M. Silver Nanoparticles with High Loading Capacity of Amphotericin B: Characterization, Bactericidal and Antifungal Effects. *Curr. Drug Deliv.* **2018**, *15*, 850–859. [CrossRef]
80. Lotfali, E.; Toreyhi, H.; Makhdoomi Sharabiani, K.; Fattahi, A.; Soheili, A.; Ghasemi, R.; Keymaram, M.; Rezaee, Y.; Iranpanah, S. Comparison of Antifungal Properties of Gold, Silver, and Selenium Nanoparticles Against Amphotericin B-Resistant Candida Glabrata Clinical Isolates. *Avicenna J. Med. Biotechnol.* **2021**, *13*, 47–50. [CrossRef] [PubMed]
81. Soliman, A.M.; Abdel-Latif, W.; Shehata, I.H.; Fouda, A.; Abdo, A.M.; Ahmed, Y.M. Green Approach to Overcome the Resistance Pattern of Candida Spp. Using Biosynthesized Silver Nanoparticles Fabricated by Penicillium Chrysogenum F9. *Biol. Trace Elem. Res.* **2021**, *199*, 800–811. [CrossRef]
82. Zhang, C.; Chen, M.; Wang, G.; Fang, W.; Ye, C.; Hu, H.; Fa, Z.; Yi, J.; Liao, W.-Q. Pd@Ag Nanosheets in Combination with Amphotericin B Exert a Potent Anti-Cryptococcal Fungicidal Effect. *PLoS ONE* **2016**, *11*, e0157000. [CrossRef]
83. Anwar, A.; Siddiqui, R.; Raza Shah, M.; Ahmed Khan, N. Gold Nanoparticles Conjugation Enhances Antiacanthamoebic Properties of Nystatin, Fluconazole and Amphotericin B. *J. Microbiol. Biotechnol.* **2019**, *29*, 171–177. [CrossRef]

84. Kumar, P.; Shivam, P.; Mandal, S.; Prasanna, P.; Kumar, S.; Prasad, S.R.; Kumar, A.; Das, P.; Ali, V.; Singh, S.K.; et al. Synthesis, Characterization, and Mechanistic Studies of a Gold Nanoparticle-Amphotericin B Covalent Conjugate with Enhanced Antileishmanial Efficacy and Reduced Cytotoxicity. *Int. J. Nanomed.* **2019**, *14*, 6073–6101. [CrossRef]
85. Patra, J.K.; Baek, K.-H. Green Biosynthesis of Magnetic Iron Oxide (Fe_3O_4) Nanoparticles Using the Aqueous Extracts of Food Processing Wastes under Photo-Catalyzed Condition and Investigation of Their Antimicrobial and Antioxidant Activity. *J. Photochem. Photobiol. B* **2017**, *173*, 291–300. [CrossRef] [PubMed]
86. Almansob, A.; Bahkali, A.H.; Ameen, F. Efficacy of Gold Nanoparticles against Drug-Resistant Nosocomial Fungal Pathogens and Their Extracellular Enzymes: Resistance Profiling towards Established Antifungal Agents. *Nanomaterials* **2022**, *12*, 814. [CrossRef]
87. Gedda, M.R.; Madhukar, P.; Vishwakarma, A.K.; Verma, V.; Kushwaha, A.K.; Yadagiri, G.; Mudavath, S.L.; Singh, O.P.; Srivastava, O.N.; Sundar, S. Evaluation of Safety and Antileishmanial Efficacy of Amine Functionalized Carbon-Based Composite Nanoparticle Appended with Amphotericin B: An in Vitro and Preclinical Study. *Front. Chem.* **2020**, *8*, 510. [CrossRef]
88. Wu, W.; Wieckowski, S.; Pastorin, G.; Benincasa, M.; Klumpp, C.; Briand, J.-P.; Gennaro, R.; Prato, M.; Bianco, A. Targeted Delivery of Amphotericin B to Cells by Using Functionalized Carbon Nanotubes. *Angew. Chem. Int. Ed Engl.* **2005**, *44*, 6358–6362. [CrossRef]
89. Benincasa, M.; Pacor, S.; Wu, W.; Prato, M.; Bianco, A.; Gennaro, R. Antifungal Activity of Amphotericin B Conjugated to Carbon Nanotubes. *ACS Nano* **2011**, *5*, 199–208. [CrossRef]
90. Prajapati, V.K.; Awasthi, K.; Gautam, S.; Yadav, T.P.; Rai, M.; Srivastava, O.N.; Sundar, S. Targeted Killing of Leishmania Donovani in Vivo and in Vitro with Amphotericin B Attached to Functionalized Carbon Nanotubes. *J. Antimicrob. Chemother.* **2011**, *66*, 874–879. [CrossRef] [PubMed]
91. Chaurasia, M.; Singh, P.K.; Jaiswal, A.K.; Kumar, A.; Pawar, V.K.; Dube, A.; Paliwal, S.K.; Chourasia, M.K. Bioinspired Calcium Phosphate Nanoparticles Featuring as Efficient Carrier and Prompter for Macrophage Intervention in Experimental Leishmaniasis. *Pharm. Res.* **2016**, *33*, 2617–2629. [CrossRef] [PubMed]
92. Niemirowicz, K.; Durnaś, B.; Tokajuk, G.; Głuszek, K.; Wilczewska, A.Z.; Misztalewska, I.; Mystkowska, J.; Michalak, G.; Sodo, A.; Wątek, M.; et al. Magnetic Nanoparticles as a Drug Delivery System That Enhance Fungicidal Activity of Polyene Antibiotics. *Nanomed. Nanotechnol. Biol. Med.* **2016**, *12*, 2395–2404. [CrossRef]
93. Iqbal, K.; Abdalla, S.A.O.; Anwar, A.; Iqbal, K.M.; Shah, M.R.; Anwar, A.; Siddiqui, R.; Khan, N.A. Isoniazid Conjugated Magnetic Nanoparticles Loaded with Amphotericin B as a Potent Antiamoebic Agent against Acanthamoeba Castellanii. *Antibiotics* **2020**, *9*, 276. [CrossRef] [PubMed]
94. Kumar, R.; Pandey, K.; Sahoo, G.C.; Das, S.; Das, V.; Topno, R.K.; Das, P. Development of High Efficacy Peptide Coated Iron Oxide Nanoparticles Encapsulated Amphotericin B Drug Delivery System against Visceral Leishmaniasis. *Mater. Sci. Eng. C Mater. Biol. Appl.* **2017**, *75*, 1465–1471. [CrossRef]
95. Saldanha, C.A.; Garcia, M.P.; Iocca, D.C.; Rebelo, L.G.; Souza, A.C.O.; Bocca, A.L.; Santos, M.d.F.M.A.; Morais, P.C.; Azevedo, R.B. Antifungal Activity of Amphotericin B Conjugated to Nanosized Magnetite in the Treatment of Paracoccidioidomycosis. *PLoS Negl. Trop. Dis.* **2016**, *10*, e0004754. [CrossRef] [PubMed]
96. Abdelnasir, S.; Anwar, A.; Kawish, M.; Anwar, A.; Shah, M.R.; Siddiqui, R.; Khan, N.A. Metronidazole Conjugated Magnetic Nanoparticles Loaded with Amphotericin B Exhibited Potent Effects against Pathogenic Acanthamoeba Castellanii Belonging to the T4 Genotype. *AMB Express* **2020**, *10*, 127. [CrossRef] [PubMed]
97. Balabathula, P.; Whaley, S.G.; Janagam, D.R.; Mittal, N.K.; Mandal, B.; Thoma, L.A.; Rogers, P.D.; Wood, G.C. Lyophilized Iron Oxide Nanoparticles Encapsulated in Amphotericin B: A Novel Targeted Nano Drug Delivery System for the Treatment of Systemic Fungal Infections. *Pharmaceutics* **2020**, *12*, E247. [CrossRef]
98. Lee, J.-H.; El-Fiqi, A.; Jo, J.-K.; Kim, D.-A.; Kim, S.-C.; Jun, S.-K.; Kim, H.-W.; Lee, H.-H. Development of Long-Term Antimicrobial Poly(Methyl Methacrylate) by Incorporating Mesoporous Silica Nanocarriers. *Dent. Mater. Off. Publ. Acad. Dent. Mater.* **2016**, *32*, 1564–1574. [CrossRef]
99. Sharma, N.; Jandaik, S.; Kumar, S. Synergistic Activity of Doped Zinc Oxide Nanoparticles with Antibiotics: Ciprofloxacin, Ampicillin, Fluconazole and Amphotericin B against Pathogenic Microorganisms. *An. Acad. Bras. Cienc.* **2016**, *88*, 1689–1698. [CrossRef]
100. Ahmadpour Kermani, S.; Salari, S.; Ghasemi Nejad Almani, P. Comparison of Antifungal and Cytotoxicity Activities of Titanium Dioxide and Zinc Oxide Nanoparticles with Amphotericin B against Different Candida Species: In Vitro Evaluation. *J. Clin. Lab. Anal.* **2021**, *35*, e23577. [CrossRef]
101. Chintalacharuvu, K.R.; Matolek, Z.A.; Pacheco, B.; Carriera, E.M.; Beenhouwer, D.O. Complexing Amphotericin B with Gold Nanoparticles Improves Fungal Clearance from the Brains of Mice Infected with Cryptococcal Neoformans. *Med. Mycol.* **2021**, *59*, 1085–1091. [CrossRef]
102. Patra, J.K.; Baek, K.-H. Comparative Study of Proteasome Inhibitory, Synergistic Antibacterial, Synergistic Anticandidal, and Antioxidant Activities of Gold Nanoparticles Biosynthesized Using Fruit Waste Materials. *Int. J. Nanomed.* **2016**, *11*, 4691–4705. [CrossRef]
103. Souza, J.A.S.; Alves, M.M.; Barbosa, D.B.; Lopes, M.M.; Pinto, E.; Figueiral, M.H.; Delbem, A.C.B.; Mira, N.P. Study of the Activity of Punica Granatum-Mediated Silver Nanoparticles against Candida Albicans and Candida Glabrata, Alone or in Combination with Azoles or Polyenes. *Med. Mycol.* **2020**, *58*, 564–567. [CrossRef]

104. Sadat Akhavi, S.; Moradi Dehaghi, S. Drug Delivery of Amphotericin B through Core-Shell Composite Based on PLGA/Ag/Fe$_3$O$_4$: In Vitro Test. *Appl. Biochem. Biotechnol.* **2020**, *191*, 496–510. [CrossRef]
105. Trikeriotis, M.; Ghanotakis, D.F. Intercalation of Hydrophilic and Hydrophobic Antibiotics in Layered Double Hydroxides. *Int. J. Pharm.* **2007**, *332*, 176–184. [CrossRef]
106. Yu, D.; Wang, L.; Zhou, H.; Zhang, X.; Wang, L.; Qiao, N. Fluorimetric Detection of Candida Albicans Using Cornstalk N-Carbon Quantum Dots Modified with Amphotericin B. *Bioconjug. Chem.* **2019**, *30*, 966–973. [CrossRef]
107. Gudz, K.Y.; Permyakova, E.S.; Matveev, A.T.; Bondarev, A.V.; Manakhov, A.M.; Sidorenko, D.A.; Filippovich, S.Y.; Brouchkov, A.V.; Golberg, D.V.; Ignatov, S.G.; et al. Pristine and Antibiotic-Loaded Nanosheets/Nanoneedles-Based Boron Nitride Films as a Promising Platform to Suppress Bacterial and Fungal Infections. *ACS Appl. Mater. Interfaces* **2020**, *12*, 42485–42498. [CrossRef]
108. Hwang, I.; Hwang, J.H.; Choi, H.; Kim, K.-J.; Lee, D.G. Synergistic Effects between Silver Nanoparticles and Antibiotics and the Mechanisms Involved. *J. Med. Microbiol.* **2012**, *61*, 1719–1726. [CrossRef]
109. Jamaran, S.; Zarif, B.R. Synergistic Effect of Silver Nanoparticles with Neomycin or Gentamicin Antibiotics on Mastitis-Causing Staphylococcus Aureus. *Open J. Ecol.* **2016**, *6*, 452–459. [CrossRef]
110. Durán, N.; Marcato, P.D.; Durán, M.; Yadav, A.; Gade, A.; Rai, M. Mechanistic Aspects in the Biogenic Synthesis of Extracellular Metal Nanoparticles by Peptides, Bacteria, Fungi, and Plants. *Appl. Microbiol. Biotechnol.* **2011**, *90*, 1609–1624. [CrossRef]
111. Janik, S.; Grela, E.; Stączek, S.; Zdybicka-Barabas, A.; Luchowski, R.; Gruszecki, W.I.; Grudzinski, W. Amphotericin B-Silver Hybrid Nanoparticles Help to Unveil the Mechanism of Biological Activity of the Antibiotic: Disintegration of Cell Membranes. *Molecules* **2023**, *28*, 4687. [CrossRef]
112. Paulo, C.S.O.; Lino, M.M.; Matos, A.A.; Ferreira, L.S. Differential Internalization of Amphotericin B--Conjugated Nanoparticles in Human Cells and the Expression of Heat Shock Protein 70. *Biomaterials* **2013**, *34*, 5281–5293. [CrossRef]
113. Paulo, C.S.O.; Vidal, M.; Ferreira, L.S. Antifungal Nanoparticles and Surfaces. *Biomacromolecules* **2010**, *11*, 2810–2817. [CrossRef] [PubMed]
114. Lino, M.M.; Paulo, C.S.O.; Vale, A.C.; Vaz, M.F.; Ferreira, L.S. Antifungal Activity of Dental Resins Containing Amphotericin B-Conjugated Nanoparticles. *Dent. Mater. Off. Publ. Acad. Dent. Mater.* **2013**, *29*, e252–e262. [CrossRef] [PubMed]
115. Alshahrani, S.M.; Khafagy, E.-S.; Riadi, Y.; Al Saqr, A.; Alfadhel, M.M.; Hegazy, W.A.H. Amphotericin B-PEG Conjugates of ZnO Nanoparticles: Enhancement Antifungal Activity with Minimal Toxicity. *Pharmaceutics* **2022**, *14*, 1646. [CrossRef]
116. Sreeharsha, N.; Chitrapriya, N.; Jang, Y.J.; Kenchappa, V. Evaluation of Nanoparticle Drug-Delivery Systems Used in Preclinical Studies. *Ther. Deliv.* **2021**, *12*, 325–336. [CrossRef]
117. Luo, M.; Boudier, A.; Clarot, I.; Maincent, P.; Schneider, R.; Leroy, P. Gold Nanoparticles Grafted by Reduced Glutathione with Thiol Function Preservation. *Colloid Interface Sci. Commun.* **2016**, *14*, 8–12. [CrossRef]
118. Hafner, A.; Lovrić, J.; Lakoš, G.P.; Pepić, I. Nanotherapeutics in the EU: An overview on current state and future directions. *Int. J. Nanomed.* **2014**, *9*, 1005–1023. [CrossRef]
119. Allen, T.M.; Cullis, P.R. Liposomal drug delivery systems: From concept to clinical applications. *Adv. Drug Deliv. Rev.* **2013**, *65*, 36–48. [CrossRef] [PubMed]
120. Bobo, D.; Robinson, K.J.; Islam, J.; Thurecht, K.J.; Corrie, S.R. Nanoparticle-Based Medicines: A Review of FDA-Approved Materials and Clinical Trials to Date. *Pharm. Res.* **2016**, *33*, 2373–2387. [CrossRef] [PubMed]
121. Anselmo, A.C.; Mitragotri, S. Nanoparticles in the clinic: An update. *Bioeng. Transl. Med.* **2019**, *4*, e10143. [CrossRef]
122. Anselmo, A.C.; Mitragotri, S. Nanoparticles in the clinic. *Bioeng. Transl. Med.* **2016**, *1*, 10–29. [CrossRef]
123. Weissig, V.; Pettinger, T.K.; Murdock, N. Nanopharmaceuticals (part 1): Products on the market. *Int. J. Nanomed.* **2014**, *9*, 4357–4573. [CrossRef] [PubMed]
124. Sosnik, A.; Carcaboso, A.M. Nanomedicines in the future of pediatric therapy. *Adv. Drug Deliv. Rev.* **2014**, *73*, 140–161. [CrossRef] [PubMed]

Disclaimer/Publisher's Note: The statements, opinions and data contained in all publications are solely those of the individual author(s) and contributor(s) and not of MDPI and/or the editor(s). MDPI and/or the editor(s) disclaim responsibility for any injury to people or property resulting from any ideas, methods, instructions or products referred to in the content.

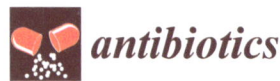

Article

Synergistic Antibacterial Effects of Gallate Containing Compounds with Silver Nanoparticles in Gallate Crossed Linked PVA Hydrogel Films

John Jackson [1,*] and Claudia Helena Dietrich [2]

1. Faculty of Pharmaceutical Sciences, University of British Columbia, 2405 Wesbrook Mall, Vancouver, BC V6T1Z3, Canada
2. Department of Pathology and Laboratory Medicine, University of British Columbia, Vancouver, BC V6T1Z7, Canada; claudinha.dietrich@gmail.com
* Correspondence: jackson@mail.ubc.ca

Abstract: Currently available silver-based antiseptic wound dressings have limited patient effectiveness. There exists a need for wound dressings that behave as comfortable degradable hydrogels with a strong antibiotic potential. The objectives of this project were to investigate the combined use of gallates (either epi gallo catechin gallate (EGCG), Tannic acid, or Quercetin) as both PVA crosslinking agents and as potential synergistic antibiotics in combination with silver nanoparticles. Crosslinking was assessed gravimetrically, silver and gallate release was measured using inductively coupled plasma and HPLC methods, respectively. Synergy was measured using 96-well plate FICI methods and in-gel antibacterial effects were measured using planktonic CFU assays. All gallates crosslinked PVA with optimal extended swelling obtained using EGCG or Quercetin at 14% loadings (100 mg in 500 mg PVA with glycerol). All three gallates were synergistic in combination with silver nanoparticles against both gram-positive and -negative bacteria. In PVA hydrogel films, silver nanoparticles with EGCG or Quercetin more effectively inhibited bacterial growth in CFU counts over 24 h as compared to films containing single agents. These biocompatible natural-product antibiotics, EGCG or Quercetin, may play a dual role of providing stable PVA hydrogel films and a powerful synergistic antibiotic effect in combination with silver nanoparticles.

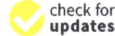

Citation: Jackson, J.; Dietrich, C.H. Synergistic Antibacterial Effects of Gallate Containing Compounds with Silver Nanoparticles in Gallate Crossed Linked PVA Hydrogel Films. *Antibiotics* **2024**, *13*, 312. https://doi.org/10.3390/antibiotics13040312

Academic Editor: Anisha D'Souza

Received: 8 March 2024
Revised: 23 March 2024
Accepted: 27 March 2024
Published: 29 March 2024

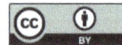

Copyright: © 2024 by the authors. Licensee MDPI, Basel, Switzerland. This article is an open access article distributed under the terms and conditions of the Creative Commons Attribution (CC BY) license (https:// creativecommons.org/licenses/by/ 4.0/).

Keywords: gallate; antibacterial; polyvinyl alcohol; synergy; silver nanoparticles

1. Introduction

The optimal features of a wound dressing are to provide an immediate anti-infective environment in a long-lasting hydrogel that may be easily removed from the wound by rinsing when required. Poly vinyl alcohol (PVA) has been extensively studied as a potential wound dressing material since it is biocompatible and may be provided as a drug-loaded, thin flexible film that quickly swells in water to form a hydrogel. The material is inexpensive and is used in existing commercial medical orthopedic devices [1,2]. PVA is generally available with high (99%) or low (under 90%) degrees of hydrolyzation which renders the material almost insoluble and fully soluble, respectively. For wound dressing applications, some control of the degradation rate of the PVA is preferred, leading many workers to describe crosslinking methods to prevent PVA dissolution including the use of borates [3], citric acid [4] or glutaraldehyde [5,6]. Our group previously investigated heat crosslinking of PVA (88% hydrolyzed) in the presence of silver nitrate or the simple ratio blending of 99% and sub 90% hydrolyzation level PVA polymers [7,8] to control degradation. Such PVA films allow for reasonable control of swelling and degradation while allowing the encapsulation and release of anti-infective silver salts or nanoparticles.

Silver is a well-established antibacterial agent used in numerous wound dressings. Silver sulfadiazine creams (prescription or online orders) have been used topically for many years and silver containing dressing materials such as Acticoat ᵗᵐ (silver nanoparticles) or Aquacel Ag ᵗᵐ are applied for longer-term treatment of wounds. Despite widespread use globally, the efficacy of these wound dressings is limited [9,10]. The improved antibacterial effect of nanoparticulate silver over ionic silver is now well established with a mechanism of action that may be additive when used with other antibiotics, especially in drug-resistant settings [11]. This additive or synergistic antibiotic effect against gram-positive and -negative bacteria of silver nitrate or silver nanoparticles in combination with existing antibiotics is well established [12–15]. Despite these known effects, there still remains a need for dual-drug-loaded anti-infective wound dressings, especially as drug resistant problems increase in clinics.

Gallate-containing molecules such as Tannic acid, Quercetin, and epigallocatechin gallate (EGCG) are polyphenols found in many plants and are known to have mild antibiotic effects against both gram-positive and -negative bacteria with minimal inhibitory concentrations determined in this laboratory of the order of 100 µg/mL as compared to silver nanoparticles at 2.5 µg/mL. The gallate-containing molecule Tannic acid, used for centuries to stabilize collagen in hides to produce leather, has been shown to create extensive hydrogen bonds with 99% hydrolyzed PVA to strengthen the polymer [16–18]. Similarly, unpurified tea polyphenol extracts which contain gallates have also been used with PVA in both a strengthening and antibacterial role [19–21]. Coincidentally, gallates (including Tannic acid, tea polyphenols, Quercetin, and EGCG) may act as "green" reducing agents to convert silver salts into stronger anti-infective silver nanoparticles [22–33]. This allows for the green and inexpensive creation of silver nanoparticles within gallate-containing, PVA cast films for a possible dual antibacterial drug composition for the treatment of wounds.

Although there is generally an improved antibiotic effect from using the dual-loaded compositions (silver with Tannic acid [23,24], Quercetin [29,33], and a minor effect with EGCG [34]), these previous studies usually show minor levels of inhibition and are complicated by the absence of compositions with silver nanoparticles alone. Almost all "green" synthesis studies do not allow for studies with silver nanoparticles alone since they are made in situ with the gallates present. Furthermore, most workers report the gallates form a stabilizing coating on the surface of the silver nanoparticles (e.g., Tannic acid [22,25], Quercetin [27–30], and EGCG [31] which may inhibit the normal antibiotic effect of the silver nanoparticles [26,31].

To overcome this problem of "green" synthesis gallate-capping of silver nanoparticles, we have investigated the use of premanufactured silver nanoparticles (AGNP) incorporated into gallate-containing PVA (88% hydrolyzed) cast films. By using fully water-soluble (88% hydrolyzed) PVA, the possible controlled crosslinking and aqueous degradation of the PVA films was explored. The antibacterial effects (against gram-positive and -negative bacteria) of all agents (gallate alone, silver nanoparticles alone, or gallate with silver nanoparticles) was measured using 96-well plate FICI synergy assays. Furthermore, for PVA films containing agents, CFU counting methods following 24 h incubations of bacteria with swollen films were used.

2. Materials and Methods

Poly (vinyl alcohol) (Selvol 540, 88 mole% hydrolyzed, Mw~150,000) was purchased from Sekisui Specialty Chemical Company (Dallas, TX, USA). Silver nanoparticles (10 nm Biopure-citrate) were purchased from Nanocomposix (San Diego, CA, USA). Tannic acid, Quercetin, glycerol, and silver salts (>99.0%) were purchased from Sigma-Aldrich (St. Louis, MO, USA). Epigallocatechin-gallate (EGCG > 94%) was purchased as a product, Teavigo, from DSM (Cambridge, ON, Canada). All solvents and other chemicals were purchased from Fisher scientific. Deionized water was used in the preparation of all formulations.

2.1. Manufacture of PVA Films

Film Preparation (Solvent-Cast PVA)

PVA solutions were prepared as a 2.5% w/w stock solution by slowly adding PVA powder to rapidly stirred water, followed by continued stirring and heating to 95 °C for approximately 60 min. When a clear solution had formed, the contents were cooled. Solutions with silver nanoparticles were prepared by adding known volumes of the stock solution to 20 mL volumes of PVA solution with or without glycerol (20% final concentration to PVA). Films were cast in 60 mm × 15 mm disposable polystyrene Petri dishes. The solutions in Petri dishes were left in a 37 °C oven overnight, in order for the water to evaporate. All dried films were stored in a dark cupboard before evaluation. Films were easily removed from Petri dishes with forceps after the rim coating on the vertical side of the Petri dish was cracked.

PVA films contained 500 mg of PVA and 100 mg of glycerol (where applicable). EGCG and Tannic acid films contained 0.04% Silver (to PVA) or 200 µg of silver, and Quercetin films contained 0.02% silver (to PVA) or 100 µg of silver. Silver salt solutions were prepared at 10 mg/mL concentrations in water and stored covered with aluminum foil in a dark cupboard until required.

2.2. Swelling Determinations

Film Swelling Studies

Film sections weighing 50 mg were placed on moistened 0.45 um filter discs (S Pak HA membrane 47 mm diameter, Millipore, Billerica, MA, USA) and weighed. The films and filters were covered with approximately 0.5 mL of water. After set time periods, the filter discs and adherent PVA-gallate gel were moved to a Millipore vacuum apparatus and vacuum was applied to draw all excess water from the filter over approximately 5 s. This was enough to remove all surface and loose water but not shrink the gels. The combined PVA gel and filter were reweighed and then placed back in water. The weight gain (termed swelling) was then calculated as a percentage of the original dry film weight.

2.3. Drug Release Studies and Characterization

Films (100 mg) containing EGCG, Tannic acid, or Quercetin along with silver nanoparticles were placed in 10 mM Hepes buffer (pH 7.3) (5 mL) and all this buffer was removed at regular intervals for silver analysis by Inductively Coupled Plasma (ICP Agilent, Santa Clara, CA, USA) analysis and gallate analysis by HPLC analysis. The 5 mL of Hepes buffer was then replaced with 5 mL of fresh buffer added to the films. Experiments were performed using triplicate samples.

Silver calibration standards (10 to 2000 ng/mL) were run every 30 samples. The ICP instrument displayed reproducible standard curves, over 75 sequential rounds of silver analysis with detection limits as low as 10 ng/mL. Each release study was run in triplicate for at least two weeks and the results plotted as the calculated percentage of silver released as a function of time. A Waters Acquity HPLC system (Milford, MA, USA) with Empower software version 1 and UV/VIS analysis was used for both Quercetin and EGCG quantitation. For EGCG, the mobile phase was a gradient of acidified water (glacial acetic acid 0.5%) and acetonitrile from 90:10 to 80:20 over 6 min followed by 6 more min with the 80:20 mobile phase and detection at 293 nm. For Quercetin, the mobile phase was isocratic using 0.5% acetic acid and acetonitrile at a 65:35 ratio and detection at 375 nm.

2.4. Bacterial Studies

The bacteria used were Methicillin-resistant *Staphylococcus aureus* (MRSA (USA 300)) (gram-positive) and *Escherichia coli* (*E. coli.* K12) (gram-negative) and were grown in lysogeny broth. These bacteria represent difficult-to-treat bacteria from the gram-positive and -negative categories are the go-to standard bacteria used by most groups in the microbiological field.

2.5. 96-Well Plate Checkerboard Assays

EGCG, Quercetin, or silver (expressed as the concentration of silver, not salt) were serially diluted 2-fold (using silver along one axis and EGCG or Quercetin along the other) across the 96-well plate. This was then followed by the addition of 100 uL of bacterial culture with an OD_{600} of 0.0025 to all wells. Plates were then wrapped with foil and incubated for 24 h at 37 °C. The turbidity in each well was then analyzed using a microplate reader at OD_{600}. Control lanes containing drugs alone and no bacteria were also run to check for background interference.

2.6. Fractional Inhibitory Concentration Index (FICI) Determination

The FICI was calculated using values of the turbidity of the wells adjusted to background interference. The FICI of each agent (e.g., Silver or EGCG) was determined as the minimal inhibitory concentration (MIC) of one agent divided by the MIC of the other agent to the MIC of that agent alone. FICI was then computed as the sum of each agent's FIC. The FICI values were then interpreted as follows: FICI $\leq$ 0.5, synergy; FICI 0.5–$\leq$0.75 partial synergy; FICI 0.75–$\leq$1.0, additive effect; FICI >1.0–$\leq$4.0, indifference; and FICI > 4.0, antagonism as similarly described by others [35–37].

2.7. Colony Forming Unit, Kill-Curve Test

PVA films (12.5 mg) were placed in 20 mL flat-bottomed screw cap glass vials. Then, 1 mL of bacterial culture at OD_{600} of 0.005 in Lysogeny broth (LB) medium was added to the film which then swelled. The vials were left in the dark at 37 °C for 24 h. Samples of 100 uL were extracted from each tube at 24 h followed by 10-fold serial dilutions in small tubes. Then, 10 uL of each dilution was taken and pipetted onto LB agar plates. These plates were then incubated for 24 h at 37 °C. Colonies were counted using a low magnification optical microscope and the counts presented in log CFU/mL.

2.8. Statistics

The students T test (unpaired) was used to determine significance with a p value of less than 0.05.

3. Results

PVA films containing Tannic acid or EGCG at lower concentrations were generally clear and strong. With the addition of glycerol, the films were very flexible but did not break under pressure. Films containing Quercetin were only clear at low concentrations (up to 100 mg in 500 mg PVA) but dried films were cloudy after that. The cloudiness in films probably arose from the reducing solubility of Quercetin, EGCG, and Tannic acid in the drying water cast film so that as the water evaporated, the agents precipitated. The final composition of the major films (termed EGCG 75, EGCG 100, Quercetin 100, and Quercetin 200) is shown in Table 1.

Table 1. Composition of major films (weight %).

Title	PVA %	Gallate %	AGNP %	Glycerol %
EGCG 75	74	11	0.03	15
EGCG 100	71	14	0.03	14.3
Quercetin 100	71	14	0.014	14.3
Quercetin 200	63	25	0.012	12.5

3.1. Swelling Studies

PVA films with or without glycerol and just silver or no drugs dissolved almost immediately and fully in less than two hours. Films were manufactured using 500 mg of PVA (20 mL of 2.5% w/v) with various amounts of Tannic acid, EGCG, or Quercetin between 50 mg and 500 mg. All films were made with or without the plasticizing agent glycerol. Swelling data (at 5 min, 1 day and 4 days) are shown for all films containing glycerol in Table 2. Because these studies included 20 samples, only single samples were used and measured over multiple time points. The experiments were repeated twice and demonstrated the same concentration-dependent crosslinking effect of the gallates on PVA.

Table 2. Swelling data were collected for PVA films all with 20% glycerol, containing different amounts of EGCG, tannic acid, or quercetin in an initial film with 500 mg of PVA. Films with EGCG or tannic acid also had 0.04% silver nanoparticles and quercetin films had 0.02% silver nanoparticles. The films were monitored over time, similar to Figures 1 and 2. PVA-only films dissolved in under 2 h. Tannic acid films, despite initial swelling, did not stay swollen for 24 h. EGCG at 75 and 100 mg or quercetin at 100 or 200 mg (initially in 500 mg PVA films) which remained swollen for four days were used for further studies.

	Swelling Studies (%)		
		Incubation Time	
500 mg PVA films with 20% glycerol (100 mg) and gallates	5 min	1 day	4 days
EGCG 50 mg	345	352	−54
EGCG 75 mg	286	370	91
EGCG 100 mg	271	220	260
EGCG 200 mg	112	152	216
EGCG 300 mg	84	92	88
EGCG 400 mg	114	120	126
EGCG 500 mg	90	92	94
Tannic 50 mg	151	180	35
Tannic 75 mg	147	82	57
Tannic 100 mg	147	74	27
Tannic 200 mg	135	45	35
Tannic 300 mg	154	59	55
Tannic 400 mg	159	69	79
Tannic 500 mg	179	70	76
Quercetin 50 mg	154	14	4
Quercetin 75 mg	798	256	170
Quercetin 100 mg	710	268	220
Quercetin 200 mg	404	402	400
Quercetin 300 mg	256	264	290

More detailed examples of the time courses of swelling for Tannic acid, EGCG, and Quercetin (all 100 mg in 500 mg PVA) are shown in Figures 1 and 2.

Films containing Tannic acid swelled rapidly (15 min) to levels between 200 and 300% which remained swollen for 3 to 4 h before slowly breaking down over 24 h. The was little impact from the concentration of Tannic acid in the PVA or the inclusion of glycerol in these swelling studies (Figure 1).

Swelling for EGCG-loaded PVA films was similarly largely unaffected by the inclusion of glycerol and was more robust and long-lasting than that observed for Tannic acid. When 100 mg of EGCG in 500 mg PVA was used, swelling was stable at approximately 300% for 14 days (Figure 1). Using 50 mg of EGCG brought high initial levels of swelling that did not last, and when 200 to 500 mg of EGCG was used, swelling levels were constant over 4 days at around 100% (Table 2).

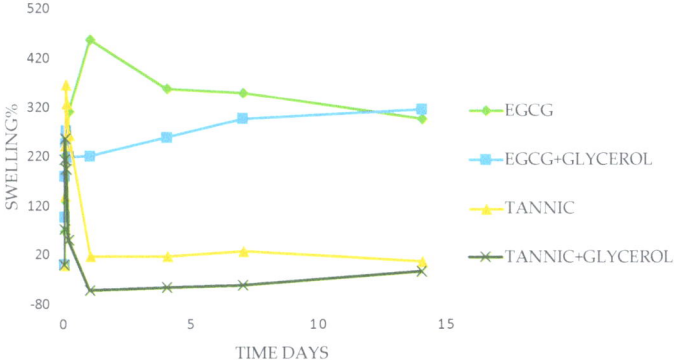

Figure 1. Swelling studies. PVA films (50 mg), with +/− 20% glycerol to PVA, and 0.04% silver nanoparticles, were tested for swelling in water. Initial films contained 100 mg EGCG in 500 mg PVA. Glycerol had no effect on swelling. Durable swelling was observed for EGCG, but only short-lived for tannic acid.

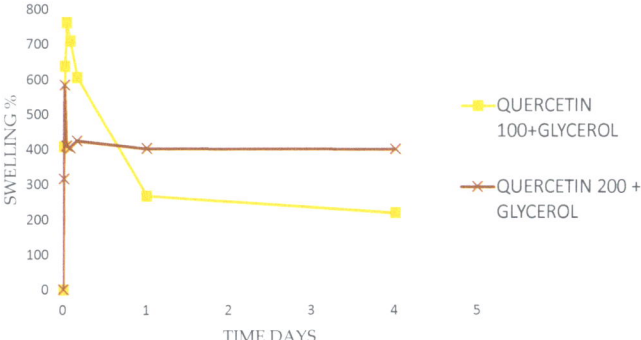

Figure 2. Swelling studies. PVA films (50 mg) each with 20% glycerol to PVA were tested for swelling in water. These films also contained silver nanoparticles at 0.02% (w/w to PVA). The initial films were loaded with either 100 mg or 200 mg of quercetin in 500 mg of PVA. It was noted that the films loaded with 100 mg and 200 mg of quercetin showed durable swelling.

For Quercetin, swelling levels were initially higher but soon dropped down to stabilize in the 200 to 400% swelling range at 4 days (Table 2 and Figure 2). Quercetin could not be loaded uniformly in PVA films at levels higher than 300 mg in 500 mg PVA.

3.2. Drug Release Studies

Release studies were performed with PVA films containing concentrations of EGCG at 75 mg or 100 mg or Quercetin at 100 mg or 200 mg (to 500 mg of PVA) containing glycerol (20%) with or without silver nanoparticles. These films showed prolonged swelling times in the swelling studies (Table 2). Tannic acid loaded films were not studied because swelling did not prolong past 1 day. These films (EGCG 75 and 100 or Quercetin 100 and 200) were considered the most clinically relevant and release studies were only performed at 37 °C, also to match clinically relevant conditions.

EGCG released from films with a burst phase over one day followed by a more sustained release over the next six days (Figure 3). All samples reached approximately 40% of encapsulated EGCG released by day 7. The 75 mg EGCG no-silver sample released a little over 50% of drug but the release data were not significantly different to the other samples. Interestingly, one residual film for the 75 mg EGCG no-silver sample was broken down (polytron homogenizer with ethanol extraction) and showed 47% of the initially loaded EGCG still present in agreement with the data in Figure 3.

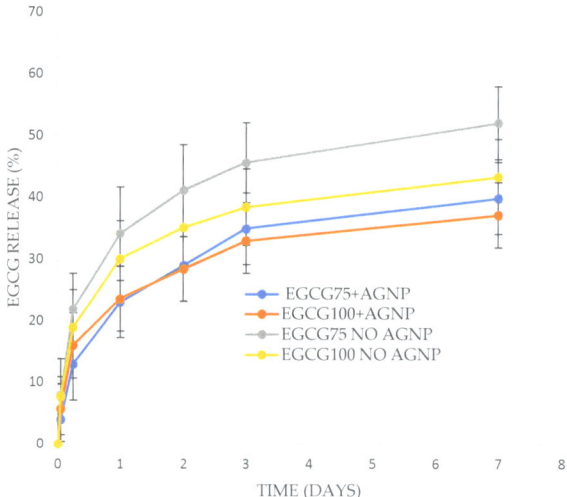

Figure 3. EGCG release from PVA films +/− silver nanoparticles (AGNP). Each film containing 75 or 100 mg of EGCG (to 500 mg of PVA in the initial film), along with 20% glycerol to PVA and 0.04% silver nanoparticles to PVA.

Quercetin released from the PVA films in a similar profile to EGCG with a burst phase over the first day followed by a slow release over the next six days. There was no significant difference between samples. However, the amount of Quercetin released was much lower than for EGCG films, reaching only six to ten percent release by 1 day and only minor (but measurable) release after that time (Figure 4). One film loaded with Quercetin at 100 mg (no silver) was broken down after 7 days and showed 94% remaining drug in approximate agreement with released data showing less than 10% drug release.

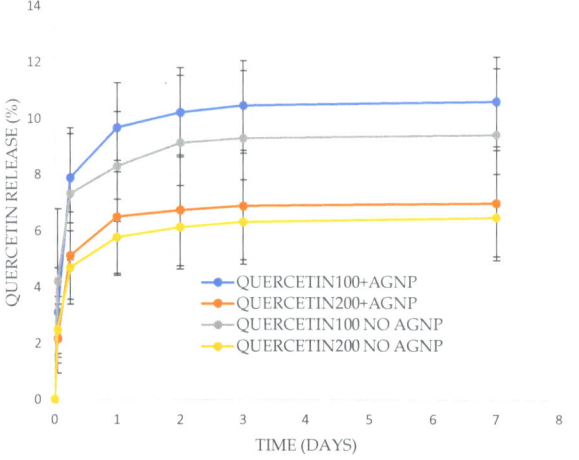

Figure 4. Quercetin release from PVA films +/− silver nanoparticles (AGNP). Each film containing 100 mg or 200 mg Quercetin (to 500 mg of PVA in the initial film), along with 20% glycerol to PVA and 0.02% silver nanoparticles to PVA.

3.3. Silver Release Study

Silver released from the PVA films more rapidly than EGCG and Quercetin released from the same films. For EGCG loaded films, silver nanoparticles released with a large burst phase for the 100 mg EGCG films but a smaller burst phase for the 75 mg EGCG loaded films (Figure 5). After five hours the release rate for both the 75 and 100 mg EGCG films was steady and sustained, reaching full release for the 100 mg films (measured at over 100%) at 7 days and 66% released for the 75 mg films. These release values were significantly different on day 3 and day 7 but not on day 2. Silver released from Quercetin loaded films without a burst phase but rather a steady release of approximately 55% by day 3 and a minor but measurable release by day 7 (Figure 6). There was no significant difference in release rates between the 100 mg and 200 mg (to 500 mg PVA) Quercetin-loaded films.

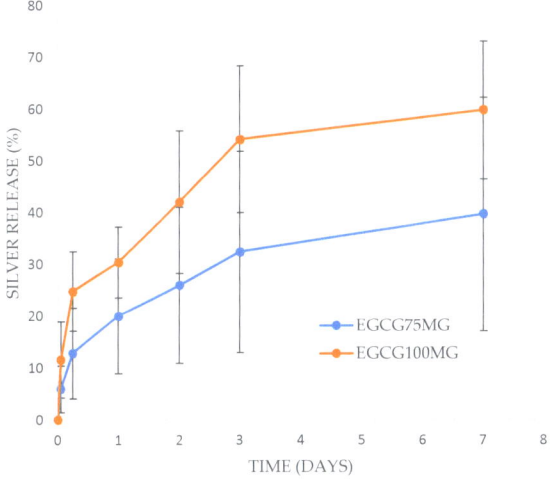

Figure 5. Silver nanoparticles released from EGCG-loaded PVA films. All films contained 20% glycerol and 0.04% silver nanoparticles. EGCG was loaded at either 75 mg (11% of PVA) or 100 mg (14% of PVA) to 500 mg PVA.

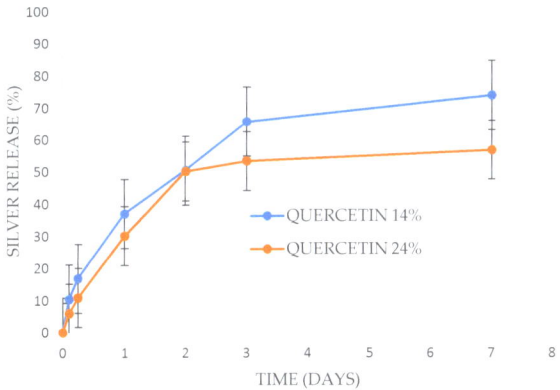

Figure 6. Silver nanoparticles released from Quercetin-loaded PVA films. All films contained 20% glycerol and 0.02% silver nanoparticles. Quercetin was loaded at either 100 mg (14% of PVA) or 200 mg (24% of PVA).

3.4. Fractional Inhibitory Concentration Index (FICI) Determinations

The minimal inhibitory concentrations (MIC) for EGCG, Tannic acid, and Quercetin against MRSA and *E. coli* were in the range of 50 to 100 μg/mL as seen in Table 3. The MIC for silver nanoparticles was much lower at 2.5 μg/mL. When placed in combination against these bacteria, the FICI values for all combinations were less than 0.5 (range 0.14 to 0.43) establishing that these combinations of antibiotics are synergistic. The same experiments were run using silver nitrate in place of silver nanoparticles. The MIC of silver nitrate against both bacteria was the same as for nanoparticles at 2.5 μg/mL. The FICI values against MRSA were 0.5 (EGCG), 0.75 (Tannic acid), and 0.62 (Quercetin). For *E. coli* the FICI values were 0.31 (EGCG), 0.56 (Tannic acid), and 0.56 (Quercetin). Therefore, silver nitrate is fully synergistic with EGCG for both bacteria and partially synergistic for Tannic acid and Quercetin (FICI of 0.75 or less).

Table 3. Final FICI scores (MIC mean combination) for gallate synergy with silver nanoparticles in bacterial studies against gram-positive (MRSA) or gram-negative (*E. coli*) bacteria.

Gallate	MRSA			E. coli		
	MIC Alone(μg/mL)	MIC (Mean) Combination	St. Dev.	MIC Alone(μg/mL)	MIC (Mean) Combination	St. Dev.
EGCG	50	0.35	0.16	100	0.3	0.22
Tannic acid	50	0.197	0.057	50	0.43	0.18
Quercetin	50	0.147	0.05	100	0.43	0.11
Silver nanoparticles	2.5			2.5		

3.5. In-PVA Gel Antibacterial Testing

When PVA films were placed in a small volume of broth containing bacteria, they swelled and formed robust gels, mimicking application to a wound with exudate. Films containing EGCG or Quercetin at two concentrations with or without silver nanoparticles along with control (no drug) or silver nanoparticles alone were compared for their ability to inhibit bacterial growth at 24 h using either MRSA or *E. coli*. Experiments were performed on three separate occasions, and all showed the same effect. The mean value of the three is shown, but because of different initial inoculum counts, error bars are not included.

3.6. EGCG with MRSA

After 24 h, the untreated bacteria proliferated from approximately 10^6 CFU/mL to approximately 10^{10} CFU/mL. All films containing agents inhibited such growth (Figure 7A). The single agents alone (silver nanoparticles or EGCG) reduced bacterial growth to the order of 10^8 to 5×10^6 CFU/mL, but the combinations of EGCG and silver nanoparticles inhibited bacterial growth, restricting it below the original 10^6 CFU/mL level with the higher EGCG loaded film killing all bacteria. The order of inhibition was EGCG100 + AGNP > EGCG75 + AGNP > EGCG100 > EGCG75 > AGNP.

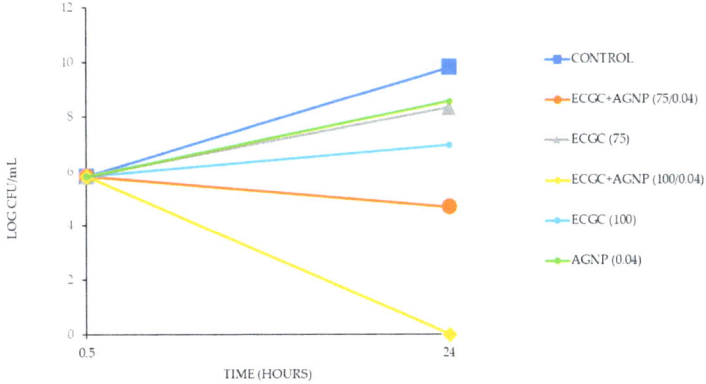

A. EGCG-MRSA

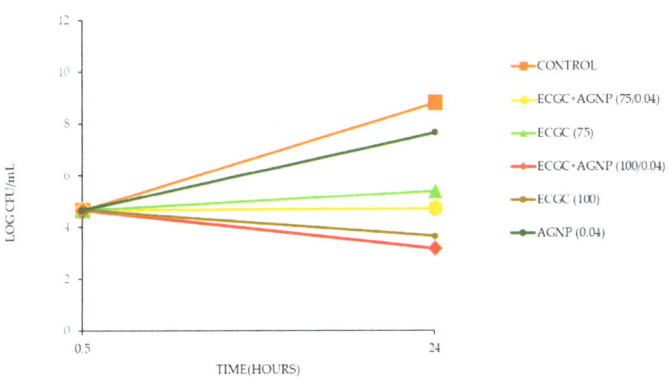

B. EGCG-*E.coli*

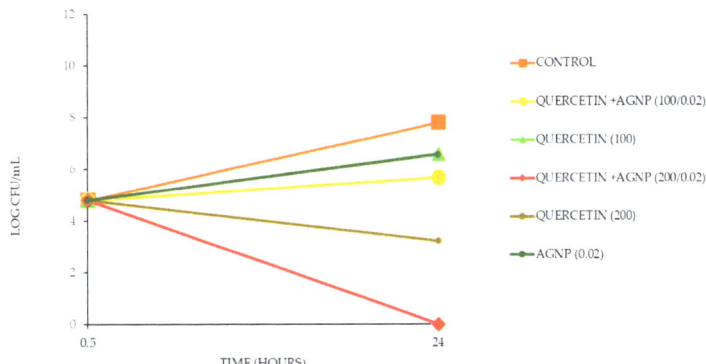

C. QUERCETIN-MRSA

Figure 7. *Cont.*

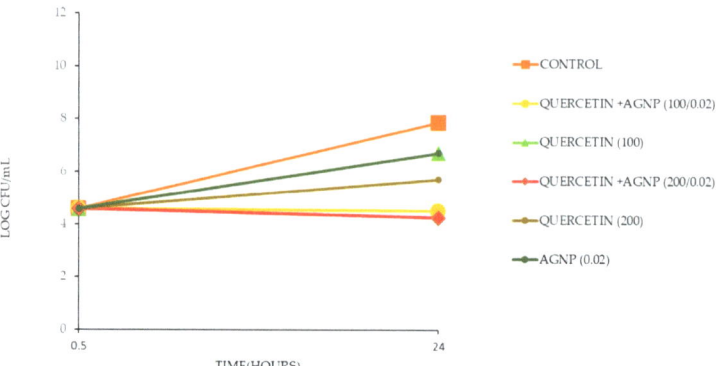

D. QUERCETIN-*E.coli*

Figure 7. CFU bacterial studies. (**A**) 12.5 mg films soaked in 1 mL MRSA broth for 24 h, then CFU counted. All films contained 20% glycerol. Films contained EGCG at 75 mg or 100 mg (in 500 mg PVA) +/− silver nanoparticles (AGNP) at 0.04%. Control films contained PVA alone. (**B**) 12.5 mg films soaked in 1 mL *E. coli* broth for 24 h, then CFU counted. All films contained 20% glycerol. Films contained EGCG at 75 mg or 100 mg (in 500 mg PVA) +/− silver nanoparticles (AGNP) at 0.04%. Control films contained PVA alone. (**C**) 12.5 mg films soaked in 1 mL MRSA broth for 24 h, then CFU counted. All films contained 20% glycerol. Films contained Quercetin at 100 mg or 200 mg (in 500 mg PVA) +/− silver nanoparticles (AGNP) at 0.02%. Control films contained PVA alone. (**D**) 12.5 mg films soaked in 1 mL *E. coli* broth for 24 h, then CFU counted. All films contained 20% glycerol. Films contained Quercetin at 100 mg or 200 mg (in 500 mg PVA) +/− silver nanoparticles (AGNP) at 0.02%. Control films contained PVA alone.

3.7. EGCG with E. coli

E. coli proliferated from an initial inoculum of approximately 10^5 CFU/mL to 5×10^9 CFU/mL after 24 h (Figure 7B). Silver nanoparticles alone only produced mild inhibition of this growth but both concentrations of EGCG-loaded films strongly inhibited the proliferation of *E. coli* bacteria. The combination of EGCG and AGNP results in increased inhibition of *E. coli* growth as compared to either agent alone.

3.8. Quercetin with MRSA

MRSA grew rapidly over 24 h from approximately 10^5 CFU/mL to approximately 10^8 CFU/mL (Figure 7C). Films loaded with either Quercetin (100) or AGNP alone inhibited bacterial proliferation mildly, whereas the film loaded with the higher concentration of Quercetin inhibited proliferation strongly. Both films containing combinations of Quercetin and AGNP inhibited proliferation more than single agents alone. Indeed, the films loaded with the high (200) loading of Quercetin killed all bacteria.

3.9. E. coli with Quercetin

After 24 h the bacteria grew from an initial approximate inoculum of 10^5/mL to approximately 10^8 CFU/Ml (Figure 7D). The film loaded with the lower concentration of Quercetin and the film with silver nanoparticles alone inhibited bacterial growth mildly. Films loaded with combinations of silver nanoparticles and Quercetin inhibited bacterial proliferation more than films loaded with each agent alone.

4. Discussion

Poly vinyl alcohol hydrogels may be suitable wound dressings because they are comfortable, easy to remove, and may contain anti-infective drugs. However, PVA films manufactured using the 99% hydrolyzed PVA do not allow for any controlled degradation since they are largely insoluble. We have previously developed crosslinked degradable PVA films using the 88% hydrolyzed form by heat treatment in the presence of silver [7]. However, heat treatment complicates the manufacturing method, and may not be suitable for certain drugs and only occurs with silver ions present.

In this study, the gallate containing compounds, EGCG, Tannic acid, and Quercetin has been shown to allow for extensive crosslinking of PVA (88% hydrolyzed) as witnessed by concentration-dependent inhibition of dissolution with certain concentrations providing well-swollen (hydrogel) films (Figures 1 and 2 and Table 2). The crosslinking is likely due to extensive hydrogen bonding between the gallate hydroxyl groups of tannic acid and the PVA hydroxyl groups on PVA and has been noted by many previous studies using 99% hydrolyzed PVA [16–18]. These previous studies sought to further strengthen PVA matrices rather than impacting dissolution in water. Similarly, tea polyphenols which contain many varieties of gallate-catechins including EGCG as well as caffeine [19,26,38] have been used to strengthen or impact the degradation of PVA films [19,20] via hydrogen bonding processes. There are limited studies using EGCG or Quercetin as singular agents directly in PVA films for mechanical or solubilization effects, although Quercetin has been used in PVA in combination with boron [39,40] and used as an antioxidant in PVA for food packaging [41]. The hydrogen bonding potential of Tannic acid and EGCG has been previously noted around drug solubilization of hydrophobic drugs [42–44].

The crosslinking effect of Tannic acid was short-lived and never lasted more than 24 h, but both EGCG and Quercetin provided swollen PVA gels at 4 days or more (Table 2). The reason for this less effective crosslinking by Tannic acid is unknown, but in terms of hydroxyl content in relation to molecular weight, then the order is EGCG > Quercetin > Tannic acid which may suggest an increased hydrogen bonding capacity of EGCG or Quercetin over Tannic acid. However, these different hydroxyl ratios are small, and the more likely influencing factor may the much larger molecular weight of Tannic acid (approximately 1700 dalton) as compared to EGCG (458) or Quercetin (302) so that steric effects may impact H bonding potential with the PVA polymer chains. Following the swelling studies, it was decided to use the EGCG (75) and EGCG (100) along with the Quercetin (100) and Quercetin (200) variants in further studies (all containing glycerol) since they allowed for swollen hydrogels with either partial or no degradation at four days (Table 2) for each crosslinking agent.

EGCG released well from the EGCG (75) and EGCG (100) PVA films with approximately 40% of the loaded drug releasing by day 3 which might provide high local concentrations of the agent on wounds for the critical first few days (Figure 3). It is likely that the unreleased fraction of the drug is more tightly bound in the PVA matrix. Quercetin released more slowly than EGCG, releasing between 6 and 10% of the loaded drug in the first three days. The minimal inhibitory concentrations of gallates against difficult-to-treat bacteria like *E. coli* and MRSA is of the order of 50–100 µg/mL (Table 3). All these films were cast in a 20 cm^2 Petri dish so that if one-quarter of a film (5 cm^2 with approximately 25 mg of gallate) was to be used for a small wound, then these rates of drug release would provide a huge excess of antibacterial agents based on these release rates. For example, the preferred care of diabetic wounds (which do have an average size of approximately 5 cm^2) is debridement with saline washing and then methods to keep the wound moist [45]. So, if a 5 cm^2 PVA-gallate film was placed on a wound with perhaps 1–2 mL of saline/exudate present in the swollen film, then the local gallate concentration would be easily sufficient as an anti-infective system.

Silver nanoparticles released more quickly from the PVA films than the gallates with approximately 50–60% of loaded silver released by two days for any films (Figures 5 and 6). These levels of drug release from a 5 cm^2 film (approximately 25–50 µg of total silver nanoparticles) placed on a wound with 2 mL of water/exudate might provide local concentrations of 6–12 µg/mL whereas the MIC of silver nanoparticles for *E. coli* and MRSA is 2.5 µg/mL (Table 3). Again, these release profiles theoretically provide sufficient drug alone for the inhibition of bacterial growth. Clearly the simultaneous release of EGCG (or Quercetin) with silver nanoparticles from these films should provide a huge excess of drug for extended periods on moist wounds.

Numerous studies have explored the antibiotic potential of gallate compositions as compared to compositions that also contain silver nanoparticles. These studies demonstrated an increased antibiotic potential over compositions containing silver or gallates alone [23,24,29,33,34]. However, these effects were not assessed by fractional inhibitory concentration index methods for synergy. In fact, although the word "synergy" is used frequently in this field, no studies measured FICI values and any reported increase in inhibitory effects were frequently small or did not include silver-alone measurements. In a study on wound closure, Kar et al. [44] demonstrated faster closure using EGCG with silver nanoparticle patches as compared to single agent patches but showed no increased inhibition in the growth of gram-positive or -negative bacteria using the combination systems. Similarly, Xiong et al. [34] described improved wound healing using EGCG plus silver nanoparticles over EGCG alone which was reported to arise from synergistic antibacterial activity (against *E. coli* and *Staph aureus*), yet improved antibacterial activity was less than 25% and silver alone was not measured. Badhwar et al. [33] demonstrated improved diabetic wound closure using Quercetin in combination with silver nanoparticles over each agent alone and mentioned synergistic effects against *E. coli* and *Staph aureus*, but the increased inhibition of bacterial growth was only measured in agar plates with only minor effects.

In this study, we have established strong antibacterial synergy among all three gallates (EGCG, Tannic acid, and Quercetin) and silver nanoparticles (Table 3). Similar results were found for the combined use of gallates with silver nitrate, whereby FICI values showed synergy (EGCG) or partial synergy (Quercetin and Tannic acid). The FICI values for silver nanoparticles were all well below 0.5 for both *E. coli* and MRSA.

These studies used the EGCG (75) and EGCG (100) or Quercetin (100) and Quercetin (200) loaded films as they had been shown to release agents well over 24 h and to allow for optimal crosslinked PVA hydrogel formation. These studies do not allow for determination of synergy but offer a suitable method for comparing the antibiotic potential of the films with individual agents or combinations of agents in a swollen aqueous setting like those found in a wound. These studies established that at all loadings of EGCG, Quercetin, and silver nanoparticles that the combined use of silver with EGCG or Quercetin provided increased inhibition of bacterial growth than films with single agents (Figure 7A–D). These data support the synergy findings established in the FICI studies (Table 2). All films had some inhibitory capacity over control films (PVA–glycerol, no drug) establishing the rationale for the use of PVA hydrogel films loaded with these drugs and especially with combinations of silver and gallates.

Author Contributions: Conceptualization, J.J.; Methodology, J.J. and C.H.D.; Investigation, J.J. and C.H.D.; Writing—original draft, J.J.; Writing—review & editing, C.H.D.; Project administration, C.H.D. All authors have read and agreed to the published version of the manuscript.

Funding: This research received no external funding.

Institutional Review Board Statement: Not applicable.

Informed Consent Statement: Not applicable.

Data Availability Statement: Data are contained within the article.

Conflicts of Interest: The authors declare no conflicts of interest.

References

1. Kobayashi, M.; Hyu, H.S. Development and evaluation of polyvinyl alcohol-hydrogels as an artificial artticular cartilage for orthopedic implants. *Materials* **2010**, *3*, 2753–2771. [CrossRef]
2. Baker, M.I.; Walsh, S.P.; Schwartz, Z.; Boyan, B.D. A review of polyvinyl alcohol and its uses in cartilage and orthopedic applications. *J. Biomed. Mater. Res. Part B Appl. Biomater.* **2012**, *100*, 1451–1457. [CrossRef]

3. Manna, U.; Patil, S. Borax mediated layer-by-layer self-assembly of neutral poly (vinyl alcohol) and chitosan. *J. Phys. Chem. B* **2009**, *113*, 9137–9142. [CrossRef] [PubMed]
4. Wali, A.; Zhang, Y.; Sengupta, P.; Higaki, Y.; Takahara, A.; Badiger, M.V. Electrospinning of non-ionic cellulose ethers/polyvinyl alcohol nanofibers: Characterization and applications. *Carbohydr. Polym.* **2018**, *181*, 175–182. [CrossRef] [PubMed]
5. Jodar, K.S.; Balcao, V.M.; Chaud, M.V.; Tubino, M.; Yoshida, V.M.; Oliveira, J.M., Jr.; Vila, M.M. Development and characterization of a hydrogel containing silver sulfadiazine for antimicrobial topical applications. *J. Pharm. Sci.* **2015**, *104*, 2241–2254. [CrossRef] [PubMed]
6. Augustine, R.; Hasan, A.; Yadu Nath, V.K.; Thomas, J.; Augustine, A.; Kalarikkal, N.; Moustafa, A.E.; Thomas, S. Electrospun polyvinyl alcohol membranes incorporated with green synthesized silver nanoparticles for wound dressing applications. *J. Mater. Sci. Mater. Med.* **2018**, *29*, 163. [CrossRef] [PubMed]
7. Jackson, J.; Burt, H.; Lange, D.; Whang, I.; Evans, R.; Plackett, D. The design, characterization and antibacterial activity of heat and silver crosslinked poly (vinyl alcohol) hydrogel forming dressings containing silver nanoparticles. *Nanomaterials* **2021**, *11*, 96. [CrossRef] [PubMed]
8. Jackson, J.; Plackett, D.; Hsu, E.; Lange, D.; Evans, R.; Burt, H. The development of solvent cast films or electrospun nanofiber membranes made from blended poly vinyl alcohol materials with different degrees of hydrolyzation for optimal hydrogel dissolution and sustained release of Anti-infective silver salts. *Nanomaterials* **2021**, *11*, 84. [CrossRef] [PubMed]
9. Khundkar, R.; Malic, C.; Burge, T. Use of Acticoat™ dressings in burns: What is the evidence? *Burns* **2010**, *36*, 751–758. [CrossRef]
10. Barnea, Y.; Weiss, J.; Gur, E. A review of the applications of the hydrofiber dressing with silver (Aquacel Ag®) in wound care. *Ther. Clin. Risk Manag.* **2010**, *6*, 21. [CrossRef]
11. Durán, N.; Durán, M.; De Jesus, M.B.; Seabra, A.B.; Fávaro, W.J.; Nakazato, G. Silver nanoparticles: A new view on mechanistic aspects on antimicrobial activity. *Nanomed. Nanotechnol. Biol. Med.* **2016**, *12*, 789–799. [CrossRef] [PubMed]
12. Jackson, J.; Lo, J.; Hsu, E.; Burt, H.M.; Shademani, A.; Lange, D. The combined use of gentamicin and silver nitrate in bone cement for a synergistic and extended antibiotic action against gram-positive and gram-negative bacteria. *Materials* **2021**, *14*, 3413. [CrossRef] [PubMed]
13. Morones-Ramirez, J.R.; Winkler, J.A.; Spina, C.S.; Collins, J.J. Silver enhances antibiotic activity against gram-negative bacteria. *Sci. Transl. Med.* **2013**, *5*, 190ra81. [CrossRef] [PubMed]
14. Hwang, I.S.; Hwang, J.H.; Choi, H.; Kim, K.J.; Lee, D.G. Synergistic effects between silver nanoparticles and antibiotics and the mechanisms involved. *J. Med. Microbiol.* **2012**, *61*, 1719–1726. [CrossRef] [PubMed]
15. Katva, S.; Das, S.; Moti, H.S.; Jyoti, A.; Kaushik, S. Antibacterial synergy of silver nanoparticles with gentamicin and chloramphenicol against Enterococcus faecalis. *Pharmacogn. Mag.* **2017**, *13* (Suppl. 4), S828.
16. Chen, W.; Li, N.; Ma, Y.; Minus, M.L.; Benson, K.; Lu, X.; Wang, X.; Ling, X.; Zhu, H. Superstrong and tough hydrogel through physical cross-linking and molecular alignment. *Biomacromolecules* **2019**, *20*, 4476–4484. [CrossRef] [PubMed]
17. Cheng, Z.; DeGracia, K.; Schiraldi, D.A. Sustainable, low flammability, mechanically-strong poly (vinyl alcohol) aerogels. *Polymers* **2018**, *10*, 1102. [CrossRef]
18. Si, C.; Tian, X.; Wang, Y.; Wang, Z.; Wang, X.; Lv, D.; Wang, A.; Wang, F.; Geng, L.; Zhao, J.; et al. A Polyvinyl Alcohol–Tannic Acid Gel with Exceptional Mechanical Properties and Ultraviolet Resistance. *Gels* **2022**, *8*, 751. [CrossRef]
19. Xu, X.J.; Huang, S.M.; Zhang, L.H. Biodegradability, antibacterial properties, and ultraviolet protection of polyvinyl alcohol-natural polyphenol blends. *Polym. Compos.* **2009**, *30*, 1611–1617. [CrossRef]
20. Liu, Y.; Wang, S.; Lan, W.; Qin, W. Development of ultrasound treated polyvinyl alcohol/tea polyphenol composite films and their physicochemical properties. *Ultrason. Sonochem.* **2019**, *51*, 386–394. [CrossRef]
21. Lan, W.; Zhang, R.; Ahmed, S.; Qin, W.; Liu, Y. Effects of various antimicrobial polyvinyl alcohol/tea polyphenol composite films on the shelf life of packaged strawberries. *Lwt* **2019**, *113*, 108297. [CrossRef]
22. Zhan, F.; Sheng, F.; Yan, X.; Zhu, Y.; Jin, W.; Li, J.; Li, B. Enhancement of antioxidant and antibacterial properties for tannin acid/chitosan/tripolyphosphate nanoparticles filled electrospinning films: Surface modification of sliver nanoparticles. *Int. J. Biol. Macromol.* **2017**, *104*, 813–820. [CrossRef] [PubMed]
23. Srikhao, N.; Theerakulpisut, S.; Chindaprasirt, P.; Okhawilai, M.; Narain, R.; Kasemsiri, P. Green synthesis of nano silver-embedded carboxymethyl starch waste/poly vinyl alcohol hydrogel with photothermal sterilization and pH-responsive behavior. *Int. J. Biol. Macromol.* **2023**, *242 Pt 3*, 125118. [CrossRef] [PubMed]
24. Liu, L.; Ge, C.; Zhang, Y.; Ma, W.; Su, X.; Chen, L.; Li, S.; Wang, L.; Mu, X.; Xu, Y. Tannic acid-modified silver nanoparticles for enhancing anti-biofilm activities and modulating biofilm formation. *Biomater. Sci.* **2020**, *8*, 4852–4860. [CrossRef] [PubMed]
25. Ranoszek-Soliwoda, K.; Tomaszewska, E.; Socha, E.; Krzyczmonik, P.; Ignaczak, A.; Orlowski, P.; Krzyzowska, M.; Celichowski, G.; Grobelny, J. The role of Tannic acid and sodium citrate in the synthesis of silver nanoparticles. *J. Nanopart. Res.* **2017**, *19*, 273. [CrossRef] [PubMed]
26. Du, L.; Li, T.; Wu, S.; Zhu, H.F.; Zou, F.Y. Electrospun composite nanofibre fabrics containing green reduced Ag nanoparticles as an innovative type of antimicrobial insole. *RSC Adv.* **2019**, *9*, 2244–2251. [CrossRef] [PubMed]
27. Chahardoli, A.; Hajmomeni, P.; Ghowsi, M.; Qalekhani, F.; Shokoohinia, Y.; Fattahi, A. Optimization of Quercetin-assisted silver nanoparticles synthesis and evaluation of their hemocompatibility, antioxidant, anti-inflammatory, and antibacterial effects. *Glob. Chall.* **2021**, *5*, 2100075. [CrossRef] [PubMed]

28. Yuan, Y.G.; Peng, Q.L.; Gurunathan, S. Effects of silver nanoparticles on multiple drug-resistant strains of Staphylococcus aureus and Pseudomonas aeruginosa from mastitis-infected goats: An alternative approach for antimicrobial therapy. *Int. J. Mol. Sci.* **2017**, *18*, 569. [CrossRef] [PubMed]
29. Vanaraj, S.; Keerthana, B.B.; Preethi, K. Biosynthesis, characterization of silver nanoparticles using Quercetin from Clitoria ternatea L to enhance toxicity against bacterial biofilm. *J. Inorg. Organomet. Polym. Mater.* **2017**, *27*, 1412–1422. [CrossRef]
30. Ahmed, B.; Hashmi, A.; Khan, M.S.; Musarrat, J. ROS mediated destruction of cell membrane, growth and biofilms of human bacterial pathogens by stable metallic AgNPs functionalized from bell pepper extract and Quercetin. *Adv. Powder Technol.* **2018**, *29*, 1601–1616. [CrossRef]
31. Meesaragandla, B.; Hayet, S.; Fine, T.; Janke, U.; Chai, L.; Delcea, M. Inhibitory Effect of Epigallocatechin Gallate-Silver Nanoparticles and Their Lysozyme Bioconjugates on Biofilm Formation and Cytotoxicity. *ACS Appl. Bio Mater.* **2022**, *5*, 4213–4221. [CrossRef] [PubMed]
32. Hussain, S.; Khan, Z. Epigallocatechin-3-gallate-capped Ag nanoparticles: Preparation and characterization. *Bioprocess Biosyst. Eng.* **2014**, *37*, 1221–1231. [CrossRef]
33. Badhwar, R.; Mangla, B.; Neupane, Y.R.; Khanna, K.; Popli, H. Quercetin loaded silver nanoparticles in hydrogel matrices for diabetic wound healing. *Nanotechnology* **2021**, *32*, 505102. [CrossRef] [PubMed]
34. Xiong, Y.; Xu, Y.; Zhou, F.; Hu, Y.; Zhao, J.; Liu, Z.; Zhai, Q.; Qi, S.; Zhang, Z.; Chen, L. Bio-functional hydrogel with antibacterial and anti-inflammatory dual properties to combat with burn wound infection. *Bioeng. Transl. Med.* **2022**, *8*, e10373. [CrossRef] [PubMed]
35. Feldman, M.; Smoum, R.; Mechoulam, R.; Steinberg, D. Potential Combinations of Endocannabinoid/ Endocannabinoid-like Compounds and Antibiotics against Methicillin-Resistant Staphylococcus Aureus. *PLoS ONE* **2020**, *15*, e0231583. [CrossRef] [PubMed]
36. Joung, D.K.; Kang, O.H.; Seo, Y.S.; Zhou, T.; Lee, Y.S.; Han, S.H.; Mun, S.H.; Kong, R.; Song, H.J.; Shin, D.W.; et al. Luteolin Potentiates the Effects of Aminoglycoside and β-Lactam Antibiotics against Methicillin-Resistant Staphylococcus Aureus in Vitro. *Exp. Ther. Med.* **2016**, *11*, 2597–2601. [CrossRef] [PubMed]
37. Bell, A. Antimalarial Drug Synergism and Antagonism: Mechanistic and Clinical Significance. *FEMS Microbiol. Lett.* **2005**, *253*, 171–184. [CrossRef] [PubMed]
38. Lin, Y.L.; Juan, I.M.; Chen, Y.L.; Liang, Y.C.; Lin, J.K. Composition of polyphenols in fresh tea leaves and associations of their oxygen-radical-absorbing capacity with antiproliferative actions in fibroblast cells. *J. Agric. Food Chem.* **1996**, *44*, 1387–1394. [CrossRef]
39. Li, X.; Yang, X.; Wang, Z.; Liu, Y.; Guo, J.; Zhu, Y.; Shao, J.; Li, J.; Wang, L.; Wang, K. Antibacterial, antioxidant and biocompatible nanosized Quercetin-PVA xerogel films for wound dressing. *Colloids Surf. B Biointerfaces* **2022**, *209*, 112175. [CrossRef]
40. Liu, K.; Dai, L.; Li, C. A lignocellulose-based nanocomposite hydrogel with pH-sensitive and potent antibacterial activity for wound healing. *Int. J. Biol. Macromol.* **2021**, *191*, 1249–1254. [CrossRef]
41. Jackson, J.K.; Letchford, K. The effective solubilization of hydrophobic drugs using epigallocatechin gallate or Tannic acid-based formulations. *J. Pharm. Sci.* **2016**, *105*, 3143–3152. [CrossRef] [PubMed]
42. Jackson, J.; Pandey, R.; Schmitt, V. Part 1. Evaluation of Epigallocatechin Gallate or Tannic Acid Formulations of Hydrophobic Drugs for Enhanced Dermal and Bladder Uptake or for Local Anesthesia Effects. *J. Pharm. Sci.* **2021**, *110*, 796–806. [CrossRef]
43. Jackson, J.; Schmitt, V. Paper 2. Epigallocatechin Gallate and Tannic Acid Based Formulations of Finasteride for Dermal Administration and Chemoembolization. *J. Pharm. Sci.* **2021**, *110*, 807–814. [CrossRef] [PubMed]
44. Kar, A.K.; Singh, A.; Dhiman, N.; Purohit, M.P.; Jagdale, P.; Kamthan, M.; Singh, D.; Kumar, M.; Ghosh, D.; Patnaik, S. Polymer-assisted in situ synthesis of silver nanoparticles with epigallocatechin gallate (EGCG) impregnated wound patch potentiate controlled inflammatory responses for brisk wound healing. *Int. J. Nanomed.* **2019**, *14*, 9837–9854. [CrossRef] [PubMed]
45. Kavitha, K.V.; Tiwari, S.; Purandare, V.B.; Khedkar, S.; Bhosale, S.S.; Unnikrishnan, A.G. Choice of wound care in diabetic foot ulcer: A practical approach. *World J. Diabetes* **2014**, *5*, 546. [CrossRef]

Disclaimer/Publisher's Note: The statements, opinions and data contained in all publications are solely those of the individual author(s) and contributor(s) and not of MDPI and/or the editor(s). MDPI and/or the editor(s) disclaim responsibility for any injury to people or property resulting from any ideas, methods, instructions or products referred to in the content.

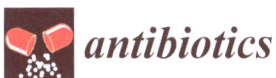 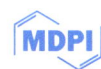

Article

Antibacterial Activity and Cytotoxicity Screening of Acyldepsipeptide-1 Analogues Conjugated to Silver/Indium/Sulphide Quantum Dots

Sinazo Z. Z. Cobongela [1,2,3,*], Maya M. Makatini [2], Bambesiwe May [3,4], Zikhona Njengele-Tetyana [1,5], Mokae F. Bambo [3] and Nicole R. S. Sibuyi [1,3,6,*]

1. Health Platform, Advanced Materials Division, Mintek, Randburg 2194, South Africa; znjengele-tetyana@wrhi.ac.za
2. Molecular Sciences Institute, School of Chemistry, University of the Witwatersrand, Johannesburg 2050, South Africa; maya.makatini@wits.ac.za
3. Department of Science and Innovation (DSI)/Mintek Nanotechnology Innovation Centre (NIC), Advanced Materials Division, Mintek, Randburg 2194, South Africa; bambesiwem@mintek.co.za (B.M.); mokaeb@mintek.co.za (M.F.B.)
4. Institute for Nanotechnology and Water Sustainability (iNanoWS), College of Science, Engineering and Technology, University of South Africa, Florida Campus, Roodepoort 1705, South Africa
5. Wits RHI, University of the Witwatersrand, Johannesburg 2050, South Africa
6. Department of Science and Innovation (DSI)/Mintek Nanotechnology Innovation Centre (NIC), Biolabels Research Node, Department of Biotechnology, University of the Western Cape, Bellville 7535, South Africa
* Correspondence: sinazoc@mintek.co.za (S.Z.Z.C.); nicoles@mintek.co.za (N.R.S.S.); Tel.: +27-117094303 (S.Z.Z.C.)

Abstract: The continuous rise in bacterial infections and antibiotic resistance is the driving force behind the search for new antibacterial agents with novel modes of action. Antimicrobial peptides (AMPs) have recently gained attention as promising antibiotic agents with the potential to treat drug-resistant infections. Several AMPs have shown a lower propensity towards developing resistance compared to conventional antibiotics. However, these peptides, especially acyldepsipeptides (ADEPs) present with unfavorable pharmacokinetic properties, such as high toxicity and low bioavailability. Different ways to improve these peptides to be drug-like molecules have been explored, and these include using biocompatible nano-carriers. ADEP1 analogues (SC005-8) conjugated to gelatin-capped Silver/Indium/Sulfide (AgInS$_2$) quantum dots (QDs) improved the antibacterial activity against Gram-negative (*Escherichia coli* and *Pseudomonas aeruginosa*), and Gram-positive (*Bacillus subtilis*, *Staphylococcus aureus* and Methicillin-resistant *Staphylococcus aureus*) bacteria. The ADEP1 analogues exhibited minimum inhibition concentrations (MIC) between 63 and 500 µM, and minimum bactericidal concentrations (MBC) values between 125 and 750 µM. The AgInS$_2$-ADEP1 analogue conjugates showed enhanced antibacterial activity as evident from the MIC and MBC values, i.e., 1.6–25 µM and 6.3–100 µM, respectively. The AgInS$_2$-ADEP1 analogue conjugates were non-toxic against HEK-293 cells at concentrations that showed antibacterial activity. The findings reported herein could be helpful in the development of antibacterial treatment strategies.

Keywords: acyldepsipeptides; antibacterial peptides; anionic peptides; palmitic acid; adamantane; nanomaterials; nano-carriers; AgInS$_2$ quantum dots

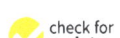

Citation: Cobongela, S.Z.Z.; Makatini, M.M.; May, B.; Njengele-Tetyana, Z.; Bambo, M.F.; Sibuyi, N.R.S. Antibacterial Activity and Cytotoxicity Screening of Acyldepsipeptide-1 Analogues Conjugated to Silver/Indium/Sulphide Quantum Dots. *Antibiotics* **2024**, *13*, 183. https://doi.org/10.3390/antibiotics13020183

Academic Editor: Anisha D'Souza

Received: 10 January 2024
Revised: 30 January 2024
Accepted: 9 February 2024
Published: 13 February 2024

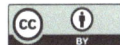

Copyright: © 2024 by the authors. Licensee MDPI, Basel, Switzerland. This article is an open access article distributed under the terms and conditions of the Creative Commons Attribution (CC BY) license (https:// creativecommons.org/licenses/by/ 4.0/).

1. Introduction

In recent years, nanotechnology has attracted significant interest, especially in the pharmaceutical industry. Nanomaterials have been explored as promising tools for biomedical applications such as biosensors, drug delivery, and imaging, amongst others [1]. Nanomaterials are very small, usually ranging from 1 to 100 nm, and have a larger surface area.

Importantly, nanomaterials can be easily functionalized by conjugating compounds of interest [2]. Properties of nanomaterials such as size, chemical composition, shape, and surface structure can significantly influence how they interact with other molecules. For instance, the surface functionalization of core nanomaterials with various ligands can lead to their use in different biological applications. Due to their small size, nanomaterials can passively diffuse through cell membrane pores and ion channels via endocytosis. In addition, active targeting can be achieved by attaching ligands to the nanomaterials to facilitate internalization by specific cells [3]. Nanomaterials are therefore good drug delivery systems that can improve existing drugs to achieve desirable therapeutic efficacy. The conjugation of pharmaceutically active compounds with poor pharmacokinetic properties to nanomaterials has been shown to increase drug solubility, bioavailability, and decrease enzyme susceptibility [4–6]. Nanomaterials can reduce toxicity and adverse side effects of conventional drug molecules by increasing drug selectivity and improving permeability across membranes, including the blood–brain barrier [7].

Nanomaterial have also been shown to play a pivotal role in enhancing the antimicrobial activity of antimicrobial peptides (AMPs) [8]. AMPs are promising antibiotic agents with the potential to treat drug-resistant infections. Several AMPs have shown a lower propensity towards developing resistance compared to conventional antibiotics [9]. However, these peptides, especially acyldepsipeptides (ADEPs) present with unfavourable pharmacokinetic properties such as high toxicity and low bioavailability [10]. ADEPs are a class of AMPs that target the bacterial ClpP protease and have great potential as antibiotics. The ADEPs bind and dysregulate the bacterial caseinolytic protease (ClpP), which is responsible for the overall bacterial cell protein homeostasis. Different ways to improve ADEPs to be drug-like molecules have been explored; however, the interventions compromise the antimicrobial potency of the peptides. In a recent study, ADEP1 analogues showed poor antibacterial activity with a minimum inhibitory concentrations (MIC) of ≥ 63 µM against Gram-positive bacteria and ≥ 125 µM against Gram-negative bacterial strains [11]. These analogues are derivatives of highly potent ADEP1 (ADEP A54556A). The conjugation of such potential drug molecules to biocompatible nano-carriers, such as quantum dots (QDs), would increase the desired biological activity.

QDs have gained traction in medicine as bio-imaging tools, drug delivery systems, and in-sensor applications [12]. QDs used as nano-carriers of drugs have been reported to improve bioavailability, biocompatibility, and the efficacy of drugs [13,14]. Conjugation of doxorubicin to ZnO QDs for the treatment of lung cancer is one example that highlights the effectiveness of using nanomaterials as drug delivery systems [15]. In this study, gelatin-capped Silver/Indium/Sulfide (AgInS$_2$) QDs were utilized as nano-carriers for antimicrobial ADEP1 analogues, previously reported by Cobongela et al., [11]. AgInS$_2$ QDs are known I-III-VI semiconductors that also exhibit a long-term photoluminescence decay lifetime [16]. Due to their remarkable photoluminescence properties and low cytotoxicity, they have found use in bio-imaging and cell targeting [17–19]. AgInS$_2$ QDs were conjugated to ADEP1 analogues (Scheme 1) to improve their antibacterial efficacy.

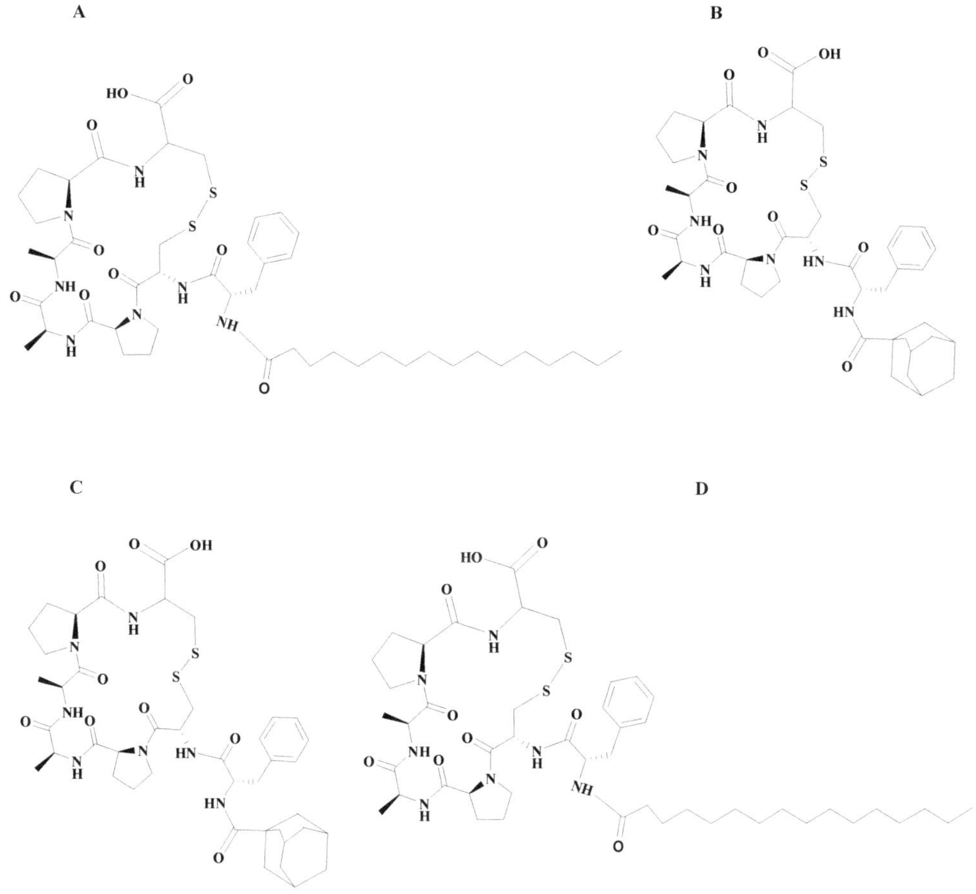

Scheme 1. Disulphide bond cyclized ADEP1 analogues. (**A**)—SC005 (Palmitic acid-FCPAAPC; D-form amino acids); (**B**)—SC006 (Adamantane-FCPAAPC; D-form amino acids); (**C**)—SC007 (Adamantane-FCPAAPC; L-form amino acids); (**D**)—SC008 (Palmitic acid-FCPAAPC; L-form amino acids) [11].

2. Results and Discussion

2.1. Characterization of AgInS$_2$ QDs

The HR-TEM in Figure 1 confirmed a successful synthesis of gelatin-capped AgInS$_2$ QDs. The micrograph shows that the AgInS$_2$ QDs are evenly dispersed and spherical in shape with a core size of 5.27 ± 1.68 nm. The elemental analysis of gelatin-capped AgInS$_2$ QDs was performed using ED-XRF and confirmed the presence of Ag, In, and S; with their percentage and ratio shown in Table 1. The gelatin on the surface of the QDs accounted for the majority of the components of AgInS$_2$ QDs.

Table 1. Elemental analysis of gelatin-capped AgInS$_2$ QDs.

Elements	Ag	In	S
%	0.8	1.6	14.4
Ratio	1	2	18

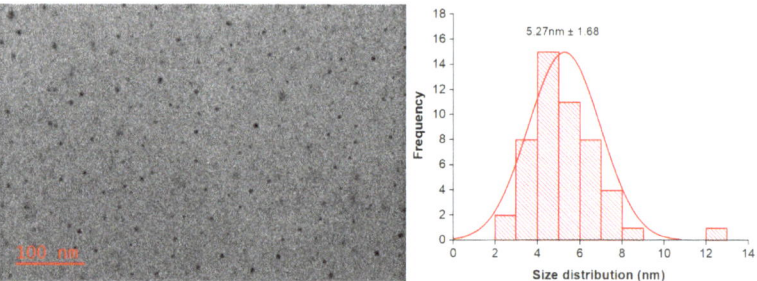

Figure 1. TEM image and size distribution of gelatin-capped AgInS$_2$ QDs.

2.2. Functionalization of AgInS$_2$ QDs with ADEP1 Analogues

Gelatin-capped AgInS$_2$ QDs were functionalized with ADEP1 analogues via EDC/sulfo-NHS coupling chemistry, as demonstrated in Scheme 2. The carboxylic groups of the ADEP1 analogues were activated in the absence of the gelatin-capped AgInS$_2$ QDs. The gelatin contains an amine (NH$_3^+$) which is readily available to form an amide bond with the activated COO$^-$ end of the ADEP1 analogues. Treatment of the ADEP1 analogues with EDC/sulfo-NHS in the presence of gelatin-capped AgInS$_2$ QDs could potentially result in intramolecular coupling between these carboxylic groups and the amine groups on the gelatin. The conjugation utilized the gelatin lysine amino group on the surface of the AgInS$_2$ QDs and the carboxylic group on the C-terminal of the ADEP1 analogues to form an amide bond [20].

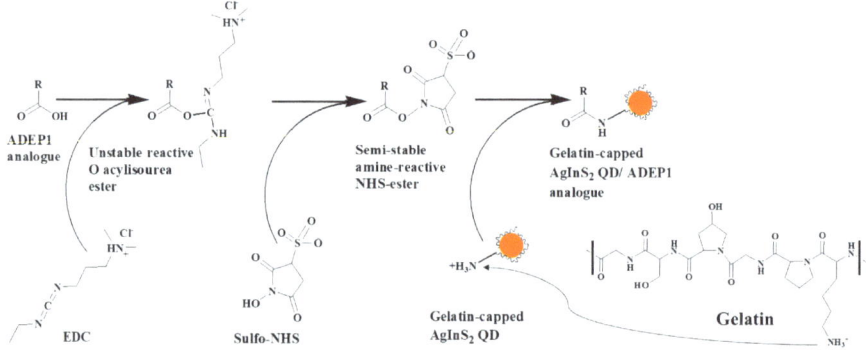

Scheme 2. Conjugation of ADEP1 analogues to gelatin-capped AgInS$_2$ QDs via EDC/sulfo-NHS coupling-chemistry. R = peptide sequence.

The conjugation of SC005-8 ADEP1 analogues increased the size of the AgInS$_2$ QDs (Figure 2A–D). The size distribution of palmitic acid-containing (SC005 and SC008) conjugates changed to 11.6 and 12.3 nm, respectively, whereas the adamantane-containing (SC006 and SC007) conjugates had average size of 6.9 and 7.7 nm, respectively. The increase in the size distribution of the conjugates is an indication of changes on the surface of the QDs. Other studies have also noted an increase in nanomaterial and QD size upon conjugation with biomolecules, such as peptides [21–23]. Optical properties were measured using photoluminescence spectroscopy with emission wavelengths between 400 and 700 nm. Luminescent QDs, such as AgInS$_2$ QDs, have long-lived excited states; therefore, the excitation wavelength was marginalized [24]. The gelatin-capped AgInS$_2$ QDs had an emission peak at 603 nm while the AgInS$_2$ QD-ADEP1 analogue conjugates shifted the emission to lower wavelengths. AgInS$_2$ QDs conjugated to the pal-containing ADEP1 analogues (i.e., SC005 and SC008) absorbed at 595 nm while ada-containing ADEP1 analogues (i.e., SC006 and SC007) absorbed at 599 nm (Figure 3). Conjugation added a coating on the surface of the AgInS$_2$ QDs, this in turn shielded the surface of the QDs. In addition, the shift in emission wavelength might be a result of increased size and the change in surface properties of the AgInS$_2$ QDs post conjugation.

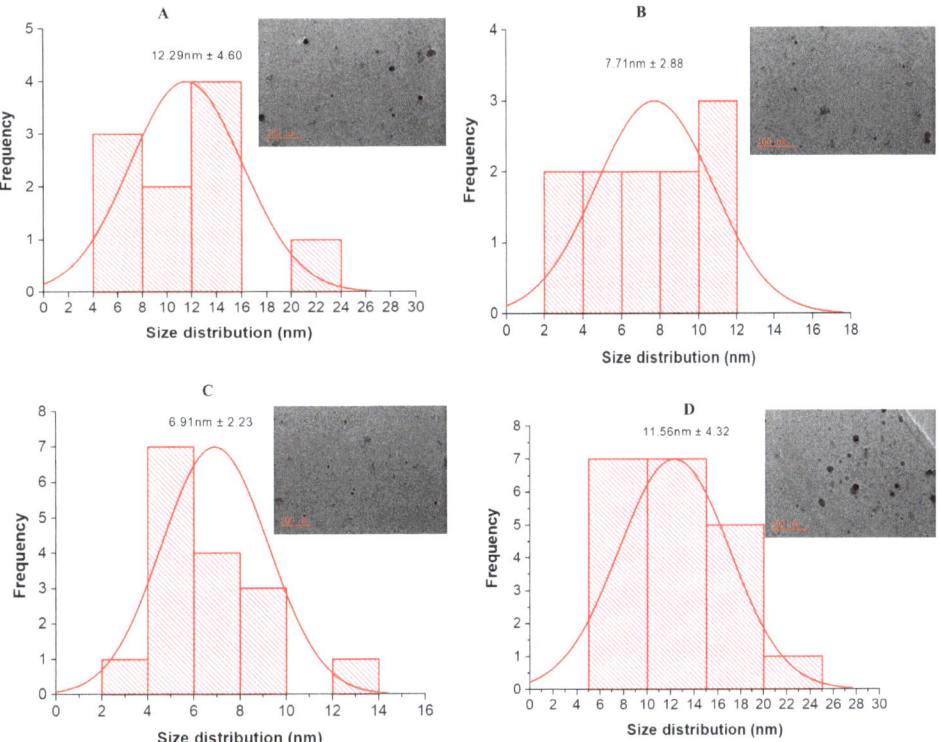

Figure 2. Core size distribution and TEM images of gelatin-capped AgInS$_2$ QDs-ADEP1 analogue conjugates and their (**A**): AgInS$_2$ QD-SC005; (**B**): AgInS$_2$ QD-SC006; (**C**): AgInS$_2$ QD-SC007; (**D**): AgInS$_2$ QD-SC008.

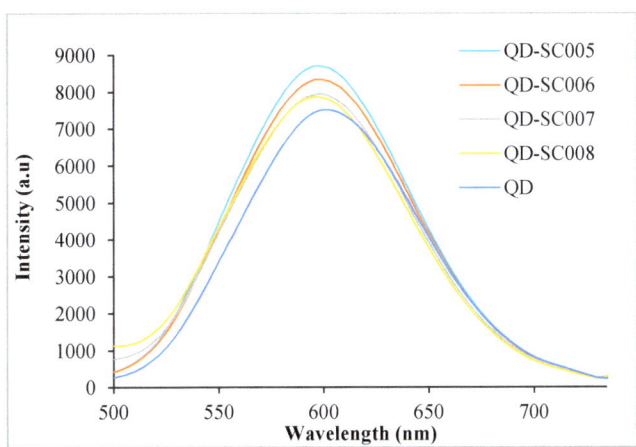

Figure 3. Photoluminescence properties of gelatin-capped AgInS$_2$ QDs and AgInS$_2$ QDs-ADEP1 analogue conjugates.

The AgInS$_2$ QDs-ADEP1 analogue conjugates were further characterized using zetasizer and DLS to determine their surface charge and hydrodynamic size. Table 2 shows the zeta potential values of the ADEP1 analogues before and after conjugation. The AgInS$_2$ QDs had a zeta potential value of -3.69 ± 0.9 mV. The ADEP1 analogues also had negative net charges ranging between -7.2 and -3.8 mV prior to conjugation. This confirmed the anionic state of the ADEP1 analogues, which is a result of the carboxylic anion (COO$^-$) at physiological pH. Anionic peptides have a disadvantage in penetrating bacterial cells, as they are made up of negatively charged polysaccharides, while cationic peptides have been commended for their cell permeability capability [25]. ADEP1 analogues lack the cationic advantage, which may lead to poor cell permeability and bioavailability. Therefore, to mitigate the challenges of poor pharmacokinetic properties associated with ADEPs, the analogues were conjugated to AgInS$_2$ QDs. The DLS results showed an increased diameter of AgInS$_2$ QDs (36.7 ± 2.8) nm compared to the particle diameter measured by TEM. The conjugation also led to an increased hydrodynamic diameter of the AgInS$_2$ QDs (Table 2), with palmitic acid-containing ADEP1 analogues being slightly bigger than the adamantane-containing ADEP1 analogues. These results showed that the conjugation of the ADEP1 analogues to AgInS$_2$ QDs resulted in a positive net charge, which could enhance the cell permeability properties of the peptides.

Table 2. Zeta potential values and hydrodynamic size of the ADEP1 analogues before and after conjugation to AgInS$_2$ QDs.

ADEP1 Analogue	Zeta Potential (mV) before Conjugation	Zeta Potential (mV) after Conjugation	Hydrodynamic Diameter (nm)
AgInS$_2$ QDs	-3.7 ± 0.9	-	36.7 ± 2.8
SC005	-7.2 ± 1.6	1.46 ± 0.02	49.6 ± 1.6
SC006	-3.8 ± 1.1	1.38 ± 0.06	44.2 ± 1.4
SC007	-3.9 ± 0.8	1.00 ± 0.15	44.4 ± 0.7
SC008	-6.9 ± 1.5	1.39 ± 0.09	50.3 ± 1.6

The FTIR spectra revealed the functional groups present on gelatin, the surface of the AgInS$_2$ QDs, ADEP1 analogues, and AgInS$_2$ QDs-ADEP1 analogue conjugates (Figure 4). There were similarities and shifts in the peaks of these molecules that suggested that gelatin was part of the AgInS$_2$ QDs, and that the ADEP1 analogues were successfully incorporated in the AgInS$_2$ QDs.

As shown in Table 3, gelatin showed broad associated N-H$_{str}$ absorption signals for secondary (2°) amine between 3700 and 3000, peaking at 3300 cm^{-1}, small sharp peaks at 2860 and 2920 cm^{-1} for symmetry and asymmetry saturated hydrocarbon (C-H$_{str}$), small multiplet signals between 1700 and 1000 cm^{-1} for C=O$_{str}$ (amide band I and II, 1625, 1525, respectively), 1450 and 1275 cm^{-1} for C-N$_{str}$, 1050 cm^{-1} for C-O$_{str}$ and the absence of peaks between 1000 and 500 cm^{-1}. After the interaction of ADEP1 analogues with AgInS$_2$, a new peak appeared at 575 cm^{-1} with a shoulder at 675 cm^{-1}, corresponding to N-H$_{bend}$ out-of-plane, implying complexation with the metal ions on the surface of the QDs. The increase in the intensities of the amino (N-H) and carbonyl (C=O) groups and a shift to a higher frequency (wavenumber) in AgInS$_2$ QDs-ADEP1 analogue conjugates further confirmed the complexation of the QDs with the ADEP1 analogues. Generally, after conjugation of the ADEP1 analogues to the QDs, peak intensities of all functional groups associated with AgInS$_2$ QDs were reduced. The initial C-H$_{str}$, C-O$_{str}$, and N-H$_{bend}$ peaks of the ADEP analogues were also replaced with those of the AgInS$_2$ QDs. All of this information confirmed the coupling of the AgInS$_2$ QDs with the ADEP1 analogues to form the hybrid material.

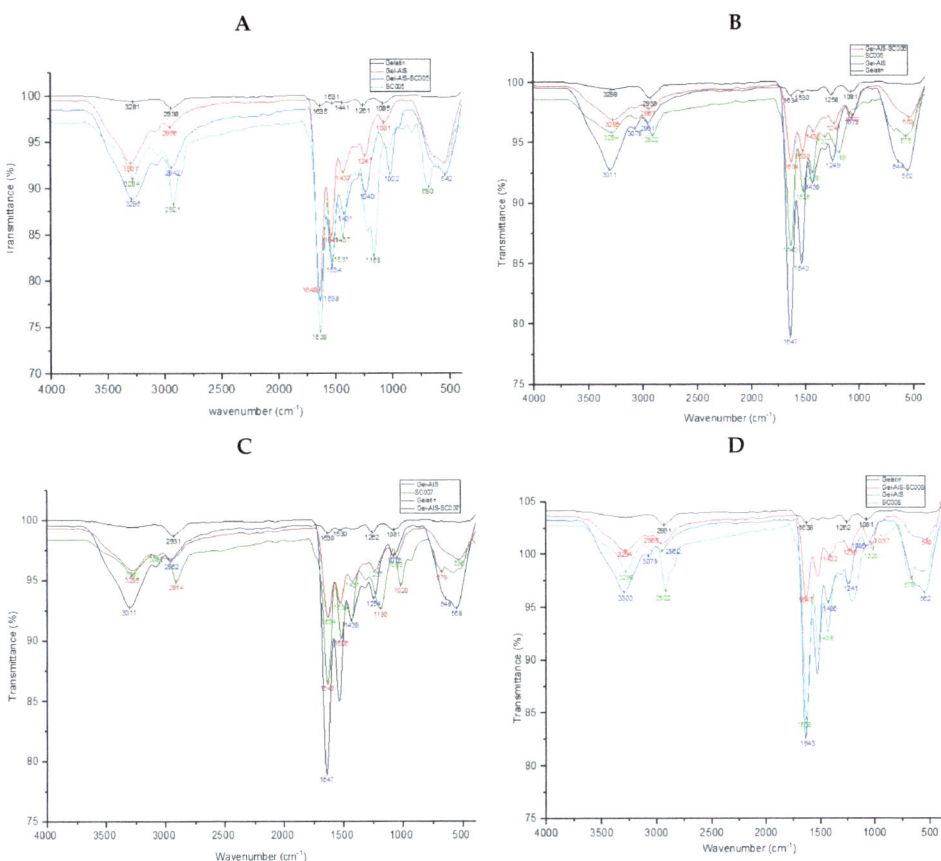

Figure 4. FTIR analysis of functional groups involved in gelatin capping of AgInS$_2$ QDs, and AgInS$_2$ QDs conjuction with ADEP1 analogues. (**A**) SC005, (**B**) SC006, (**C**) SC007 and (**D**) SC008.

Table 3. FTIR data for gelatin, AgInS$_2$ QDs and AgInS$_2$ QDs-ADEP1 analogue conjugates.

Functional Groups	Gelatin	AgInS$_2$-QDs	ADEP1 Analogues	AgInS$_2$ QDs-ADEP1 Analogues
N-Hstr	3300	3300	3300	3300
C-Hstr	2920–2860	2960–2875	2920–2860	2960–2875
C=Ostr (Amide band I, Amide band II)	1625, 1525	1637, 1537	1625, 1525	1637, 1537
C-Nstr	1450, 1390	1450, 1400	1450	1450, 1400
C-Nstr	1275, 1390	1237, 1337	1237, 1337	1237, 1337
C-Ostr	1050	1090	1190	1090
N-Hbend (out-of-plane)	x	575, 675	700	575, 675

2.3. Antibacterial Activity of AgInS$_2$ QDs-ADEP1 Analogue Conjugates

Following the successful synthesis of the gelatin-capped AgInS$_2$ QDs and their subsequent conjugation to the ADEP1 analogues, the antibacterial activity of the conjugates was tested against three Gram-positive (*B. subtilis*, *S. aureus* and Methicillin-resistant *S. aureus*) and two Gram-negative (*E. coli* and *P. aeruginosa*) bacterial strains. The MICs and MBCs of the AgInS$_2$ QDs-ADEP1 analogue conjugates were evaluated. On their own, the AgInS$_2$ QDs did not show any antibacterial activity against the selected bacterial strains at the tested concentrations. The ADEP1 analogues, as reported in [11], had MIC and MBC values that were between 63 and 500 μM and 125 and 750 μM, respectively. However, upon conjugation to the ADEP1 analogues, the antibacterial activity was significantly improved. The MIC and MBC values of the AgInS$_2$ QDs-ADEP1 analogue conjugates on the tested strains ranged from 1.6 to 25 μM and 6.3 to 100 μM, respectively (Table 4).

Table 4. MIC and MBC values of the AgInS$_2$ QD-ADEP1 analogue conjugates and ADEP1 analogues.

Treatments	B. subtilis		S. aureus		MRSA		P. aeruginosa		E. coli	
	MIC μM	MBC μM	MIC μM	MBC μM	MIC μM	MBC μM	MIC μM	MBC μM	MIC μM	MBC μM
QD-SC005	6.3	25.0	6.3	25.0	12.5	50.0	25.0	100.0	1.6	6.3
SC005	125	125	63	125	125	250	125	250	500	750
QD-SC006	6.3	25.0	6.3	25.0	12.5	50.0	25.0	100.0	1.6	6.3
SC006	250	250	63	125	250	250	125	250	500	750
QD-SC007	6.3	25.0	6.3	25.0	12.5	50.0	25.0	100.0	1.6	6.3
SC007	125	125	63	125	250	500	125	250	500	750
QD-SC008	6.3	25.0	6.3	25.0	12.5	50.0	25.0	100.0	1.6	6.3
SC008	125	125	63	125	250	500	125	250	500	750
Gentamicin	26.1	52.3	0.5	1.0	26.2	52.4	419	838	NT	NT
Ampicillin	NT	NT	NT	NT	NT	NT	NT	NT	2862	5724

The most susceptible bacterium to the AgInS$_2$ QD-ADEP1 analogue conjugates was E. coli with an MIC of 1.6 μM, followed by B. subtilis and S. aureus with MIC values of 6.3 μM, MRSA at 12.5 μM and lastly, P. aeruginosa at 25 μM. These results showed that the AgInS$_2$ QD-ADEP1 analogue conjugates were effective against both Gram-positive and Gram-negative bacteria. A study conducted by Cobongela et al. [11] reported that the Gram-negative bacterial strains (E. coli and P. aeruginosa) showed resistance against the ADEP1 analogues with MIC and MBC values of 500 and 750 μM, respectively. These observations were in line with previous studies, which reported a higher ADEP1 activity against Gram-positive bacteria compared to Gram-negative bacteria [26]. These new findings showed that conjugating the ADEP1 analogues to the AgInS$_2$ QDs helped overcome the resistance that was exhibited by E. coli against these peptides. Previous studies have discovered that peptides conjugated to nanomaterials show increased activity due to a re-binding mechanism to the target, which then increases the retention time of the peptide within the target [27]. The re-binding or reassociation mechanisms of nano-conjugates is enhanced by the slow dissociation rate of conjugates compared to free drug molecules. In addition, the increased density of the conjugate compared to either the nanomaterial or peptide alone exhibits increased binding affinity due to steric hindrance introduced upon binding to the target [28,29].

2.4. Cytotoxicity Screening of AgInS$_2$ QDs-ADEP1 Analogue Conjugates

The cytotoxicity of the AgInS$_2$ QDs-ADEP1 analogue conjugates was evaluated on HEK-293 cells using the MTS assay. The HEK-293 cells originate from the kidney, which is one of the organs in the excretory or renal system and is responsible for the removal of unwanted or toxic materials from the body [30]. Evaluating cytotoxicity is of utmost importance, especially if the materials are to be used in biological applications. For this assay, the HEK-293 cells were exposed to the AgInS$_2$ QDs-ADEP1 analogue conjugates (loaded with ~1.2–150 μM of ADEP1 analogues) for 72 h. The results presented in Figure 5A show cell viability greater than 80% for all of the tested concentrations of the AgInS$_2$ QDs and AgInS$_2$ QDs-ADEP1 analogue conjugates. In a study by Oluwafemu et al., a similar trend in cell viability was observed when the similar QDs variant, AgInS$_2$/ZnS core/shell, were tested against baby hamster kidney cells [18]. The AgInS$_2$ QDs used in the current study are regarded environmentally friendly as they are capped with gelatin, an animal product that is also used in food.

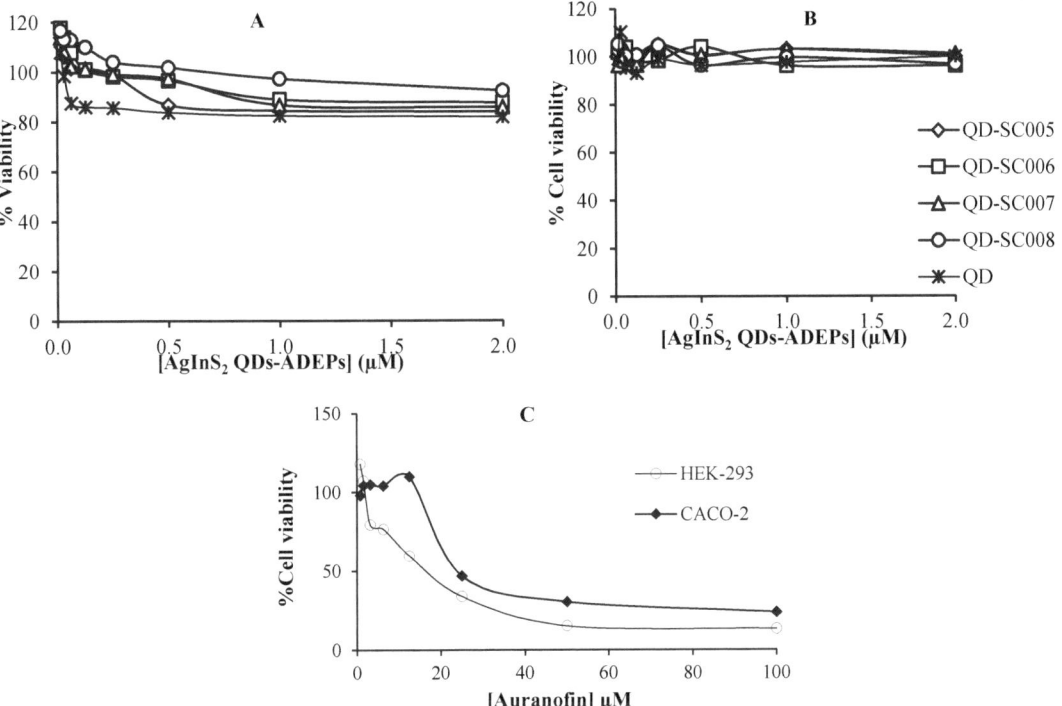

Figure 5. Effect of AgInS$_2$ QD-ADEP1 analogue conjugates (**A**) on HEK-293 and (**B**) Caco-2 cell viability. Cells treated with auranofin (**C**) were used as a positive control.

3. Materials and Methods

3.1. Materials

ADEP1 analogues (SC005-8) were synthesized in-house, as described by Cobongela et al., [11]. 1-Ethyl-3-(3-dimethylaminopropyl) carbodiimide (EDC), N-hydroxysuccinimide (sulfo-NHS), dimethyl sulfoxide (DMSO), thioglycolic acid (TGA), silver nitrate (AgNO$_3$), sodium sulfide (Na$_2$S·xH$_2$O), gelatin, Dulbecco's Modified Eagle Medium (DMEM), phosphate, trypsin, penicillin-streptomycin, fetal bovine serum (FBS), 3-(4,5-dimethylthiazol-2-yl)-5-(3-carboxymethoxyphenyl)-2-(4-sulfophenyl)-2H-tetrazolium (MTS dye), and trypan blue stain dye were all purchased from Sigma (St Louis, MO, USA). *Bacillus subtilis* American Type Culture Collection (ATCC) 11774, *Staphylococcus aureus* ATCC 25,923 and Methicillin-resistant *Staphylococcus aureus* (MRSA) ATCC 43300, and two Gram-negative (*Escherichia coli* ATCC 33,876 and *Pseudomonas aeruginosa* ATCC 15,442 were purchased from ATCC (Manassas, VA, USA). Human embryonic kidney 293 (HEK-293) cells were purchased from Cellonex (Randburg, Gauteng Province, South Africa).

3.2. Synthesis of AgInS$_2$ QDs

The AgInS$_2$ QDs were synthesized using a procedure reported by May et al., 2019 [31], with some modifications. In a typical synthesis, 0.25 mmol (0.0753 g) of In (NO$_3$)$_3$, 0.438 mmol TGA, 0.0625 mmol of silver nitrate, 0.2941 g of gelatin, and 0.406 mmol of Na$_2$S.9H$_2$O were added to 100 mL of deionized water with stirring (Ag:In:S:gelatin:TGA mole ratio of 1:4:6.5:16:7, respectively). The pH was adjusted to 6. The mixture was refluxed at 95 °C for 1 h to produce the gelatin-capped AgInS$_2$ QDs. The QDs were precipitated with ethanol and air dried.

3.3. Conjugation of AgInS$_2$ QDs to ADEP1 Analogues

The ADEP1 analogues were synthesized using the Fmoc solid peptide synthesis strategy, as previously described [11]. ADEP1 analogues (600 µM) dissolved in 5 mL of dimethyl formamide were treated with EDC (0.75 µM) and sulfo-NHS (0.3 µM), and the reaction was left shaking for 3 h at room temperature. Concurrently, 8 mg/mL of AgInS$_2$ QDs were dissolved in 10 mL of boiling water. Upon cooling down, the AgInS$_2$ QDs were added to the ADEP1 analogues solution, and the reaction was left shaking for 3 h at room temperature. The AgInS$_2$-ADEP1 analogue conjugates were precipitated with ethanol and lyophilized (LyoQuest, Telstar, Terrassa, Barcelona). The powder was re-suspended in phosphate buffered saline (PBS; pH 7.4) to a final concentration of 4 mg/mL AgInS$_2$-ADEP1 analogue conjugates with 200 µM ADEP1 analogues.

3.4. Characterization of QDs, AgInS$_2$-ADEP1 Analogue Conjugates, and ADEP1 Analogues

A Spectro Xepos-05 energy-dispersive X-ray fluorescence (ED-XRF, Rigaku, TX, USA) instrument was used to determine the Ag, In, and S concentrations in the gelatin-capped AgInS$_2$ QD powder. The core sizes of AgInS$_2$ QDs and AgInS$_2$-ADEP1 analogue conjugates were analyzed by the high-resolution transmission electron microscope (HR-TEM, JEOL, Tokyo, Japan). Fourier transform infrared spectroscopy (FTIR) spectra were recorded using a Perkin Elmer Spectrum Two UATR-FTIR spectrometer (PerkinElmer, Buckinghamshire, UK). The Hitachi F-2700FL spectrofluorophotometer (Hitachi, Tokyo, Japan) was used for the fluorescence measurements. Malvern system 4700 zetasizer (Malvern, Great Malvern, UK) together with a dynamic light scattering (DLS) technique were used to determine the zeta potential and particle hydrodynamic size of the AgInS$_2$ QDs and AgInS$_2$-ADEP1 analogue conjugates using.

3.5. Antibacterial Activity of AgInS$_2$-ADEP1 Analogue Conjugates

The MIC and MBC of the AgInS$_2$-ADEP1 analogue conjugates against *B. subtilis*, *S. aureus*, MRSA, *P. aeruginosa* and *E. coli* was determined using the broth microdilution susceptibility assay, following a previously described protocol [11]. Briefly, overnight-grown bacterial cultures were adjusted to approximately 1.5×10^8 CFU/mL in a sterile Luria–Bertani broth. The concentration of ADEP1 on AgInS$_2$-ADEP1 analogue conjugates was calculated based on the ADEP1 analogues calibration curve. AgInS$_2$-ADEP1 analogue conjugates and ADEP1 analogues were diluted via 2-fold serial dilution with broth containing a final concentration range of 0.8–100 µM and 15.6–2000 µM, respectively. Gentamicin (concentration range between 0.007 and 6.7 mM) was used as a positive control for *B. subtilis*, *S. aureus*, MRSA, and *P. aeruginosa*, while ampicillin (concentration range between 0.18 and 6.7 mM) was used as a positive control for *E. coli*, and 5% DMSO was used as a negative control. The 96-well plates were then incubated overnight at 37 °C. The lowest concentration of the AgInS$_2$-ADEP1 analogue conjugates and controls that resulted in clear wells with no turbidity (i.e., no visible bacterial growth) was recorded as the MIC. The bacterial culture from the MIC wells at concentrations of AgInS$_2$-ADEP1 conjugates above the MIC were inoculated into Luria–Bertani agar plates and incubated overnight at 37 °C. The MBC was determined as the lowest concentration resulting in complete bacterial-growth inhibition.

3.6. Cytotoxicity Activity of AgInS$_2$-ADEP1 Analogue Conjugates

The cytotoxicity of the AgInS$_2$-ADEP1 analogue conjugates was assessed on HEK-293 cells (purchased from Cellonex (Randburg, Gauteng Province, South Africa)) using the MTS cell proliferation assay, as previously reported [11]. The cells were cultured in Dulbecco's Modified Eagle Medium (DMEM) consisting of 10% fetal bovine serum (FBS), 2% DMSO, and 1% penicillin–streptomycin. The cells were seeded at 1×10^5 cells/mL into a 96-well plate and incubated at 37 °C overnight in a humidified incubator at 5% CO_2. The cells were then treated with $AgInS_2$-ADEP1 analogue conjugates to attain a final concentration range of 1.2–150 µM. Auranofin was used as a positive control at a concentration range of 0.78–100 µM and DMSO (2%) was used as a negative control. After 72 h of treatment, the metabolic activity of cells was determined by adding 10% of MTS dye. The percentage cell viability was calculated using the equation below:

$$\% \text{ cell viability} = \left(\frac{\text{OD of test sample}}{\text{OD of control}}\right) \times 100 \quad (1)$$

4. Conclusions

In this study, gelatin-capped $AgInS_2$ QDs were synthesized and conjugated to novel ADEP1 analogues, with the aim of improving the antibacterial efficacy of these peptides. The conjugation of the QDs to the peptides was confirmed using multiple techniques, namely, zeta potential, PL, ED-XRF, and HR-TEM. Compared to the $AgInS_2$ QDs, which did not show any appreciable antibacterial activity, and the ADEP1 analogues, which presented moderate activity, the $AgInS_2$ QDs-ADEP1 analogue conjugates exhibited excellent antibacterial activity. The MIC values obtained for the $AgInS_2$ QDs-ADEP1 analogue conjugates were between 3- and 200-folds lower than those obtained for the ADEP1 analogues, while the MBC values were between 5- and 13-folds lower. The MIC and MBC values showed that the $AgInS_2$ QDs-ADEP1 analogue conjugates were mostly potent against *E. coli*, followed by *B. subtilis* and *S. aureus*. The $AgInS_2$ QDs-ADEP1 analogue conjugates were non-toxic to HEk-293 cells at concentrations higher than the MIC and MBC and can be considered to be biocompatible. These findings suggest that the $AgInS_2$ QDs-ADEP1 analogue conjugates could potentially be used as antibacterial agents without eliciting any significant toxic effects against mammalian cells. The photoluminescence and fluorescent properties of $AgInS_2$ QDs will be exploited in future investigations to monitor ADEP1 analogues targeting, delivery and response in real time, and further determine the antibacterial mode of action of these ADEP1 analogues.

Author Contributions: S.Z.Z.C.: Conceptualization, Methodology, Validation, Formal analysis, Data curation, Investigation, Writing—Original draft, Visualization, Project administration, Funding acquisition. M.M.M.: Conceptualization, Resources, Supervision, Project administration, Funding acquisition. B.M.: Methodology, Formal analysis, Data curation. Z.N.-T.: Methodology, Resources, Supervision. M.F.B.: Methodology. N.R.S.S.: Data curation, Writing—Review and Editing. All authors have read and agreed to the published version of the manuscript.

Funding: This work was supported by Mintek Science Vote (Grant number—ADR42304) and DSI/NIC (Grant number—ADE42305).

Institutional Review Board Statement: Not applicable.

Informed Consent Statement: Not applicable.

Data Availability Statement: The data in this study are presented as tables and figures.

Acknowledgments: The work published here is part of SZZ Cobongela's PhD theses submitted to University of the Witwatersrand, School of Chemistry, Braamfontein, South Africa.

Conflicts of Interest: The authors declare that they have no known competing financial interests or personal relationships that could have appeared to influence the work reported in this paper. S.Z.Z.C., B.M., M.F.B. and N.R.S.S. are employed by Mintek (Randburg, SA); M.M.M. is employed by University of the Witwatersrand (Johannesburg, SA), ZN-T by Wits RHI (Johannesburg, SA).

References

1. De Jong, W.H.; Borm, P.J. Drug Delivery and Nanoparticles: Applications and Hazards. *Int. J. Nanomed.* **2008**, *3*, 133–149. [CrossRef]
2. Guisbiers, G.; Mejía-Rosales, S.; Leonard Deepak, F. Nanomaterial Properties: Size and Shape Dependencies. Available online: https://www.hindawi.com/journals/jnm/2012/180976/ (accessed on 31 August 2018).

3. Mandal, A. Copper Nanomaterials as Drug Delivery System against Infectious Agents and Cancerous Cells. *J. Appl. Life Sci. Int.* **2017**, *15*, 1–8. [CrossRef]
4. Kawabata, Y.; Wada, K.; Nakatani, M.; Yamada, S.; Onoue, S. Formulation Design for Poorly Water-Soluble Drugs Based on Biopharmaceutics Classification System: Basic Approaches and Practical Applications. *Int. J. Pharm.* **2011**, *420*, 1–10. [CrossRef] [PubMed]
5. Martínez-Carmona, M.; Lozano, D.; Colilla, M.; Vallet-Regí, M. Selective Topotecan Delivery to Cancer Cells by Targeted pH-Sensitive Mesoporous Silica Nanoparticles. *RSC Adv.* **2016**, *6*, 50923–50932. [CrossRef]
6. Müller, R.H.; Jacobs, C.; Kayser, O. Nanosuspensions as Particulate Drug Formulations in Therapy. Rationale for Development and What We Can Expect for the Future. *Adv. Drug Deliv. Rev.* **2001**, *47*, 3–19. [CrossRef] [PubMed]
7. Kou, L.; Bhutia, Y.D.; Yao, Q.; He, Z.; Sun, J.; Ganapathy, V. Transporter-Guided Delivery of Nanoparticles to Improve Drug Permeation across Cellular Barriers and Drug Exposure to Selective Cell Types. *Front. Pharmacol.* **2018**, *9*. [CrossRef] [PubMed]
8. Fadaka, A.O.; Sibuyi, N.R.S.; Madiehe, A.M.; Meyer, M. Nanotechnology-Based Delivery Systems for Antimicrobial Peptides. *Pharmaceutics* **2021**, *13*, 1795. [CrossRef] [PubMed]
9. Wang, S.; Zeng, X.; Yang, Q.; Qiao, S. Antimicrobial Peptides as Potential Alternatives to Antibiotics in Food Animal Industry. *Int. J. Mol. Sci.* **2016**, *17*, 603. [CrossRef] [PubMed]
10. Goodreid, J.D.; Janetzko, J.; Santa Maria, J.P.; Wong, K.S.; Leung, E.; Eger, B.T.; Bryson, S.; Pai, E.F.; Gray-Owen, S.D.; Walker, S.; et al. Development and Characterization of Potent Cyclic Acyldepsipeptide Analogues with Increased Antimicrobial Activity. *J. Med. Chem.* **2016**, *59*, 624–646. [CrossRef] [PubMed]
11. Cobongela, S.Z.Z.; Makatini, M.M.; Njengele-Tetyana, Z.; Sikhwivhilu, L.M.; Sibuyi, N.R.S. Design and Synthesis of Acyldepsipeptide-1 Analogues: Antibacterial Activity and Cytotoxicity Screening. *Arab. J. Chem.* **2023**, *16*, 105000. [CrossRef]
12. Matea, C.T.; Mocan, T.; Tabaran, F.; Pop, T.; Mosteanu, O.; Puia, C.; Iancu, C.; Mocan, L. Quantum Dots in Imaging, Drug Delivery and Sensor Applications. *Int. J. Nanomed.* **2017**, *12*, 5421–5431. [CrossRef]
13. Probst, C.E.; Zrazhevskiy, P.; Bagalkot, V.; Gao, X. Quantum Dots as a Platform for Nanoparticle Drug Delivery Vehicle Design. *Adv. Drug Deliv. Rev.* **2013**, *65*, 703–718. [CrossRef]
14. Zhao, M.-X.; Zhu, B.-J. The Research and Applications of Quantum Dots as Nano-Carriers for Targeted Drug Delivery and Cancer Therapy. *Nanoscale Res. Lett.* **2016**, *11*, 207. [CrossRef] [PubMed]
15. Cai, X.; Luo, Y.; Zhang, W.; Du, D.; Lin, Y. pH-Sensitive ZnO Quantum Dots-Doxorubicin Nanoparticles for Lung Cancer Targeted Drug Delivery. *ACS Appl. Mater. Interfaces* **2016**, *8*, 22442–22450. [CrossRef] [PubMed]
16. Jiao, M.; Li, Y.; Jia, Y.; Li, C.; Bian, H.; Gao, L.; Cai, P.; Luo, X. Strongly Emitting and Long-Lived Silver Indium Sulfide Quantum Dots for Bioimaging: Insight into Co-Ligand Effect on Enhanced Photoluminescence. *J. Colloid Interface Sci.* **2020**, *565*, 35–42. [CrossRef] [PubMed]
17. Fahmi, M.Z.; Chang, J.-Y. Forming Double Layer-Encapsulated Quantum Dots for Bio-Imaging and Cell Targeting. *Nanoscale* **2013**, *5*, 1517–1528. [CrossRef] [PubMed]
18. Oluwafemi, O.S.; May, B.M.M.; Parani, S.; Rajendran, J.V. Cell Viability Assessments of Green Synthesized Water-Soluble AgInS$_2$/ZnS Core/Shell Quantum Dots against Different Cancer Cell Lines. *J. Mater. Res.* **2019**, *34*, 4037–4044. [CrossRef]
19. Kang, X.; Yang, Y.; Wang, L.; Wei, S.; Pan, D. Warm White Light Emitting Diodes with Gelatin-Coated AgInS$_2$/ZnS Core/Shell Quantum Dots. *ACS Appl. Mater. Interfaces* **2015**, *7*, 27713–27719. [CrossRef]
20. Babel, W. Gelatine—Ein vielseitiges Biopolymer. *Chem. Unserer Zeit* **1996**, *30*, 86–95. [CrossRef]
21. Esfandyari-Manesh, M.; Mostafavi, S.H.; Majidi, R.F.; Koopaei, M.N.; Ravari, N.S.; Amini, M.; Darvishi, B.; Ostad, S.N.; Atyabi, F.; Dinarvand, R. Improved Anticancer Delivery of Paclitaxel by Albumin Surface Modification of PLGA Nanoparticles. *Daru* **2015**, *23*, 28. [CrossRef]
22. Jablonski, A.E.; Humphries, W.H.; Payne, C.K. Pyrenebutyrate-Mediated Delivery of Quantum Dots across the Plasma Membrane of Living Cells. *J. Phys. Chem. B* **2009**, *113*, 405–408. [CrossRef]
23. Katas, H.; Nik Dzulkefli, N.N.S.; Sahudin, S. Synthesis of a New Potential Conjugated TAT-Peptide-Chitosan Nanoparticles Carrier via Disulphide Linkage. *J. Nanomater.* **2012**, *2012*, e134607. [CrossRef]
24. Qian, H.S.; Guo, H.C.; Ho, P.C.-L.; Mahendran, R.; Zhang, Y. Mesoporous-Silica-Coated Up-Conversion Fluorescent Nanoparticles for Photodynamic Therapy. *Small* **2009**, *5*, 2285–2290. [CrossRef] [PubMed]
25. Almarwani, B.; Phambu, N.; Hamada, Y.Z.; Sunda-Meya, A. Interactions of an Anionic Antimicrobial Peptide with Zinc(II): Application to Bacterial Mimetic Membranes. *Langmuir* **2020**, *36*, 14554–14562. [CrossRef] [PubMed]
26. Brötz-Oesterhelt, H.; Beyer, D.; Kroll, H.-P.; Endermann, R.; Ladel, C.; Schroeder, W.; Hinzen, B.; Raddatz, S.; Paulsen, H.; Henninger, K.; et al. Dysregulation of Bacterial Proteolytic Machinery by a New Class of Antibiotics. *Nat. Med.* **2005**, *11*, 1082–1087. [CrossRef]
27. Vauquelin, G.; Charlton, S.J. Long-Lasting Target Binding and Rebinding as Mechanisms to Prolong in Vivo Drug Action. *Br. J. Pharmacol.* **2010**, *161*, 488–508. [CrossRef]
28. Mammen, M.; Choi, S.-K.; Whitesides, G.M. Polyvalent Interactions in Biological Systems: Implications for Design and Use of Multivalent Ligands and Inhibitors. *Angew. Chem. Int. Ed. Engl.* **1998**, *37*, 2754–2794. [CrossRef]
29. Mesquita, B.S.; Fens, M.H.A.M.; Di Maggio, A.; Bosman, E.D.C.; Hennink, W.E.; Heger, M.; Oliveira, S. The Impact of Nanobody Density on the Targeting Efficiency of PEGylated Liposomes. *Int. J. Mol. Sci.* **2022**, *23*, 14974. [CrossRef]

30. Boroushaki, M.T.; Arshadi, D.; Jalili-Rasti, H.; Asadpour, E.; Hosseini, A. Protective Effect of Pomegranate Seed Oil Against Acute Toxicity of Diazinon in Rat Kidney. *Iran. J. Pharm. Res.* **2013**, *12*, 821–827. [PubMed]
31. May, B.M.M.; Parani, S.; Oluwafemi, O.S. Detection of Ascorbic Acid Using Green Synthesized AgInS$_2$ Quantum Dots. *Mater. Lett.* **2019**, *236*, 432–435. [CrossRef]

Disclaimer/Publisher's Note: The statements, opinions and data contained in all publications are solely those of the individual author(s) and contributor(s) and not of MDPI and/or the editor(s). MDPI and/or the editor(s) disclaim responsibility for any injury to people or property resulting from any ideas, methods, instructions or products referred to in the content.

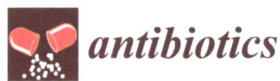 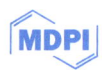

Article

Characteristics and Antimicrobial Activities of Iron Oxide Nanoparticles Obtained via Mixed-Mode Chemical/Biogenic Synthesis Using Spent Hop (*Humulus lupulus* L.) Extracts

Jolanta Flieger [1,*], Sylwia Pasieczna-Patkowska [2], Natalia Żuk [1], Rafał Panek [3], Izabela Korona-Głowniak [4], Katarzyna Suśniak [4], Magdalena Pizoń [1] and Wojciech Franus [3]

[1] Department of Analytical Chemistry, Medical University of Lublin, Chodźki 4A, 20-093 Lublin, Poland; natalia.zuk@umlub.pl (N.Ż.); magdalena.pizon@umlub.pl (M.P.)
[2] Faculty of Chemistry, Department of Chemical Technology, Maria Curie Skłodowska University, Pl. Maria Curie-Skłodowskiej 3, 20-031 Lublin, Poland; sylwia.pasieczna-patkowska@mail.umcs.pl
[3] Department of Geotechnics, Civil Engineering and Architecture Faculty, Lublin University of Technology, Nadbystrzycka 40, 20-618 Lublin, Poland; rapanek@gmail.com (R.P.); w.franus@pollub.pl (W.F.)
[4] Department of Pharmaceutical Microbiology, Medical University of Lublin, Chodźki 1 St., 20-093 Lublin, Poland; izabela.korona-glowniak@umlub.pl (I.K.-G.); katarzyna.susniak@umlub.pl (K.S.)
* Correspondence: j.flieger@umlub.pl

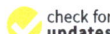

Citation: Flieger, J.; Pasieczna-Patkowska, S.; Żuk, N.; Panek, R.; Korona-Głowniak, I.; Suśniak, K.; Pizoń, M.; Franus, W. Characteristics and Antimicrobial Activities of Iron Oxide Nanoparticles Obtained via Mixed-Mode Chemical/Biogenic Synthesis Using Spent Hop (*Humulus lupulus* L.) Extracts. *Antibiotics* **2024**, *13*, 111. https://doi.org/10.3390/antibiotics13020111

Academic Editor: Anisha D'Souza

Received: 23 December 2023
Revised: 19 January 2024
Accepted: 22 January 2024
Published: 23 January 2024

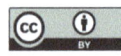

Copyright: © 2024 by the authors. Licensee MDPI, Basel, Switzerland. This article is an open access article distributed under the terms and conditions of the Creative Commons Attribution (CC BY) license (https://creativecommons.org/licenses/by/4.0/).

Abstract: Iron oxide nanoparticles (IONPs) have many practical applications, ranging from environmental protection to biomedicine. IONPs are being investigated due to their high potential for antimicrobial activity and lack of toxicity to humans. However, the biological activity of IONPs is not uniform and depends on the synthesis conditions, which affect the shape, size and surface modification. The aim of this work is to synthesise IONPs using a mixed method, i.e., chemical co-precipitation combined with biogenic surface modification, using extracts from spent hops (*Humulus lupulus* L.) obtained as waste product from supercritical carbon dioxide hop extraction. Different extracts (water, dimethyl sulfoxide (DMSO), 80% ethanol, acetone, water) were further evaluated for antioxidant activity based on the silver nanoparticle antioxidant capacity (SNPAC), total phenolic content (TPC) and total flavonoid content (TFC). The IONPs were characterised via UV-vis spectroscopy, scanning electron microscopy (SEM), energy-dispersive spectrometry (EDS) and Fourier-transform infrared (FT-IR) spectroscopy. Spent hop extracts showed a high number of flavonoid compounds. The efficiency of the solvents used for the extraction can be classified as follows: DMSO > 80% ethanol > acetone > water. FT-IR/ATR spectra revealed the involvement of flavonoids such as xanthohumol and/or isoxanthohumol, bitter acids (i.e., humulones, lupulones) and proteins in the surface modification of the IONPs. SEM images showed a granular, spherical structure of the IONPs with diameters ranging from 81.16 to 142.5 nm. Surface modification with extracts generally weakened the activity of the IONPs against the tested Gram-positive and Gram-negative bacteria and yeasts by half. Only the modification of IONPs with DMSO extract improved their antibacterial properties against Gram-positive bacteria (*Staphylococcus epidermidis*, *Staphylococcus aureus*, *Micrococcus luteus*, *Enterococcus faecalis*, *Bacillus cereus*) from a MIC value of 2.5–10 mg/mL to 0.313–1.25 mg/mL.

Keywords: nanoparticles; iron oxide; *Humulus lupulus* L.; spent hops; antimicrobial effect

1. Introduction

There are many nanoparticles containing iron (Fe), including nano zero-valent iron (NZVI), oxides, hydroxides and oxyhydroxides of iron (II) and iron (III), e.g., $Fe(OH)_3$, $Fe(OH)_2$, ferrihydryt ($Fe_5HO_8 \cdot 4H_2O$), Fe_3O_4, FeO, five polymorphs of FeOOH and four of Fe_2O_3 [1]. The most common iron oxides that occur naturally are magnetite (Fe_3O_4), maghemite (γ-Fe_2O_3) and hematite (α-Fe_2O_3). Fe can also be present in nanomaterials in the form of nanoalloys or core–shell nanoparticles [2,3].

Depending on the type, iron nanoparticles (INPs) have found many different applications. Their electrical applications are mainly due to their high magnetism, good thermal and electrical conductivity and high microwave adsorption capacity [4,5]. Due to their catalytic activity and large surface area, they are used in catalytic reactions. As INPs are non-toxic and have high dimensional stability, they have found many biomedical applications, such as magnetic resonance imaging, drug delivery and gene therapy [4,6]. Magnetic and superparamagnetic iron oxide nanoparticles (IONPs) have been used for drug delivery in cancer treatments [7,8]. INPs have been used to remove organic and inorganic pollutants from water, soil and sediments in the natural environment [9–11]. Examples include the use of NZVI, which can destroy chlorinated organic hydrocarbons such as trichloroethylene [12], trichloroethene (TCE) [13–15] and dibenzo-p-dioxin [11]; reduce chlorinated ethanes [16]; and remove nitrites [17]. There is great interest in the possibility of using iron oxide nanoparticles to remove pollutants from the environment, e.g., phenol [18], oxyanions, including arsenite, arsenate, chromate, vanadate and phosphate, or remove toxic metal ions, e.g., for the adsorption of lead (II) [19] and arsenic [20–26]. An example is magnetic iron oxide modified with 1,4,7,10-tetraazacyclododecane (Fe_3O_4@SiO_2-cyclen), which is able to selectively sorb heavy metal ions Cd^{2+}, Pb^{2+} and Cu^{2+} [27].

The preparation of INPs, like other nanomaterials, can be achieved through "top-down methods", in which the material is ground to nanosize [28–32], and "bottom-up methods" [33], in which the synthesis involves the self-organisation of atoms into new nuclei [31,34] as a result of aerosol, sol-gel processes, spinning, co-precipitation [35], mineralisation, sonochemical synthesis, microemulsion, etc. [4,34]. The use of a "bottom-up" method requires the purification of the nanoparticles and their separation from the reaction mixture [4,36].

NPs prepared using chemical and physical methods tend to form larger aggregates [37–41], which requires the addition of stabilisers in the form of polymers (PEG, polyacrylic acid, 4-butanediphosphonic acid and methoxyethoxyethoxyacetic acid (MEEA)) or surfactants [42]. Chitosan (CTS) is an example of a non-toxic, biocompatible, biodegradable natural polymer that can be used to coat magnetic nanoparticles. It is a hydrophilic polymer of a cationic nature that also has antibacterial properties [43–45].

Another possibility for bottom-up production is the so-called green synthesis, which is an attractive alternative to the above-mentioned methods due to its simplicity, cheapness and ecological safety using biological materials for the synthesis [34,46,47]. Green synthesis involves mixing appropriate precursors, most commonly aqueous solutions of iron salts (II) and (III), i.e., chlorides, sulphates (VI) and nitrates (V), in low concentrations ranging from 0.01 to 0.1 M [4,34,46,48], with material derived from bacteria, fungi, algae and plants [34,49,50]. The ecological synthesis of iron nanoparticles is preceded by the preparation of extracts containing bioactive compounds. It is known that many natural antioxidants and secondary metabolites, i.e., polyphenols, flavonoids, tannic acids, terpenoids, carboxylic acids, carotenoids, alkaloids, glycosides, vitamins and phenolic acids, have the ability not only to reduce iron ions but also to stabilise nanoparticles by binding to their surface [51–54].

The use of extracts has been described in the literature, such as the use of tea extract (polyphenols) as both a reducing and stabilising agent [55]. Iron oxide nanoparticles synthesised from clove and green coffee extracts showed a sorption capacity for divalent metal ions Cd^{2+} and Ni^{2+} and a broad spectrum of antibacterial activity against Gram-positive *Staphylococcus aureus* (*S. aureus*) and Gram-negative *Escherichia coli* (*E. coli*) bacteria [56]. Iron nanoparticles prepared from cloves had a MIC of 62.5 µg/mL against *S. aureus* and 125 against *E. coli* and were more effective against the tested pathogens than those prepared from green coffee with MIC values of 125 and 150 µg/mL, respectively [56]. Experimental studies have confirmed that superparamagnetic iron oxide nanoparticles obtained using this co-precipitation method, in which CTS protects the surface, have excellent antibacterial activity against the Gram-negative bacteria *Pseudomonas aeruginosa* (*P. aeruginosa*) and *E. coli* [57]. Spinach leaf extract and banana peel have also been considered for the preparation of iron nanoparticles [58]. The synthesised nanoparticles exhibited antimicrobial activity against two foodborne bacteria, i.e., *Bacillus subtilis* (*B. subtilis*) and *E. coli*, while remaining non-toxic against *Drosophila melanogaster* (*D. melanogaster*) in vivo.

In a study by Das et al. [59], *Humulus lupulus* extract was used for the first time for the green synthesis of silver nanoparticles, which showed antibacterial and anticancer activity with minimal genotoxicity and haemolysis.

Hops (*Humulus lupulus* L., Cannabaceae) are grown throughout the world as a raw material for beer production. The biological properties of this plant are related to the content of active compounds extracted from hop cones [60]. Hop cone extracts have antioxidant [61], antimicrobial and anti-inflammatory properties, as well as antimutagenic, antiallergic, neuroprotective and estrogenic properties [62,63]. The chemical compositions of the extracts vary and depend mainly on the variety and the growing environment [64]. The most important components of extracts for the industry are polyphenols, essential oils and alpha and beta acids. The phenolic fraction consists mainly of flavonoids, including xanthohumol [63] with high antimicrobial and antioxidant potential [65,66]. Also, α acids (humulones, i.e., cohumulone, humulone and adhumulone) and β-acids (lupulones, i.e., colupulone, lupulone and adlupulone) have confirmed antimicrobial activity [63]. α-acids are isomerised at high temperature to iso-α-acids, which also have antibacterial activity, mainly against Gram-positive bacteria [67,68]. Studies have confirmed the antibacterial, antiviral, antifungal and antiparasitic properties of compounds found in female cones and leaves [60,69,70]. Drug-resistant strains of *Staphylococcus aureus*, *Trypanosoma brucei* and *Leishmanis mexicana* were found to be sensitive to xanthohumol and lupulone administered in synergy with antibiotics [69,71].

Currently, the industrial production of hop extracts is carried out using the supercritical CO_2 method (30 MPa, 50 °C) [72,73]. In Poland, this method is used by the Institute of Fertilisers in Puławy. The extracts are rich in soft and hard resins [74]. About 1000 tonnes of hop waste are produced annually, containing substances that are poorly soluble in non-polar supercritical CO_2. Hops, therefore, contain valuable polar substances, i.e., proteins, amino acids, mineral salts, vitamins, proteins, sugars, polyphenols including prenylflavonoids (xanthohumol) and salts.

Spent hops left over from supercritical carbon dioxide extraction are treated as a source of xanthohumol, which has anti-cancer and antioxidant properties. Spent hops are also used as a feed additive. In a 2008 study [75], the total content of hop acids in extracted hop kernels was determined to be 1.051 µg/g (222 µg bitter isohumulones and 757 µg humulones per g). About 1000 prenylated flavonoids have been identified [76], occurring in several plant families that use these compounds in defence against pathogens and stress caused by unfavourable environmental conditions. Prenylated flavonoids include isoxanthohumol (IXN), xanthohumol (XN) and 8-prenylnaringenin (8PN), which are found in hops and hop waste remaining after extractions with supercritical carbon dioxide.

The increasing number of infections that are resistant to treatment with known antimicrobial agents stimulates the search for new compounds as alternatives to antibiotics [77–80]. The most dangerous are nosocomial infections caused by the formation of a bacterial biofilm composed of Gram-negative bacteria, namely *Pseudomonas aeruginosa* (*P. aeruginosa*) and *Escherichia coli* (*E. coli*) [81,82]. Taking into account the above needs and in cultivating a green approach to biotechnology, we designed a synthesis of iron oxide nanoparticles (IONPs) modified with the extract of wasted and unusable spent hops, which are a by-product of supercritical carbon dioxide extraction.

Not without significance is the fact that superparamagnetic iron oxide nanoparticles (SPIONPs), such as magnetite (Fe_3O_4), have antibacterial properties [83] and are biocompatible (BC) with the human body [1]. However, it is known that the observed activity of nanomagnetites is variable and depends on their size and shape and the type of stabilisers used [84]. Therefore, the synthesis procedure determines the final properties of the nanoparticles.

In this work, iron oxide nanoparticles (IONPs) modified with extracts from spent hops were obtained for the first time using a hybrid method, combining the chemical method of IONP synthesis through the co-precipitation of mixed ferrous and ferric salts from a solution in an alkaline medium with modification using plant extracts.

Initially, hop extracts were tested for their antioxidant activity. The final product was tested for antimicrobial activity against Gram-positive and Gram-negative bacteria and yeasts.

2. Results

2.1. Spent Hop Extract Characteristics

The total polyphenols and flavonoids, expressed as vitamin C equivalents, are summarised in Table 1. Regarding the content of each group of compounds, all types of extracts showed a greater amount of total flavonoid compounds than polyphenols. The potency of the extraction solvents used can be ranked from the most effective to the least effective for the extraction of flavonoids as follows: DMSO > 80% ethanol > acetone > water.

Table 1. Total polyphenols and flavonoids and the total antioxidant capacity (TAC) values expressed as mg mL^{-1} or mM of the vit. C equivalent obtained using the SNPAC method for the *Humulus lupulus* L. extracts.

Parameter	Extraction Solvent			
	80% EtOH	Acetone	DMSO	H$_2$O
		TPC		
Abs.Mean (n = 3)	0.8823	0.6763	0.8983	0.3843
Std. Dev.	0.0031	0.0021	0.0006	0.0012
mg vit. C mL^{-1}	0.0296	0.0247	0.0655	0.0140
		TFC		
Abs.Mean (n = 3)	0.8757	0.8233	1.2173	0.5077
Std. Dev.	0.0006	0.0025	0.0029	0.0006
mg vit. C mL^{-1}	0.0247	0.0232	0.0340	0.0146
		SNPAC		
Abs.Mean (n = 3)	0.2772	0.1404	0.5301	0.3260
Std. Dev.	0.0021	0.0061	0.0012	0.0002
TAC (μM)	16.012	8.092	30.636	18.844

Abbreviations: vit. C—ascorbic acid equivalents; TAC—the total antioxidant capacity expressed as vit. C equivalents; EtOH—ethanol; Std. Dev.—the standard deviation of three independent measurements; Abs.—absorbance measured spectrophotometrically at 423 nm.

The total antioxidant capacity (TAC) should be understood as a net measure of all redox substances present in biological materials [85]. The TAC for complex mixtures is additive.

In order to compare TAC values for different samples using the chosen assay, it is necessary to consider the range of concentrations at which a linear relationship occurs.

The evaluation of the TAC using the SNPAC method is based on the plotting of a calibration curve for the antioxidant, i.e., the relationship between absorbance and concentration. The molar absorbance (ε) is estimated from the slope of the calibration curve.

The samples were prepared by mixing an initial solution of AgNPs with the citrate capping agent with different volumes of the standard or extracts (5–795 μL) and water. Figure 1 shows the changes in absorbance of the mixture with an increasing volume of the extract or standard. The absorbance value corresponding to the plasmon resonance of the AgNPs was linearly dependent on the antioxidant concentration/volume. It can be seen that the reducing potential of all mixtures increases, indicating a high concentration of antioxidants [86–88].

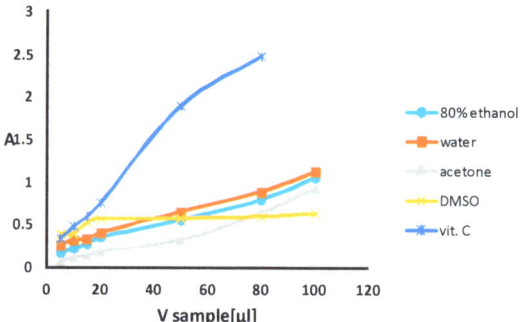

Figure 1. Absorbance (A) measured at 423 nm versus the volume of the extracts or standard antioxidant (vit. C) added to the test tubes with the initial solution of AgNPs with the citrate capping agent.

The plasmon absorbances of the AgNPs were perfectly linear ($R^2 > 0.99$), but in different ranges depending on the type of extraction solvent, i.e., from 5 to 100 µL for all extracts except DMSO extract, from 5 to 20 µL of extract for DMSO extract and from 5 to 50 µL for the antioxidant standard (vit. C) with a concentration of 1 mg mL^{-1}, i.e., in the concentration range from $10{,}139 \times 10^{-6}$ to $101{,}386 \times 10^{-6}$ M vit. C (final concentrations in the mixture and molar absorption capacity $\varepsilon = 1.73 \times 10^4$ L mol^{-1} cm^{-1}).

The obtained relationships are in agreement with the observation of Eustis et al., who claimed that among the various factors influencing the absorption of SPR (surface plasmon resonance absorption) by AgNPs, the reaction stoichiometry, particle morphology and dielectric constants of the surrounding medium are crucial [89].

The addition of DMSO to the reaction system used in the SNPAC method affects the A423 nm versus volume of extract added. The inhibition of absorbance after the addition of 20 µL of DMSO extract is analogous to the observed slowing of the increase in the fluorescence of fluorescent probes in the vicinity of this solvent, as described by Setsukinai et al. [90]. The tighter solvation of silver cations by DMSO, combined with the strong Lewis basicity of this solvent and the low medium effect (-5.11) [91], slows down the reduction of silver ions. The silver cations in DMSO can form di- and tetrasolvated species [Ag(DMSO)2]+ and [Ag(DMSO)4]+, as reported by Ahrland et al. [92]. Rodríguez-Gattorno et al. confirmed that the reaction to form AgNPs in DMSO is slow and practically impossible without the addition of citrate as a reducing and stabilising agent [93]. The oxidation of DMSO leads to the formation of dimethylsulphone ($CH_3)_2SO_2$. However, DMSO does not reduce various silver salts such as nitrate, perchlorate and metavanadate, even when heated to 80 °C. This reaction occurs only when trisodium citrate is added, which is responsible for the reduction of silver even at room temperature. Also, the ζ-potential, tested in different solvents, shows the highest value in water (-26.5 mV) and the lowest in DMSO (-15.8 mV) [94]. Furthermore, according to recent findings, the sizes of NPs such as magnetite particles decrease with increasing concentrations of DMSO [95].

The above findings may explain the unusual behaviour of the relationship between the absorbance and volume of extract obtained for DMSO compared to those obtained for extracts prepared with water and 80% ethanol. As can be seen in Figure 1, despite the rich content of flavonoids and polyphenols in the extract prepared with DMSO, the reduction of silver ions is inhibited after the addition of 20 µL of DMSO.

With regard to the total antioxidant capacity (TAC) of the extracts evaluated via SNPAC, the highest reducing power was observed for the DMSO extract, followed by water and 80% ethanol, and the lowest, for the acetone extract. The vitamin C equivalent antioxidant capacity (TAC) of a given extract is the ratio of its absorbance from the linearity region (observed after the addition of 15 µL of extract) to the molar extinction coefficient (ε) value of vitamin C under the same SNPAC test conditions [96].

2.2. Humulus Lupulus–Iron Oxide NP Characteristics

2.2.1. UV-Vis Analysis

As a result of the chemical synthesis, nanoparticles were created, which were visible as a colour change from yellowish to intense black. Under the influence of an external magnetic field, the nanoparticles could be separated from the solution (Figure 2).

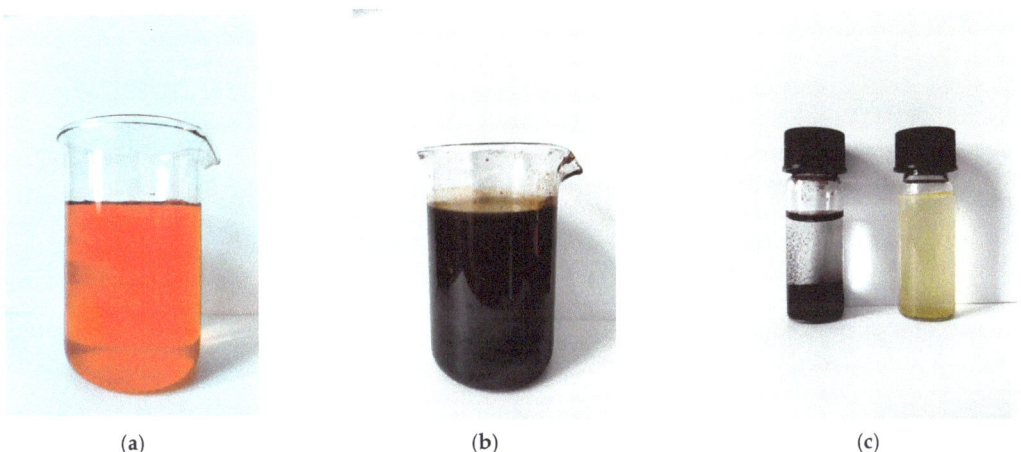

(a)   (b)   (c)

Figure 2. The visible colour change of the precursor solution FeCl$_3$ (**a**) into synthesised IONPs (**b**). The prepared IONPs were added to an aqueous solution of plant extract and separated using a magnet (**c**).

The UV-vis spectra recorded in the 330–600 nm range are shown in Figure 3. A spectrophotometric analysis of the ferric chloride solution showed characteristic absorption bands around 340 nm. The reduction of iron was confirmed using UV-vis spectra and is shown in Figure 3a. The reaction product is visible as the colour of the reaction mixture changes from yellow orange to dark black. In addition, the UV-vis spectra after the reaction showed a broad absorption at a higher wavelength and no sharp absorptions at lower wavelengths. Similar results have been obtained by other researchers [55,97–103]. A slight variation in the wavelengths of the peaks visible in the spectrum may be due to different measurement conditions, different materials used for synthesis, etc. Figure 3b shows the absorption spectra of the extracts before and after sorption with IONPs. As can be seen, the UV-vis spectrum of the extract has a broad band below 330 nm, confirming the high content of polyphenolic compounds [86]. After the addition of IONPs, a loss of colour of the extract and a decrease of absorbance in the range of 330–600 nm were observed. The decrease in the absorbance of the extract after the addition of IONPs confirms the sorption of the active components of the extract by the nanoparticles.

2.2.2. FT-IR Measurements

The FT-IR/ATR spectra of the studied samples, i.e., aqueous and alcoholic spent hop extracts, pristine IONPs and IONPs with adsorbed aqueous and alcoholic extracts, are presented in Figure 4.

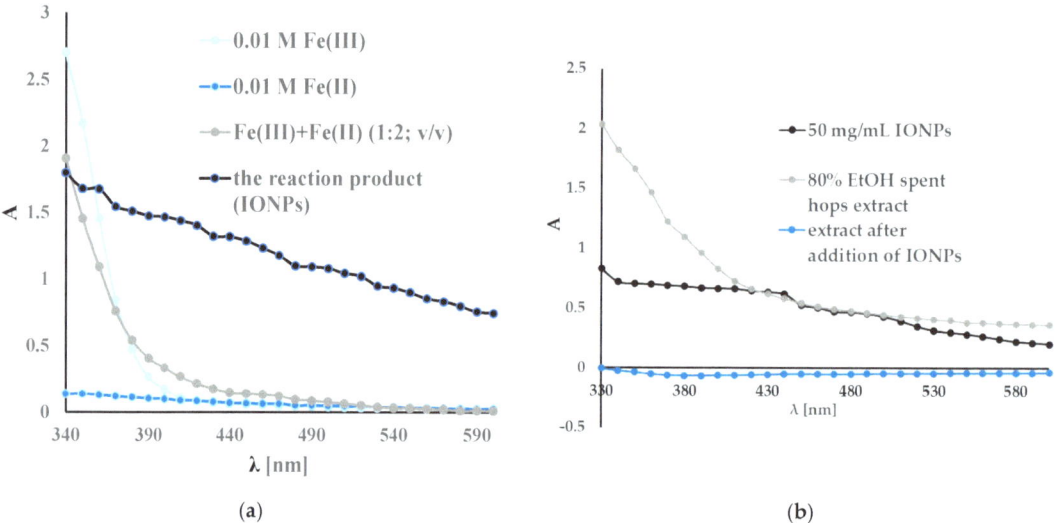

Figure 3. The UV-vis spectra recorded in the range of 330–600 nm during chemical synthesis: initial iron ion solution and IONPs (**a**) and during the modification of the IONPs using plant extract (**b**).

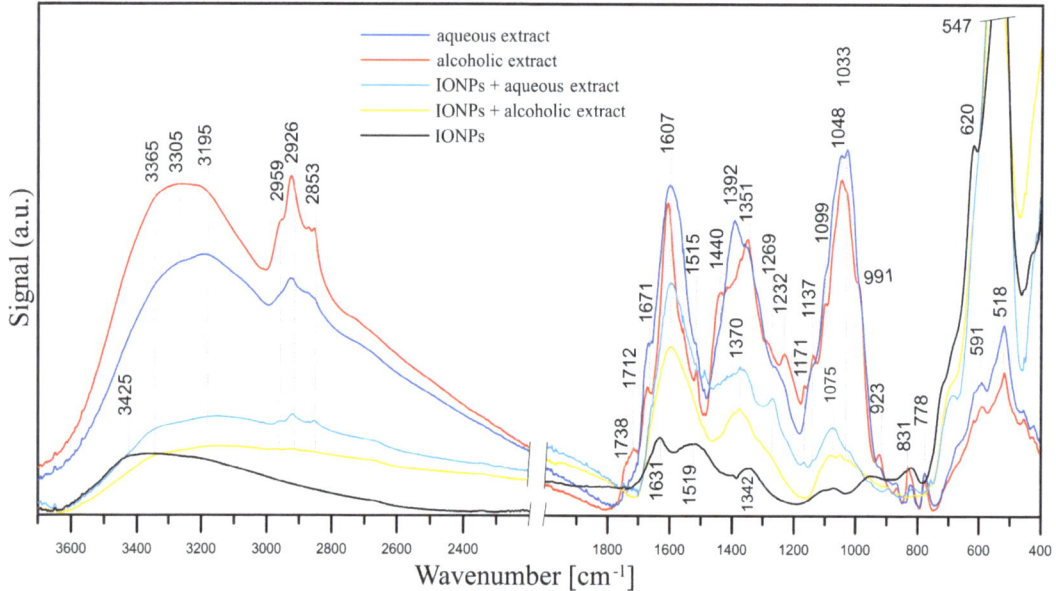

Figure 4. FT-IR/ATR spectra of studied samples: spent hop aqueous and alcoholic extracts, IONPs and IONPs with adsorbed *Humulus lupulus* aqueous and alcoholic extracts.

An analysis of the FT-IR spectrum of the IONPs confirmed that they are iron oxide nanoparticles [104]. The spectrum of pristine IONPs shows well-defined peaks at 3425, 1631, 1342, 938, 620 and 547 cm^{-1}. The two peaks at 620 and 547 cm^{-1} result from the presence of iron-oxygen (Fe–O) bonds. The peaks at 3425 and 1631 cm^{-1} are the result of bending vibrations of hydroxyl –OH groups and adsorbed water, respectively. The bands at 1342, ~1090, 938 and 830 cm^{-1} may indicate the presence of nitrate groups (precursors of iron ions).

Hops contain more than 1000 various chemical substances, i.e., flavonoids, volatile oils, hop acids and proteins [105,106]; hence, the compositions of both the aqueous and alcoholic hop extracts are complex [107–109]. In analysing the FT-IR/ATR spectra of the aqueous and alcoholic extracts, it can be concluded that their chemical compositions are similar, but not identical. Bands with maxima at ~3305 and 3195 cm^{-1} represent the stretching vibrations of both the hydroxyl –OH groups and N–H in amino groups. Stretching vibrations of aliphatic C–H were observed within 2960–2853 cm^{-1} and ~1440–1350 cm^{-1}. These bands indicate the presence of i.a. polysaccharides, proteins and phenolic compounds in the hop extracts.

The bands at 1738 and 1712 cm^{-1} indicate the presence of C=O (carboxylic acids, esters, aldehydes and ketones), while the band at 1671 cm^{-1} may indicate both C=O stretching vibrations in flavones and quinones, amides (C=O in amide I) and C=C stretching and C=N stretching vibrations [110]. The band at 1607 cm^{-1} may be responsible for C=N and C=C (also a ring stretching vibration in aromatic structures). However, the band at ~1607 cm^{-1} in the extract spectra may also be assigned to asymmetric COO– stretching, while the peak at ~1392 cm^{-1} may point to COO– symmetric stretching. The latter peak can also be assigned to C–OH stretching vibrations of the phenolic and/or alcoholic groups. Peaks within 1270–1230 cm^{-1} may be responsible for C–O stretching vibrations in the phenols. Bands within the 1100–1030 cm^{-1} range are attributed to C–O–C stretching vibrations of aromatic ethers and carbohydrates. The presence of carbohydrates is also indicated by the peak at 991 cm^{-1} of CH$_2$OH in carbohydrates (shoulder, visible only in the alcoholic extract spectrum). The peak at ~1137 cm^{-1} may be attributed to the C–N stretching vibration of aromatic primary and secondary amines, and the bands within 930–600 cm^{-1} correspond to primary and secondary amines and amides (–NH$_2$ wagging) and/or C–O and C–O–C symmetric stretching. The bands at ~591 cm^{-1} and ~518 cm^{-1} are C–CO–C and C–CO in-plane deformation vibrations in the ketone groups, respectively [110]. In summary, all these bands indicate the presence of flavonoids such as xantohumol and/or isoxantohumol [105] as well as bitter acids (i.e., humulones, lupulones) and proteins in the extracts.

As it was mentioned, the FT-IR/ATR spectra of aqueous and alcoholic extracts are similar, although there are some differences in the positions and intensities of the peaks. In the spectrum of the alcoholic extract, the peaks of the C=O bands at 1738 and 1712 cm^{-1} have much higher intensities, which may indicate a higher amount of carboxylic acids, esters, aldehydes and ketones. The peaks of aliphatic C–H groups within 2960–2853 cm^{-1} also have higher intensities.

The adsorptions of both the alcoholic and aqueous extracts in the IONPs are visible in the form of bands that were absent in the spectrum of pure IONPs (Figure 4). In the spectrum of IONPs with adsorbed *Humulus lupulus* aqueous extract, bands for the hydroxyl –OH groups and N–H in amino groups (3365–3195 cm^{-1}) and C–H groups appear (2960–2853 cm^{-1}). The C–H bands have higher intensities in the spectrum of IONPs with adsorbed aqueous extract. The adsorption of the extracts is also evidenced by bands with relatively high intensities at 1607, 1370 and 1075 cm^{-1}. In the spectrum of IONPs with adsorbed aqueous extract, there are additional bands absent or bands that have lower intensities in the spectrum with adsorbed alcoholic extract, namely 1269, 1033 and bands in the 930–600 cm^{-1} range. The intensities of the bands in the spectrum of IONPs with adsorbed aqueous extract are higher than in the case of IONPs with adsorbed alcoholic extract, which may indicate a greater adsorption of compounds from the aqueous extract. Nevertheless, the analysis of the FT-IR/ATR spectra allows us to confirm the adsorption of compounds present in both the aqueous and alcoholic extracts on the IONPs.

2.2.3. Scanning Electron Microscopy (SEM) with Energy-Dispersive X-ray Spectroscopy (EDX)

SEM images of the IONPs obtained via chemical synthesis using the co-precipitation method showed a granular, uniform, spherical structure with a diameter ranging from 81.16 nm to 142.5 nm, as shown in Figure 5a. An initial measurement of the sizes of the nanoparticles using the Malvern Zetasizer Nano ZS with the DLS technique showed a size of 293.13 nm ± 18.50 with a PDI of 0.58 ± 0.09 (Figure 6). This higher value is probably due to the aggregation of the NPs in an aqueous environment visible on the SEM image (Figure 7a).

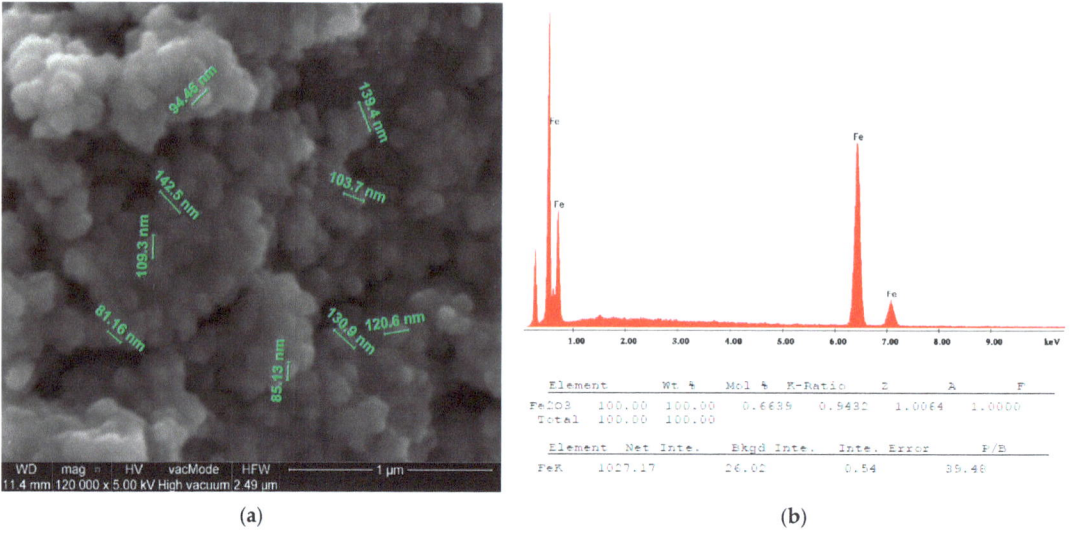

(a)   (b)

Figure 5. SEM image (**a**) with EDS analysis (**b**) of IONPs.

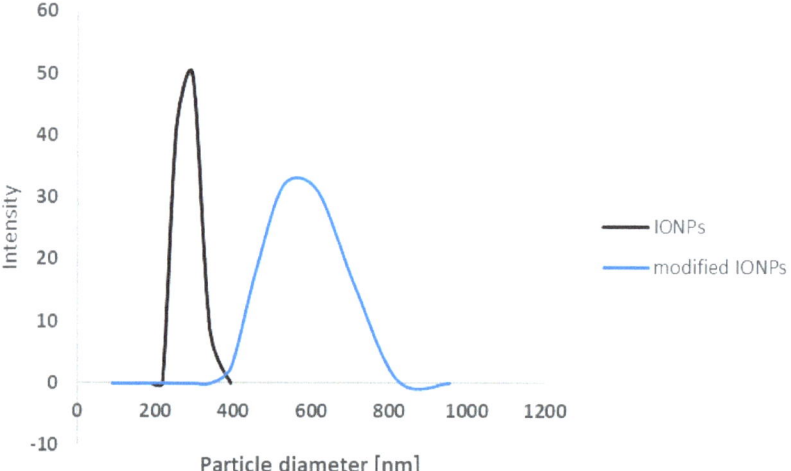

Figure 6. The hydrodynamic particle diameter of biosynthesised IONPs.

However, it can be seen that the synthesised IONPs are more clearly separated and can be better distinguished. After modification with the extract, the NPs appear to be more viscous and aggregated (Figure 7b). This change is reflected in the size of the NPs measured via DLS (Figure 6). As can be seen, after the modification, the size increases almost twice that of an average value of 544.66 21.02 nm. In addition, EDS was used to provide information on the chemical compositions of the identified nanostructures. The amplitude of the spectrum showed the presence of several characteristic iron peaks in the range of about 0.5 to 7 keV, as shown in Figure 5b.

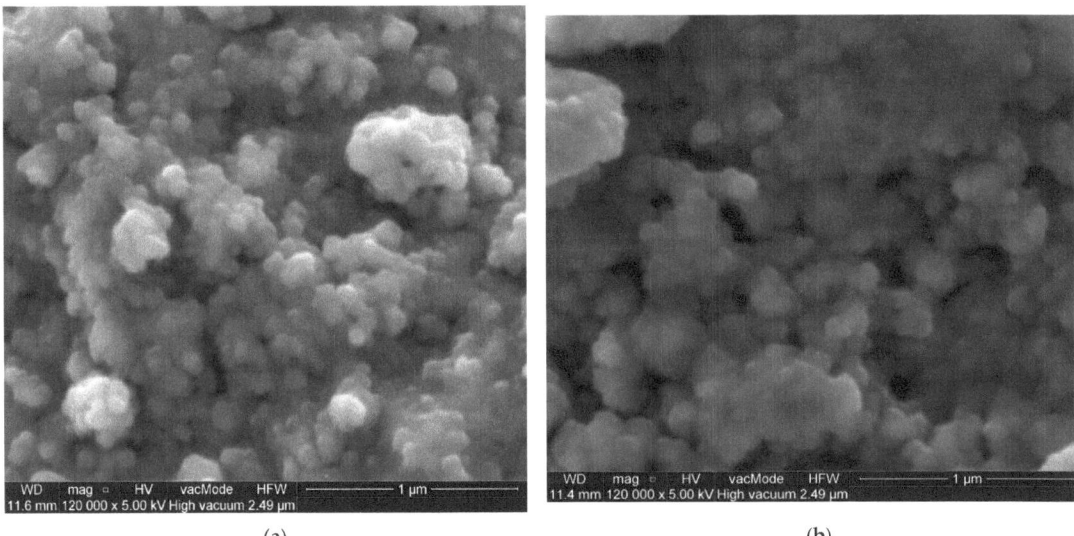

(a)　　　　　　　　　　　　　　　　　(b)

Figure 7. SEM images of IONPs (**a**) and IONPs modified using *Humulus lupulus* aqueous extract (**b**).

2.3. Antimicrobial Activity

The antimicrobial activities of the extracts were tested against selected Gram-positive and Gram-negative bacteria and yeasts. The bioactivity results are presented in Table 2 as minimum inhibitory concentration (MIC) and minimum bactericidal concentration (MBC) values. Water extract showed weak bioactivity (MIC 5–10 mg/mL) against the tested reference strains, whereas ethanol extract showed moderate bioactivity against Gram-positive bacteria. The DMSO extract showed the highest activity against Gram-positive bacteria.

Table 2. Antimicrobial activity of the spent hop extracts, IONPs and spent hop-modified IONPs obtained via mix-mode chemical/biogenic synthesis presented as minimal inhibitory concentration (MIC) and minimal bactericidal concentration (MBC) values in mg L^{-1} or as the dissolution ratio of the initial extract in the case of DMSO.

Microorganism	IONPs + Water Extract		IONPs + 80% Ethanol Extract		IONPs + DMSO Extract		IONPs		Water Extract		80% Ethanol Extract		DMSO Extract	
	MIC	MBC	MIC	MBC	MIC	MBC	MIC	MBC	MIC	MBC	MIC	MBC	MIC	MBC
					Gram-positive bacteria									
Staphylococcus aureus ATCC 25923	>10	Nd	>10	Nd	1.25	5	5	>10	5	10	0.313	0.625	1:3200	1:400
Staphylococcus aureus ATCC BA1707	>10	Nd	>10	Nd	0.625	2.5	>10	>10	5	10	0.313	0.625	1:6400	1:800
Staphylococcus epidermidis ATCC 12228	10	>10	10	>10	1.25	5	5	>10	5	10	0.156	2.5	1:3200	1:100
Micrococcus luteus ATCC 10240	10	>10	2.5	10	0.625	0.625	2.5	5	0.313	2.5	0.078	0.078	1:6400	1:200
Bacillus cereus ATCC 10876	>10	Nd	10	>10	0.313	0.313	5	>10	5	>10	0.156	5	1:12,800	1:3200
Enterococcus faecalis ATCC 29212	>10	Nd	5	>10	0.625	10	5	>10	10	>10	5	10	1:12,800	1:100

Table 2. Cont.

Microorganism	IONPs + Water Extract		IONPs + 80% Ethanol Extract		IONPs + DMSO Extract		IONPs		Water Extract		80% Ethanol Extract		DMSO Extract	
	MIC	MBC	MIC	MBC	MIC	MBC	MIC	MBC	MIC	MBC	MIC	MBC	MIC	MBC
Gram-negative bacteria														
Salmonella typhimurium ATCC 14028	10	>10	10	>10	>10	Nd	5	>10	>10	>10	5	>10	>1:5	Nd
Escherichia coli ATCC 25922	>10	Nd	>10	Nd	>10	Nd	5	>10	5	10	5	5	>1:5	Nd
Proteus mirabilis ATCC 12453	>10	Nd	>10	Nd	>10	Nd	>10	>10	5	10	5	10	>1:5	Nd
Klebsiella pneumoniae ATCC 13883	10	>10	>10	Nd	>10	Nd	5	>10	5	5	5	2.5	>1:5	Nd
Pseudomonas aeruginosa ATCC 9027	10	>10	10	>10	>10	Nd	5	10	5	5	5	5	>1:5	Nd
Yeasts														
Candida glabrata ATCC 90030	10	10	10	10	10	10	5	5	5	5	5	5	1:10	1:10
Candida albicans ATCC 102231	5	10	5	10	10	10	2.5	5	5	5	2.5	5	1:20	1:10
Candida parapsilosis ATCC 22019	10	10	5	10	10	10	2.5	5	5	5	2.5	5	1:80	1:10

IONP surface modification did not increase the bioactivity of the new preparations. The antifungal (against *C. albicans*, *C. parapsilosis* and *C. glabrata*) and antibacterial bioactivities of the modified IONPs were weak and usually lower or equal to those of the extracts themselves.

Only surface modification with DMSO extract improved the activity of the IONPs against Gram-positive bacteria. While unmodified IONPs have MIC values in the range of 2.5–10 mg/mL, IONPs modified with DMSO extract have MIC values many times lower in the range of 0.313–1.25 mg/mL.

3. Discussion

Sergey V. Gudkov tried to answer the question on whether IONPs have significant antibacterial properties in his review article in 2021 [76]. The collected research confirms the antimicrobial effect of IONPs on Gram-negative and Gram-positive bacteria and fungi, with low toxicity toward eukaryotic cells. However, the effect of IONPs varies greatly depending on the type of microorganism and the method of synthesis. A practical inhibition of bacterial growth occurs at concentrations ranging from 1–3 µg/mL against *S. mutans* [111] through 3 mg/mL against *S. aureus* [80] to 62.5 mg/mL against *Corynebacterium* sp., *K. pneumonia*, *P. aeruginosa* and *S. aureus* [112]. However, it should be emphasised that in these cases, the IONPs were obtained via biogenic synthesis or modified with diethyl lenglycol or polyvinyl alcohol (PVA).

In our work, IONPs were obtained through chemical co-precipitation. Extracts from the waste products of supercritical carbon dioxide hop extraction were used to modify the IONPs for the first time. It seems that the observed low bioactivity of IONPs is related to the phenomenon of the agglomeration of magnetic nanoparticles, which does not disappear after modification with hop extracts, except for the DMSO extract. It has been repeatedly reported that magnetic nanoparticles (mainly magnetite and maghemite) tend to form aggregates or agglomerates due to a combination of van der Waals and magnetic forces [113]. Such associations can be permanent or reversible and largely determine the properties of magnetic nanoparticles. It should be emphasised that these processes are still under investigation and not fully understood [114]. As emphasised by many authors, the sizes of aggregated clusters can even exceed 1 µm [115,116]. Therefore, the formation of clusters affects both the transport of nanoparticles and the reactivity by changing the activity of a single nanoparticle.

Not only aggregation, but also the type of materials chosen to coat IONPs fundamentally determine their cytotoxicity [117]. In our work, the surface modification of IONPs using water and 80% ethanol extracts reduced or did not change the activity of the IONPs against Gram-positive and Gram-negative bacteria and yeasts. IONPs have activity comparable to that of aqueous extract with a MIC of 5 mg/mL toward Gram-positive bacteria, whereas its activity against Gram-negative and yeasts was comparable to that of ethanol extract. IONPs modified with ethanol extract showed anti-yeast activity comparable to that of aqueous extract with a MIC value of 2.5 to 5 mg/mL. However, it should be noted that the modification reduces the activity by half of the anti-yeast activity of unmodified IONPs.

C. parapsilosis and *C. albicans* live on the surface of the skin and are the most common cause of infections in hospital intensive care units. Similar to other Candida microorganisms, their main virulence factor is the ability to colonise artificial surfaces. The ability to colonise is determined by the ability to grow in the form of a biofilm. Therefore, unmodified IONPs have the potential to be used in anti-yeast preparations for topical applications. Furthermore, taking into account the fact that IONPs possess magnetic abilities, this can be used to hold them on artificial surfaces to protect against colonisation.

In our work, the ability of IONPs to inhibit the growth of Gram-positive bacteria (*S. epidermidis*, *S. aureus*, *M. luteus*, *E. faecalis*, *B. cereus*) increases from a MIC value of 2.5–10 mg/mL to 0.313–1.25 mg/mL after their modification with DMSO hop extract. This seems to be reasonable since the DMSO spent hop extract showed the highest values of TPC, TFC and TAC evaluated using the SNPAC method.

4. Materials and Methods

4.1. Materials

Ascorbic acid (vitamin C, vit. C), silver nitrate ($AgNO_3$) and dimethyl sulfoxide (DMSO) were purchased from Sigma-Aldrich Inc., St. Louis, MO, USA. Ethanol was purchased from E.Merck (Darmstadt, Germany). Water with a resistivity of 18.2 MΩ cm was obtained from an ULTRAPURE Millipore Direct-Q 3UV-R (Merck, Darmstadt, Germany).

4.2. Extraction of Spent Hops

Hop cones (*Humulus lupulus*) were grown in the Lublin region (Chmielnik near Lublin). Spent hops (of the Marynka variety), which were subjected to supercritical CO_2 extraction, were obtained from the Fertiliser Research Centre of the Institute of New Chemical Synthesis of the Łukasiewicz Research Network in Puławy, Poland. The spent hops were extracted with different solvents, i.e., water, 80% ethanol and DMSO. For the extraction, 5 g of dried plant material was suspended in 100 mL of solvent in a 250 mL Erlenmeyer flask and sonicated for 60 min in an ultrasonic bath (ultrasonic power 1200 W, frequency 35 kHz), a Bandelin Sonorex RK 103 H (Bandelin Electronics, Berlin, Germany), at 80 °C. After cooling, the extracts were centrifuged at 11,000 rpm for 15 min to precipitate traces of solids from the extract. The supernatants were collected, filtered through Whatman No. 1 filter paper and evaporated under vacuum. The residue was dissolved in 5 mL of water.

4.3. Total Flavonoid Content (TFC)

The total flavonoid content (TFC) was determined spectrophotometrically using a Genesys 20 spectrophotometer (The ThermoSpectronic, Waltham, MA, USA) according to Lamaison and Carnat [118]. Briefly, 1.0 mL of 1.2% aluminium chloride ($AlCl_3$) in water was mixed with 100 µL of extract and 900 µL of water. Absorbance at 415 nm was measured against a blank (water) after 30 min.

The total flavonoid content was expressed as the mg reference equivalent (vit. C) per 1 mL^{-1} of extract. Quantification was evaluated using a linear curve of ascorbic acid used as a standard at concentrations ranging from 0.0625 to 1.00 mg mL^{-1}. The calibration curve was generated from six standard solutions with concentrations of 0.0625, 0.125, 0.25, 0.5, 0.75 and 1.00 mg mL^{-1}. The equation of the calibration curve was as follows:

$$1.837\ (\pm 0.065)x - 0.029\ (\pm 0.036),\ R^2 = 0.9950,\ F = 800.64,\ se = 0.05 \tag{1}$$

4.4. Total Phenolic (TPC)

The total phenolic content (TPC) was determined using the Folin–Ciocalteu method [119]. Briefly, 250 µL of extracts diluted 1:10 and 1000 µL of Folin–Ciocalteu phenol reagent diluted 1:10 (Sigma-Aldrich, St. Louis, MO, USA) were added to flasks and mixed thoroughly. Then, 1.0 mL of 10% Na_2CO_3 solution was added, and the mixture was kept in the dark for 2 h at room temperature. The absorbance was then read at 765 nm.

The total phenolic content was expressed as milligrams of the reference equivalent (vit. C) per 1 mL^{-1} of extract. Quantification was evaluated using a linear curve of the ascorbic acid used as the standard at concentrations ranging from 3.9063 to 125.00 µg mL^{-1}. The calibration curve was constructed from six standard solutions with concentrations of 3.91, 7.81, 15.63, 31.25, 62.50 and 125.00 µg mL^{-1}. The equation of the calibration curve was as follows:

$$7.6201\ (\pm 0.2136)x + 0.0707\ (\pm 0.126),\ R^2 = 0.9969,\ F = 1272.60,\ se = 0.02 \tag{2}$$

4.5. Silver Nanoparticle Antioxidant Capacity (SNPAC)

SNPAC measurements were performed according to Özyürek et al. [96]. The procedure has been described in detail previously [86,87]. The initial solution of silver nanoparticles (AgNPs) was prepared by mixing 5 mL of 1% aqueous tripotassium citrate solution with 50 mL of 1 mM $AgNO_3$ at an elevated temperature (around 90 °C). The test samples were prepared by mixing 2 mL AgNPs, standard or tested extract (x) and (0.8 − x) mL water. After storage in the dark for 30 min, the mixtures were measured spectrophotometrically at 423 nm, which is characteristic of the surface plasmon resonance of AgNPs [87]. The calibration curve showed the relationship between the absorbance (A) and the final micromolar concentration of the standard antioxidant (vit. C). The calibration curve was linear from 10.16 to 101.39 µM (10.139; 20.277; 30.416; 40.554; 101.386 µM). The equation for the calibration curve was as follows:

$$A_{423nm} = 0.0173\ (\pm 0.00075)c_{\mu M} + 0.112\ (\pm 0.039),\ R^2 = 0.9944,\ F = 537.77,\ se = 0.05 \tag{3}$$

The total antioxidant capacity in µM (TAC) of the extracts was calculated by dividing the observed absorbance at λ = 423 nm for 15 µL of added sample by the molar absorptivity (ε) of vitamin C, which can be obtained from the slope of the calibration curve. The method is effective for antioxidants with a standard potential of less than 0.8 V due to E Ag(I), Ag° = 0.8 V.

4.6. Synthesis of IONPs

0.1 M $FeCl_3$ and 0.1 M $FeSO_4$ were mixed in a volume ratio of 2:1. 25 mL of 25%. NH_3 was added dropwise to the solution with constant stirring. A black precipitate formed. It was separated using an external magnetic field and washed several times with deionised water until the solution above the precipitate reached pH 7. The IONPs were prepared according to the following reaction:

$$FeCl_2 \times 4H_2O + 2FeCl_3 \times 6H_2O \rightarrow 8NaCl + Fe_3O_4 + 14H_2O \tag{4}$$

4.7. Modification of the NP Surfaces Using Plant Extracts

The dried extracts (aqueous and 80% EtOH) were dissolved in 5 mL of water. Then 3 g of dried IONPs were added and conditioned at room temperature for 3 days; after which, the IONPs were separated using a magnet, and the supernatant was removed. The modified nanoparticles were washed several times with small volumes of deionised water and allowed to dry. The powders were then stored in airtight glass vials at 4 °C until further analysis.

4.8. Characterization of AgNPs

4.8.1. UV-Vis Spectroscopy, SEM, EDS and DLS

IONPs were characterised spectrophotometrically using a Genesys 20 spectrophotometer (The ThermoSpectronic, Waltham, MA, USA).

The morphology and chemical composition of the IONPs were investigated using a Quanta 250 FEG scanning electron microscope from FEI (Almelo, The Netherlands) equipped with a FEG electron source and energy-dispersive X-ray spectroscopy (EDS). The experiment was carried out in the same conditions as previously described [87]. Observations were made using accelerating voltages ranging from 10 to 15 keV.

The Malvern Zetasizer Nano ZS (Malvern Instruments Ltd. (Malvern, UK), GB) with the DLS technique was used to measure the size of the nanoparticles.

4.8.2. FT-IR

Fourier-transform infrared–attenuated total reflectance (FT-IR/ATR) spectra were recorded in the 3700–400 cm^{-1} range, resolution 4 cm^{-1}, at room temperature using a Nicolet 6700 spectrometer (Thermo Fisher Scientific Inc., Waltham, MA, USA) and a Meridian Diamond ATR accessory (Harrick Scientific Products, Inc., Pleasantville, NY, USA). Interferograms of 512 scans were averaged for each spectrum. Dry potassium bromide (48 h, 105 °C) was used as a reference material to collect the ATR spectra. No smoothing functions were applied. All spectral measurements were performed at least in triplicate. Raw spectra were processed using OMNIC™ software (Thermo Fisher Scientific Inc., USA) version 8.2.387.

4.9. Antimicrobial Activity Assay

Suspensions of all compounds in DMSO were screened for antibacterial and antifungal activities using the 2-fold microdilution broth method. The detailed procedure of the assay was previously described [120]. The minimal inhibitory concentrations (MIC) of the tested compounds were evaluated for the following panel of reference yeasts: *Candida parapsilosis* ATCC 22019, *Candida glabrata* ATCC 90030 and *Candida albicans* ATCC 102231. The panel of reference Gram-positive bacteria included *Staphylococcus epidermidis* ATCC 12228, *Staphylococcus aureus* ATCC 25923, *S. aureus* ATCC BAA-1707, *Micrococcus luteus* ATCC 10240, *Enterococcus faecalis* ATCC 29212 and *Bacillus cereus* ATCC 10876. The Gram-negative bacteria panel included *Escherichia coli* ATCC 25922, *Proteus mirabilis* ATCC 12453, *Salmonella Typhimurium* ATCC 14028, *Pseudomonas aeruginosa* ATCC 9027 and *Klebsiella pneumoniae* ATCC 13883.

5. Conclusions

This work describes for the first time the possibility of obtaining IONPs using a method that combines chemical synthesis with modification using plant extracts. The waste product remaining after the supercritical carbon dioxide extraction of hop cones was used to obtain the extracts. Among the different solvents used for extraction, the modification of IONPs with DMSO extract improved their antibacterial properties against Gram-positive bacteria almost tenfold, from a MIC of 2.5–10 mg/mL to 0.313–1.25 mg/mL. This is the first study to use spent hop extract to modify IONPs. The results obtained show the great potential of the waste material (spent hops), which should be further investigated for use in the biogenic synthesis of nanoparticles of other metals and their activity toward microorganisms as well as cancer cell lines.

Author Contributions: Conceptualization, J.F. and S.P.-P.; methodology, N.Ż., R.P. and K.S.; software, R.P., S.P.-P. and I.K.-G.; validation, N.Ż., M.P. and K.S.; formal analysis, N.Ż. and W.F.; investigation, N.Ż.; resources, M.P.; data curation, S.P.-P.; writing—original draft preparation, J.F. and S.P.-P.; writing—review and editing, J.F.; visualization, N.Ż.; supervision, W.F. and I.K.-G.; project administration, W.F.; funding acquisition, J.F. and W.F. All authors have read and agreed to the published version of the manuscript.

Funding: This research received no external funding.

Institutional Review Board Statement: Not applicable.

Informed Consent Statement: Not applicable.

Data Availability Statement: The data are available for request from Prof. J. Flieger.

Conflicts of Interest: The authors declare no conflicts of interest.

References

1. Lattuada, M.; Hatton, T.A. Functionalization of monodisperse magnetic nanoparticles. *Langmuir* **2007**, *23*, 2158–2168. [CrossRef] [PubMed]
2. Kharisov, B.I.; Kharissova, O.V.; Rasika Dias, H.V.; Méndez, U.O.; de la Fuente, I.G.; Peña, Y.; Dimas, A.V. *Iron-Based Nanomaterials in the Catalysis*; Advanced Catalytic Materials—Photocatalysis and Other Current Trends; InTech.: Rijeka, Croatia, 2016. [CrossRef]
3. Kharisov, B.I.; Rasika Dias, H.V.; Kharissova, O.V.; Jiménez-Pérez, V.M.; Olvera Pérez, B.; Muñoz Flores, B. Iron-containing nanomaterials: Synthesis, properties, and environmental applications. *RSC Adv.* **2012**, *2*, 9325–9358. [CrossRef]
4. Ebrahiminezhad, A.; Zare-Hoseinabadi, A.; Sarmah, A.K.; Taghizadeh, S.; Ghasemi, Y.; Berenjian, A. Plant-Mediated Synthesis and Applications of Iron Nanoparticles. *Mol. Biotechnol.* **2018**, *60*, 154–168. [CrossRef] [PubMed]
5. Batool, F.; Iqbal, M.S.; Khan, S.U.D.; Khan, J.; Ahmed, B.; Qadir, M.I. Biologically Synthesized Iron Nanoparticles (FeNPs) from Phoenix dactylifera Have Anti-Bacterial Activities. *Sci. Rep.* **2021**, *11*, 22132. [CrossRef] [PubMed]
6. Huber, D.L. Synthesis, Properties, and Applications of Iron Nanoparticles. *Small* **2005**, *1*, 482–501. [CrossRef]
7. Peng, X.H.; Qian, X.; Mao, H.; Wang, A.Y.; Chen, Z.G.; Nie, S.; Shin, D.M. Targeted magnetic iron oxide nanoparticles for tumor imaging and therapy. *Int. J. Nanomed.* **2008**, *3*, 311–321. [CrossRef]
8. Yu, M.K.; Park, J.; Jeong, Y.Y.; Moon, W.K.; Jon, S. Integrin-targeting thermally cross-linked superparamagnetic iron oxide nanoparticles for combined cancer imaging and drug delivery. *Nanotechnology* **2010**, *21*, 415102. [CrossRef]
9. Xu, W.; Yang, T.; Liu, S.; Du, L.; Chen, Q.; Li, X.; Dong, J.; Zhang, Z.; Lu, S.; Gong, Y.; et al. Insights into the Synthesis, types and application of iron Nanoparticles: The overlooked significance of environmental effects. *Environ. Int.* **2022**, *158*, 106980. [CrossRef]
10. Gutierrez, A.M.; Dziubla, T.D.; Hilt, J.Z. Recent advances on iron oxide magnetic nanoparticles as sorbents of organic pollutants in water and wastewater treatment. *Rev. Environ. Health* **2017**, *32*, 111–117. [CrossRef]
11. Hoch, L.B.; Mack, E.J.; Hydutsky, B.W.; Hershman, J.M.; Skluzacek, J.M.; Mallouk, T.E. Carbothermal synthesis of carbon-supported nanoscale zero-valent iron particles for the remediation of hexavalent chromium. *Environ. Sci. Technol.* **2008**, *42*, 2600–2605. [CrossRef]
12. Huang, K.C.; Ehrman, S.H. Synthesis of iron nanoparticles via chemical reduction with palladium ion seeds. *Langmuir* **2007**, *23*, 1419–1426. [CrossRef] [PubMed]
13. Huang, Q.; Shi, X.; Pinto, R.A.; Petersen, E.J.; Weber, W.J., Jr. Tunable synthesis and immobilization of zero-valent iron nanoparticles for environmental applications. *Environ. Sci. Technol.* **2008**, *42*, 8884–8889. [CrossRef] [PubMed]
14. Guo, L.; Huang, Q.J.; Li, X.Y.; Yang, S. PVP-coated iron nanocrystals: Anhydrous synthesis, characterization, and electrocatalysis for two species. *Langmuir* **2006**, *22*, 7867–7872. [CrossRef] [PubMed]
15. Kanel, S.R.; Goswami, R.R.; Clement, T.P.; Barnett, M.O.; Zhao, D. Two dimensional transport characteristics of surface stabilized zero-valent iron nanoparticles in porous media. *Environ. Sci. Technol.* **2008**, *42*, 896–900. [CrossRef] [PubMed]
16. Liu, Y.; Lowry, G.V. Effect of particle age (Fe0 content) and solution pH on NZVI reactivity: H2 evolution and TCE dechlorination. *Environ. Sci. Technol.* **2006**, *40*, 6085–6090. [CrossRef] [PubMed]
17. He, F.; Zhao, D. Manipulating the size and dispersibility of zerovalent iron nanoparticles by use of carboxymethyl cellulose stabilizers. *Environ. Sci. Technol.* **2007**, *41*, 6216–6221. [CrossRef]
18. Yoon, S.U.; Mahanty, B.; Ha, H.M.; Kim, C.G. Phenol adsorption on surface-functionalized iron oxide nanoparticles: Modeling of the kinetics, isotherm, and mechanism. *J. Nanopart. Res.* **2016**, *18*, 170. [CrossRef]
19. Islama, J.; Gangulia, P.; Mondala, S.; Chaudhuri, S. Green synthesis of iron oxide magnetic nanoparticles for the adsorption of lead (II) from aqueous medium. *J. Indian Chem. Soc.* **2020**, *52*, 1854–1860.
20. Anjum, M.; Miandad, R.; Waqas, M.; Gehany, F.; Barakat, M.A. Remediation of wastewater using various nanomaterials. *Arab. J.Chem.* **2019**, *12*, 4897–4919. [CrossRef]
21. Dixit, S.; Hering, J.G. Comparison of arsenic(V) and arsenic(III) sorption onto iron oxide minerals: Implications for arsenic mobility. *Environ. Sci. Technol.* **2003**, *37*, 4182–4189. [CrossRef]

22. Hua, M.; Zhang, S.; Pan, B.; Zhang, W.; Lv, L.; Zhang, Q. Heavy metal removal from water/wastewater by nanosized metal oxides: A review. *J. Hazard. Mater.* **2012**, *211–212*, 317–331. [CrossRef] [PubMed]
23. Savage, N.; Diallo, M.S. Nanomaterials and Water Purification: Opportunities and Challenges. *J. Nanopart. Res.* **2005**, *7*, 331–342. [CrossRef]
24. Molloy, A.L.; Andrade, M.F.C.; Escalera, G.; Bohloul, A.; Avendano, C.; Colvin, V.L.; Gonzalez-Pech, N.I. The Effect of Surface Coating on Iron-Oxide Nanoparticle Arsenic Adsorption. *MRS Adv.* **2021**, *6*, 867–874. [CrossRef]
25. Ha, H.T.; Phong, P.T.; Minh, T.D. Synthesis of Iron Oxide Nanoparticle Functionalized Activated Carbon and Its Applications in Arsenic Adsorption. *J. Anal. Methods Chem.* **2021**, *2021*, 6668490. [CrossRef] [PubMed]
26. Cheng, W.; Zhang, W.; Hu, L.; Ding, W.; Wu, F.; Li, J. Etching synthesis of iron oxide nanoparticles for adsorption of arsenic from water. *RSC Adv.* **2016**, *6*, 15900–15910. [CrossRef]
27. Kulpa-Koterwa, A.; Ryl, J.; Górnicka, K.; Niedziałkowski, P. New nanoadsorbent based on magnetic iron oxide containing 1,4,7,10-tetraazacyclododecane in outer chain (Fe_3O_4@SiO_2-cyclen) for adsorption and removal of selected heavy metal ions Cd^{2+}, Pb^{2+}, Cu^{2+}. *J. Mol. Liq.* **2022**, *368*, 120710. [CrossRef]
28. Mittal, A.K.; Chisti, Y.; Banerjee, U.C. Synthesis of metallic nanoparticles using plant extracts. *Biotechnol. Adv.* **2013**, *31*, 346–356. [CrossRef]
29. Shibata, T. Method for Producing Green Tea in Microfine Powder. U.S. Patent No 6,416,803, 7 July 2002.
30. Brody, A.L.; Bugusu, B.; Han, J.H.; Sand, C.K.; McHugh, T.H. Innovative Food Packaging Solutions. *J. Food Sci.* **2008**, *73*, R107–R116. [CrossRef]
31. Jadoun, S.; Arif, R.; Jangid, N.K.; Meena, R.K. Green synthesis of nanoparticles using plant extracts: A review. *Env. Chem. Lett.* **2021**, *19*, 355–374. [CrossRef]
32. Benković, M.; Valinger, D.; Jurina, T.; Gajdoš Kljusurić, J.; Jurinjak Tušek, A. Biocatalysis as a Green Approach for Synthesis of Iron Nanoparticles—Batch and Microflow Process Comparison. *Catalysts* **2023**, *13*, 112. [CrossRef]
33. Cushen, M.; Kerry, J.; Morris, M.; Cruz-Romero, M.; Cummins, E. Nanotechnologies in the Food Industry—Recent Developments, Risks and Regulation. *Trends Food Sci. Technol.* **2012**, *24*, 30–46. [CrossRef]
34. Akintelu, S.A.; Oyebamiji, A.K.; Olugbeko, S.C.; Folorunso, A.S. Green Synthesis of Iron Oxide Nanoparticles for Biomedical Application and Environmental Remediation: A Review. *Eclet. Quim.* **2021**, *46*, 17–37. [CrossRef]
35. Ma, M.; Zhang, Y.; Yu, W.; Shen, H.-Y.; Zhang, H.-Q.; Gu, N. Preparation and characterization of magnetite nanoparticles coated by amino silane. *Colloids Surf. A Physicochem. Eng. Aspect* **2003**, *212*, 219. [CrossRef]
36. Herlekar, M.; Barve, S.; Kumar, R. Plant-Mediated Green Synthesis of Iron Nanoparticles. *J. Nanoparticles* **2014**, *2014*, 140614. [CrossRef]
37. Song, H.; Carraway, E.R. Reduction of chlorinated ethanes by nanosized zero-valent iron: Kinetics, pathways, and effects of reaction conditions. *Environ. Sci. Technol.* **2005**, *39*, 6237–6245. [CrossRef]
38. Kim, J.H.; Tratnyek, P.G.; Chang, Y.S. Rapid dechlorination of polychlorinated dibenzo-p-dioxins by bimetallic and nanosized zerovalent iron. *Environ. Sci. Technol.* **2008**, *42*, 4106–4112. [CrossRef]
39. Sarathy, V.; Tratnyek, P.G.; Nurmi, J.T.; Baer, D.R.; Amonette, J.E.; Chun, C.L.; Penn, R.L.; Reardon, E.J. Aging of Iron Nanoparticles in Aqueous Solution: Effects on Structure and Reactivity. *J. Phys. Chem. C* **2008**, *112*, 2286. [CrossRef]
40. Nadagouda, M.N.; Varma, R.S. Green and controlled synthesis of gold and platinum nanomaterials using vitamin B2: Density-assisted self-assembly of nanospheres, wires and rods. *Green Chem.* **2006**, *8*, 516. [CrossRef]
41. Raveendran, P.; Fu, J.; Wallen, S.L. Completely "green" synthesis and stabilization of metal nanoparticles. *J. Am. Chem. Soc.* **2003**, *125*, 13940–13941. [CrossRef]
42. Lee, J.; Isobe, T.; Senna, M.J. Preparation of Ultrafine Fe_3O_4 Particles by Precipitation in the Presence of PVA at High pH. *J. Colloid Interface Sci.* **1996**, *177*, 490. [CrossRef]
43. Zhao, L.; Mitomo, H.; Zhai, M.; Yushii, F.; Nagasawa, N.; Kume, T. Synthesis of antibacterial PVA/CM-chitosan blend hydrogels with electron beam irradiation. *Carbohydr. Polym.* **2003**, *53*, 439. [CrossRef]
44. Kumar, M.N.; Muzzarelli, R.A.; Muzzarelli, C.; Sashiwa, H.; Domb, A.J. Chitosan chemistry and pharmaceutical perspectives. *Chem. Rev.* **2004**, *104*, 6017–6084. [CrossRef]
45. Kim, E.H.; Ahn, Y.; Lee, H.S. Biomedical applications of superparamagnetic iron oxide nanoparticles encapsulated within chitosan. *J. Alloys Compd.* **2007**, *434–435*, 633–636. [CrossRef]
46. Asghar, M.A.; Zahir, E.; Asghar, M.A.; Iqbal, J.; Rehman, A.A. Facile, One-Pot Biosynthesis and Characterization of Iron, Copper and Silver Nanoparticles Using Syzygium cumini Leaf Extract: As an Effective Antimicrobial and Aflatoxin B1 Adsorption Agents. *PLoS ONE* **2020**, *15*, e0234964. [CrossRef]
47. Chauhan, S.; Upadhyay, L.S.B. Biosynthesis of Iron Oxide Nanoparticles Using Plant Derivatives of Lawsonia inermis (Henna) and Its Surface Modification for Biomedical Application. *Nanotechnol. Environ. Eng.* **2019**, *4*, 8. [CrossRef]
48. Machado, S.; Pinto, S.L.; Grosso, J.P.; Nouws, H.P.A.; Albergaria, J.T.; Delerue-Matos, C. Green Production of Zero-Valent Iron Nanoparticles Using Tree Leaf Extracts. *Sci. Total Environ.* **2013**, *445–446*, 1–8. [CrossRef]
49. Iravani, S.; Korbekandi, H.; Mirmohammadi, S.V.; Zolfaghari, B. Synthesis of Silver Nanoparticles: Chemical, Physical and Biological Methods. *Res. Pharm. Sci.* **2014**, *9*, 385–406.

50. Mahanty, S.; Bakshi, M.; Ghosh, S.; Gaine, T.; Chatterjee, S.; Bhattacharyya, S.; Das, S.; Das, P.; Chaudhuri, P. Mycosynthesis of Iron Oxide Nanoparticles Using Manglicolous Fungi Isolated from Indian Sundarbans and Its Application for the Treatment of Chromium Containing Solution: Synthesis, Adsorption Isotherm, Kinetics and Thermodynamics Study. *Environ. Nanotechnol. Monit. Manag.* **2019**, *12*, 100276. [CrossRef]
51. Kaur, M.; Chopra, D.S. Green Synthesis of Iron Nanoparticles for Biomedical Applications. *Glob. J. Nanomed.* **2018**, *4*, 68–77. [CrossRef]
52. Huang, L.; Weng, X.; Chen, Z.; Megharaj, M.; Naidu, R. Green Synthesis of Iron Nanoparticles by Various Tea Extracts: Comparative Study of the Reactivity. *Spectrochim. Acta. A Mol. Biomol. Spectrosc.* **2014**, *130*, 295–301. [CrossRef]
53. Harshiny, M.; Iswarya, C.N.; Matheswaran, M. Biogenic Synthesis of Iron Nanoparticles Using Amaranthus dubius Leaf Extract as a Reducing Agent. *Powder Technol.* **2015**, *286*, 744–749. [CrossRef]
54. Martínez-Cabanas, M.; López-García, M.; Barriada, J.L.; Herrero, R.; Sastre de Vicente, M.E. Green Synthesis of Iron Oxide Nanoparticles. Development of Magnetic Hybrid Materials for Efficient As(V) Removal. *Chem. Eng. J.* **2016**, *301*, 83–91. [CrossRef]
55. Nadagouda, M.N.; Castle, A.B.; Murdock, R.C.; Hussain, S.M.; Varma, R.S. In vitro biocompatibility of nanoscale zerovalent iron particles (NZVI) synthesized using tea polyphenols. *Green Chem.* **2010**, *12*, 114–122. [CrossRef]
56. Mohamed, A.; Atta, R.R.; Kotp, A.A.; Abo El-Ela, F.I.; Abd El-Raheem, H.; Farghali, A.; Alkhalifah, D.H.M.; Hozzein, W.N.; Mahmoud, R. Green synthesis and characterization of iron oxide nanoparticles for the removal of heavy metals (Cd^{2+} and Ni^{2+}) from aqueous solutions with Antimicrobial Investigation. *Sci. Rep.* **2023**, *13*, 7297. [CrossRef]
57. Shrifian-Esfahni, A.; Salehi, M.T.; Nasr-Esfahni, M.; Ekramian, E. Chitosan-modified superparamgnetic iron oxide nanoparticles: Design, fabrication, characterization and antibacterial activity. *Chemik* **2015**, *69*, 19–32.
58. Tyagi, P.K.; Gupta, S.; Tyagi, S.; Kumar, M.; Pandiselvam, R.; Daştan, S.D.; Sharifi-Rad, J.; Gola, D.; Arya, A. Green Synthesis of Iron Nanoparticles from Spinach Leaf and Banana Peel Aqueous Extracts and Evaluation of Antibacterial Potential. *J. Nanomater.* **2021**, *2021*, 4871453. [CrossRef]
59. Das, P.; Dutta, T.; Manna, S.; Loganathan, S.; Basak, P. Facile green synthesis of non-genotoxic, non-hemolytic organometallic silver nanoparticles using extract of crushed, wasted, and spent *Humulus lupulus* (hops): Characterization, anti-bacterial, and anti-cancer studies. *Environ. Res.* **2022**, *204 Pt. A*, 111962. [CrossRef]
60. Zanoli, P.; Zavatti, M. Pharmacognostic and pharmacological profile of *Humulus lupulus* L. *J. Ethnopharmacol.* **2008**, *116*, 383–396. [CrossRef]
61. Arruda, T.R.; Pinheiro, P.F.; Silva, P.I.; Bernardes, P.C. A new perspective of a well-recognized raw material: Phenolic content, antioxidant and antimicrobial activities and α- and β-acids profile of Brazilian hop (*Humulus lupulus* L.) extracts. *LWT* **2021**, *141*, 110905. [CrossRef]
62. Hrncic, M.K.; Spaninger, E.; Kosir, I.J.; Knez, Z.; Bren, U. Hop compounds: Extraction techniques, chemical analyses, antioxidative, antimicrobial, and anticarcinogenic effects. *Nutrients* **2019**, *11*, 257. [CrossRef]
63. Sanz, V.; Torres, M.D.; Vilarino, J.M.L.; Domínguez, H. What is new on the hop extraction? *Trends Food Sci. Technol.* **2019**, *93*, 12–22. [CrossRef]
64. Abram, V.; Ceh, B.; Vidmar, M.; Hercezi, M.; Lazi'c, N.; Bucik, V.; Ulrih, N.P. A comparison of antioxidant and antimicrobial activity between hop leaves and hop cones. *Ind. Crops Prod.* **2015**, *64*, 124–134. [CrossRef]
65. Formato, A.; Gallo, M.; Ianniello, D.; Montesano, D.; Naviglio, D. Supercritical fluid extraction of alfa and beta-acids from hops compared to cyclically pressurized solid—Liquid extraction. *J. Supercrit. Fluids* **2013**, *84*, 113–120. [CrossRef]
66. Larson, A.E.; Yu, R.R.Y.; Lee, O.A.; Price, S.; Haas, G.J.; Johnson, E.A. Antimicrobial activity of hop extracts against Listeria monocytogenes in media and in food. *Int. J. Food Microbiol.* **1996**, *33*, 195–207. [CrossRef]
67. Kramer, B.; Thielmann, J.; Hickisch, A.; Muranyi, P.; Wunderlich, J.; Hauser, C. Antimicrobial activity of hop extracts against foodborne pathogens for meat applications. *J. Appl. Microbiol.* **2015**, *118*, 648–657. [CrossRef]
68. Steenackers, B.; De Cooman, L.; De Vos, D. Chemical transformations of characteristic hop secondary metabolites in relation to beer properties and the brewing process: A review. *Food Chem.* **2015**, *172*, 742–756. [CrossRef]
69. Bocquet, L.; Sahpaz, S.; Bonneau, N.; Beaufay, C.; Mahieux, S.; Samaillie, S.; Rivière, C. Phenolic compounds from *Humulus lupulus* as natural antimicrobial products: New weapons in the fight against methicillin resistant Staphylococcus aureus, Leishmania mexicana and Trypanosoma brucei strains. *Molecules* **2019**, *24*, 1024. [CrossRef]
70. Betancur, M.; López, J.; Salazar, F. Antimicrobial activity of compounds from hop (*Humulus lupulus* L.) following supercritical fluid extraction: An overview. *Chil. J. Agric. Res.* **2023**, *83*, 499–509. [CrossRef]
71. Alonso-Esteban, J.I.; Pinela, J.; Barros, L.; Ćirić, A.; Soković, M.; Calhelha, R.C.; Ferreira, I.C. Phenolic composition and antioxidant, antimicrobial and cytotoxic properties of hop (*Humulus lupulus* L.) seeds. *Ind. Crops Prod.* **2019**, *134*, 154–159. [CrossRef]
72. Palmer, M.V.; Ting, S.S.T. Applications for supercritical fluid technology in food processing. *Food Chem.* **1995**, *53*, 345–352. [CrossRef]
73. Bartoli, G.; Cupone, G.; Dalpozzo, R.; De Nino, A.; Maiuolo, L.; Marcantoni, E.; Procopio, A. Cerium-Mediated Deprotection of Substituted Allyl Ethers. *Synlett* **2001**, *2001*, 1897–1900. [CrossRef]
74. Anioł, M. Extraction of Spent Hops Using Organic Solvents. *J. Am. Soc. Brew. Chem.* **2008**, *66*, 208–214. [CrossRef]
75. Żołnierczyk, A.K.; Mączka, W.K.; Grabarczyk, M.; Wińska, K.; Woźniak, E.; Anioł, M. Isoxanthohumol--Biologically active hop flavonoid. *Fitoterapia* **2015**, *103*, 71–82. [CrossRef]

76. Gudkov, S.V.; Burmistrov, D.E.; Serov, D.A.; Rebezov, M.B.; Semenova, A.A.; Lisitsyn, A.B. Do Iron Oxide Nanoparticles Have Significant Antibacterial Properties? *Antibiotics* **2021**, *10*, 884. [CrossRef]
77. Prasad, S.K.; Kumar, S.L.; Prasad, M.; Jayalakshmi, B.; Revanasiddappa, H.D. Synthesis, spectral characterization, DNA interaction studies, anthelmintic and antimicrobial activity of transition metal complexes with 3-(2-hydroxybenzylideneamino)-2-methylquinazolin-4(3 H)-one and 1,10-phenanthroline. *Biointerface Res. Appl. Chem.* **2011**, *1*, 127–138. [CrossRef]
78. Kaittanis, C.; Nath, S.; Perez, J.M. Rapid Nanoparticle-Mediated Monitoring of Bacterial Metabolic Activity and Assessment of Antimicrobial Susceptibility in Blood with Magnetic Relaxation. *PLoS ONE* **2008**, *3*, 3253. [CrossRef]
79. Taylor, E.N.; Webster, T.J. The use of superparamagnetic nanoparticles for prosthetic biofilm prevention. *Int. J. Nanomed.* **2009**, *4*, 145–152.
80. Tran, N.; Mir, A.; Mallik, D.; Sinha, A.; Nayar, S.; Webster, T.J. Bactericidal effect of iron oxide nanoparticles on Staphylococcus aureus. *Int. J. Nanomed.* **2010**, *5*, 277–283. [CrossRef]
81. Høiby, N.; Bjarnsholt, T.; Givskov, M.; Molin, S.; Ciofu, O. Antibiotic resistance of bacterial biofilms. *Int. J. Antimicrob. Agents.* **2010**, *35*, 322–332. [CrossRef]
82. Suárez, C.; Peña, C.; Tubau, F.; Gavaldà, L.; Manzur, A.; Dominguez, M.A.; Pujol, M.; Gudiol, F.; Ariza, J. Clinical impact of imipenem-resistant Pseudomonas aeruginosa bloodstream infections. *J. Infect.* **2009**, *58*, 285–290. [CrossRef]
83. Niemirowicz, K.; Markiewicz, K.H.; Wilczewska, A.Z.; Car, H. Magnetic nanoparticles as new diagnostic tools in medicine. *Adv. Med. Sci.* **2012**, *57*, 196–207. [CrossRef]
84. Zhou, Y.T.; Nie, H.L.; Branford-White, C.; He, Z.Y.; Zhu, L.M. Removal of Cu^{2+} from aqueous solution by chitosan-coated magnetic nanoparticles modified with alpha-ketoglutaric acid. *J. Colloid Interface Sci.* **2009**, *330*, 29–37. [CrossRef]
85. Apak, R.; Güçlü, K.; Demirata, B.; Özyürek, M.; Çelik, S.E.; Bektaşoğlu, B.; Berker, K.I.; Özyurt, D. Comparative Evaluation of Various Total Antioxidant Capacity Assays Applied to Phenolic Compounds with the CUPRAC Assay. *Molecules* **2007**, *12*, 1496–1547. [CrossRef]
86. Radzikowska-Büchner, E.; Flieger, W.; Pasieczna-Patkowska, S.; Franus, W.; Panek, R.; Korona-Głowniak, I.; Suśniak, K.; Rajtar, B.; Świątek, Ł.; Żuk, N.; et al. Antimicrobial and Apoptotic Efficacy of Plant-Mediated Silver Nanoparticles. *Molecules* **2023**, *28*, 5519. [CrossRef]
87. Flieger, J.; Franus, W.; Panek, R.; Szymańska-Chargot, M.; Flieger, W.; Flieger, M.; Kołodziej, P. Green Synthesis of Silver Nanoparticles Using Natural Extracts with Proven Antioxidant Activity. *Molecules* **2021**, *26*, 4986. [CrossRef]
88. Flieger, J.; Flieger, W.; Baj, J.; Maciejewski, R. Antioxidants: Classification, Natural Sources, Activity/Capacity Measurements, and Usefulness for the Synthesis of Nanoparticles. *Materials* **2021**, *14*, 4135. [CrossRef]
89. Eustis, S.; El-Sayed, M.A. Why gold nanoparticles are more precious than pretty gold: Noble metal surface plasmon resonance and its enhancement of the radiative and nonradiative properties of nanocrystals of different shapes. *Chem. Soc. Rev.* **2006**, *35*, 209–217. [CrossRef]
90. Setsukinai, K.; Urano, Y.; Kakinuma, K.; Majima, H.J.; Nagano, T. Development of novel fluorescence probes that can reliably detect reactive oxygen species and distinguish specific species. *J. Biol. Chem.* **2003**, *278*, 3170–3175. [CrossRef] [PubMed]
91. Matsuura, N.; Umemoto, K. Medium Effects for Single Ions in Dimethyl Sulfoxide, N,N'-Dimethylformamide, and Propylene Carbonate. *Bull. Chem. Soc. Jpn.* **1974**, *47*, 1334–13378. [CrossRef]
92. Rosli, I.; Zulhaimi, H.; Ibrahim, S.; Gopinath, S.; Kasim, K.; Akmal, H.; Nuradibah, M.; Sam, T. Phytosynthesis of iron nanoparticle from Averrhoa Bilimbi Linn. In *IOP Conference Series: Materials Science and Engineering, Proceedings of the Malaysian Technical Universities Conference on Engineering and Technology 2017 (MUCET 2017), Penang, Malaysia, 6–7 December 2017*; IOP Publishing: Bristol, UK; p. 012012.
93. Rodríguez-Gattorno, G.; Díaz, D.; Rendón, L.; Hernández-Segura, G.O. Metallic Nanoparticles from Spontaneous Reduction of Silver(I) in DMSO. Interaction between Nitric Oxide and Silver Nanoparticles. *J. Phys. Chem. B* **2002**, *106*, 2482–2487. [CrossRef]
94. Mohamed, H.E.A.; Afridi, S.; Khalil, A.T.; Ali, M.; Zohra, T.; Salman, M.; Ikram, A.; Shinwari, Z.K.; Maaza, M. Bio-redox potential of Hyphaene thebaica in bio-fabrication of ultrafine maghemite phase iron oxide nanoparticles (Fe_2O_3 NPs) for therapeutic applications. *Mater. Sci. Eng. C Mater. Biol. Appl.* **2020**, *112*, 110890. [CrossRef] [PubMed]
95. Gardner, D.S. Commercial Scale Extraction of Alpha-Acids and Hop Oils with Compressed CO_2. In *Extraction of Natural Products Using Near-Critical Solvents*; King, M.B., Bott, T.R., Eds.; Blackie, Academic and Professional: London, UK, 1993; pp. 84–100.
96. Özyürek, M.; Güngör, N.; Baki, S.; Güçlü, K.; Apak, R. Development of a silver nanoparticle-based method for the antioxidant capacity measurement of polyphenols. *Anal. Chem.* **2012**, *84*, 8052–8059. [CrossRef]
97. Mahdavi, M.; Namvar, F.; Ahmad, M.B.; Mohamad, R. Green biosynthesis and characterization of magnetic iron oxide (Fe3O4) nanoparticles using seaweed (*Sargassum muticum*) aqueous extract. *Molecules* **2013**, *18*, 5954–5964. [CrossRef] [PubMed]
98. Saif, S.; Tahir, A.; Asim, T.; Chen, Y.; Adil, S.F. Polymeric Nanocomposites of Iron–Oxide Nanoparticles (IONPs) Synthesized Using Terminalia chebula Leaf Extract for Enhanced Adsorption of Arsenic(V) from Water. *Colloids Interfaces* **2019**, *3*, 17. [CrossRef]
99. Veena, S.; Gopal, R.; Mini, V.; Bena Jothy, I.; Joe, H. Synthesis and characterization of iron oxide nanoparticles using DMSO as a stabilizer. *Mater. Today Proc.* **2015**, *2*, 1051–1055. [CrossRef]
100. Wu, W.; Jiang, C.Z.; Roy, V.A. Designed synthesis and surface engineering strategies of magnetic iron oxide nanoparticles for biomedical applications. *Nanoscale* **2016**, *8*, 19421–19474. [CrossRef] [PubMed]
101. Madivoli, E.S.; Kareru, P.G.; Maina, E.G.; Nyabola, A.O.; Wanakai, S.I.; Nyang'au, J.O. Biosynthesis of iron nanoparticles using Ageratum conyzoides extracts, their antimicrobial and photocatalytic activity. *SN Appl. Sci.* **2019**, *1*, 500. [CrossRef]

102. Ali, A.; Zafar, H.; Zia, M.; Ul Haq, I.; Phull, A.R.; Ali, J.S.; Hussain, A. Synthesis, characterization, applications, and challenges of iron oxide nanoparticles. *Nanotechnol. Sci. Appl.* **2016**, *9*, 49–67. [CrossRef]
103. Gobi, M.; Sujatha, M.; Pradeepa, V.; Muralidharan, M.; Venkatesan, M. Green synthesis of iron oxide nanoparticles (FeONPs) and its antibacterial effect using *Chamaecrista nigricans* (Vahl) Greene (Caesalpiniaceae). *Biomass Conv. Bioref.* **2023**, 1–8. [CrossRef]
104. Hwang, S.W.; Umar, A.; Dar, G.N.; Kim, S.H.; Badran, R.I. Synthesis and Characterization of Iron Oxide Nanoparticles for Phenyl Hydrazine Sensor Applications. *Sens. Lett.* **2014**, *12*, 97–101. [CrossRef]
105. Masek, A.; Chrzescijanska, E.; Kosmalska, A.; Zaborski, M. Characteristics of compounds in hops using cyclic voltammetry, UV–VIS, FTIR and GC–MS analysis. *Food Chem.* **2014**, *156*, 353–361. [CrossRef] [PubMed]
106. Neugrodda, C.; Gastl, M.; Becker, T. Protein Profile Characterization of Hop (*Humulus lupulus* L.) Varieties. *J. Am. Soc. Brew. Chem.* **2014**, *72*, 184–191. [CrossRef]
107. Shellie, R.A.; Poynter, S.D.; Li, J.; Gathercole, J.L.; Koutoulus, A. Varietal characterisation of hop (*Humulus lupulus*) by GC–MS analysis of hop cone extracts. *J. Sep. Sci.* **2009**, *32*, 3720–3725. [CrossRef]
108. Ocvirk, M.; Grdadolnik, J.; Košir, I.J. Determination of the botanical origin of hops (*Humulus lupulus* L.) using different analytical techniques in combination with statistical methods. *J. Inst. Brew.* **2016**, *122*, 452–461. [CrossRef]
109. Lin, M.; Xiang, D.; Chen, X.; Huo, H. Role of Characteristic Components of *Humulus lupulus* in Promoting Human Health. *J. Agric. Food Chem.* **2019**, *67*, 8291–8302. [CrossRef] [PubMed]
110. Socrates, G. *Infrared and Raman Characteristic Group Frequencies: Tables and Charts*; John Wiley & Sons, Ltd.: Chichester, UK, 2001.
111. Javanbakht, T.; Laurent, S.; Stanicki, D.; Wilkinson, K.J. Relating the surface properties of superparamagnetic iron oxide nanoparticles (SPIONs) to their bactericidal effect towards a biofilm of Streptococcus mutans. *PLoS ONE* **2016**, *11*, e0154445. [CrossRef]
112. Mousavi, S.M.; Hashemi, S.A.; Zarei, M.; Bahrani, S.; Savardashtaki, A.; Esmaeili, H.; Lai, C.W.; Mazraedoost, S.; Abassi, M.; Ramavandi, B. Data on cytotoxic and antibacterial activity of synthesized Fe_3O_4 nanoparticles using Malva sylvestris. *Data Brief.* **2019**, *28*, 104929. [CrossRef] [PubMed]
113. Vikesland, P.J.; Rebodos, R.L.; Bottero, J.Y.; Rose, J.; Masion, A. Aggregation and sedimentation of magnetite nanoparticle clusters. *Environ. Sci. Nano* **2016**, *3*, 567–577. [CrossRef]
114. Gutiérrez, L.; de la Cueva, L.; Moros, M.; Mazarío, E.; de Bernardo, S.; de la Fuente, J.M.; Morales, M.P.; Salas, G. Aggregation effects on the magnetic properties of iron oxide colloids. *Nanotechnology* **2019**, *30*, 112001. [CrossRef]
115. Rubasinghege, G.; Lentz, R.W.; Park, H.; Scherer, M.M.; Grassian, V.H. Nanorod dissolution quenched in the aggregated state. *Langmuir* **2010**, *26*, 1524–1527. [CrossRef]
116. Vikesland, P.J.; Heathcock, A.M.; Rebodos, R.L.; Makus, K.E. Particle size and aggregation effects on magnetite reactivity toward carbon tetrachloride. *Environ. Sci. Technol.* **2007**, *41*, 5277–5283. [CrossRef] [PubMed]
117. Natarajan, S.; Harini, K.; Gajula, G.P.; Sarmento, B.; Neves-Petersen, M.T.; Thiagarajan, V. Multifunctional magnetic iron oxide nanoparticles: Diverse synthetic approaches, surface modifications, cytotoxicity towards biomedical and industrial applications. *BMC Mat.* **2019**, *1*, 2. [CrossRef]
118. Lawag, I.L.; Yoo, O.; Lim, L.Y.; Hammer, K.; Locher, C. Optimisation of Bee Pollen Extraction to Maximise Extractable Antioxidant Constituents. *Antioxidants* **2021**, *10*, 1113. [CrossRef] [PubMed]
119. Mannino, G.; Campobenedetto, C.; Vigliante, I.; Contartese, V.; Gentile, C.; Bertea, C.M. The application of a plant biostimulant based on seaweed and yeast extract improved tomato fruit development and quality. *Biomolecules* **2020**, *10*, 1662. [CrossRef]
120. Widelski, J.; Okińczyc, P.; Paluch, E.; Mroczek, T.; Szperlik, J.; Żuk, M.; Sroka, Z.; Sakipova, Z.; Chinou, I.; Skalicka-Woźniak, K.; et al. The Antimicrobial Properties of Poplar and Aspen–Poplar Propolises and Their Active Components against Selected Microorganisms, including Helicobacter pylori. *Pathogens* **2022**, *11*, 191. [CrossRef]

Disclaimer/Publisher's Note: The statements, opinions and data contained in all publications are solely those of the individual author(s) and contributor(s) and not of MDPI and/or the editor(s). MDPI and/or the editor(s) disclaim responsibility for any injury to people or property resulting from any ideas, methods, instructions or products referred to in the content.

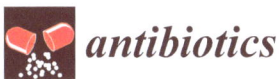

Review

From Polymeric Nanoformulations to Polyphenols—Strategies for Enhancing the Efficacy and Drug Delivery of Gentamicin

Ance Bārzdiņa [1,2,*], Aiva Plotniece [1,3], Arkadij Sobolev [3], Karlis Pajuste [3], Dace Bandere [1,2] and Agnese Brangule [1,2]

[1] Department of Pharmaceutical Chemistry, Riga Stradins University, 21 Konsula Str., LV-1007 Riga, Latvia; aiva@osi.lv (A.P.)

[2] Baltic Biomaterials Centre of Excellence, Headquarters at Riga Technical University, LV-1007 Riga, Latvia

[3] Latvian Institute of Organic Synthesis, 21 Aizkraukles Str., LV-1006 Riga, Latvia; arkady@osi.lv (A.S.); kpajuste@osi.lv (K.P.)

* Correspondence: ance.barzdina@rsu.lv

Abstract: Gentamicin is an essential broad-spectrum aminoglycoside antibiotic that is used in over 40 clinical conditions and has shown activity against a wide range of nosocomial, biofilm-forming, multi-drug resistant bacteria. Nevertheless, the low cellular penetration and serious side effects of gentamicin, as well as the fear of the development of antibacterial resistance, has led to a search for ways to circumvent these obstacles. This review provides an overview of the chemical and pharmacological properties of gentamicin and offers six different strategies (the isolation of specific types of gentamicin, encapsulation in polymeric nanoparticles, hydrophobization of the gentamicin molecule, and combinations of gentamicin with other antibiotics, polyphenols, and natural products) that aim to enhance the drug delivery and antibacterial activity of gentamicin. In addition, factors influencing the synthesis of gentamicin-loaded polymeric (poly (lactic-co-glycolic acid) (PLGA) and chitosan) nanoparticles and the methods used in drug release studies are discussed. Potential research directions and future perspectives for gentamicin-loaded drug delivery systems are given.

Keywords: gentamicin; antibacterial activity; drug delivery; nanoparticles; polyphenols; natural products; synergy

1. Introduction

Due to the alarming rate of increase in antibacterial resistance, common broad-spectrum antibiotics often fail to treat infections. More and more often opportunistic and nosocomial pathogens, especially bacterial strains with a tendency to form biofilms, like *Pseudomonas aeruginosa*, are the cause of high-morbidity and high-mortality infections that require high-dosage and longer antibacterial treatments [1–3]. This again leads to increased antibacterial resistance, creating a vicious cycle. The majority of nosocomial infections are caused by six multidrug-resistant bacteria (*Enterococcus faecium*, *Staphylococcus aureus*, *Klebsiella pneumoniae*, *Acinetobacter baumannii*, *Pseudomonas aeruginosa*, and *Enterobacter* species). This group of bacteria is commonly referred to as ESKAPE pathogens [4]. All of these bacteria can also be found on the World Health Organization's (WHO) priority list for research on and the development of new antibiotics for antibiotic-resistant bacteria at either critical or high-priority levels [5]. As there has been a serious shortage of new antimicrobials entering the market in recent years, a search for ways to enhance the efficacy and drug delivery of already known and widely used antibacterial agents like gentamicin is essential.

Gentamicin is a broad-spectrum, bactericidal, aminoglycoside antibiotic. It is effective against a wide range of aerobic Gram-negative bacteria, as well as Gram-positive *Staphylococcus* species [6]. Of special importance is its potential activity against ESKAPE pathogens. Although it was discovered in the early 1960s [7], gentamicin still is a part of the essential medicines list of the World Health Organization [8]. Because of its wide activity spectrum, gentamicin is used to treat over 40 different clinical conditions, including bacterial sepsis, peritonitis, meningitis, the urinary tract and respiratory tract, eye, ear, bone, and surgical site infections, and others, proving its important role in modern medicine [6,8–10]. Figure 1 summarizes United States (US) Food and Drug Administration (FDA) approved, prevalent indications treated with gentamicin.

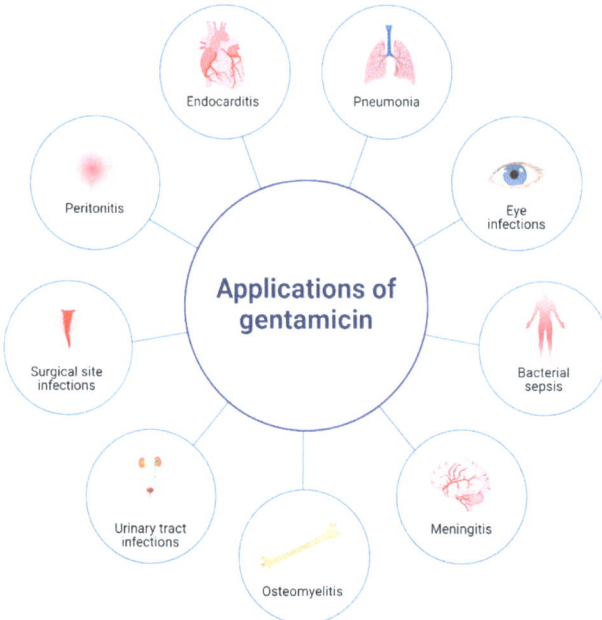

Figure 1. Applications of gentamicin. Created with BioRender.com (accessed on 29 February 2024).

Gentamicin represents class III of the Biopharmaceutical Classification System due to its high solubility in water and low cellular penetration [11]. Consequently, drug delivery of this active agent alone may be hindered. As gentamicin is used to fight serious infections, often caused by multi-drug-resistant pathogens, ways to lower the needed concentration of gentamicin and ultimately minimize the chance of the development of resistance against it are one of the top priorities.

Therefore, this review paper provides an overview of the chemical and pharmacological properties of gentamicin and offers six different strategies (the isolation of specific types of gentamicin, encapsulation in polymeric nanoformulations, hydrophobization of the gentamicin molecule, and combinations of gentamicin with other antibiotics, polyphenols, and natural products) that aim to enhance the drug delivery and antibacterial activity of gentamicin.

2. The Components and Properties of Gentamicin Complex

Gentamicin is produced by the *Micromonospora* species of bacteria, as a mixture of multiple components, but mainly consists of five structurally different C-subtypes (C1, C1a, C2, C2a, and C2b) with structural modifications at position $6'$ of moiety I (Figure 2A) [12]. The structural differences in the major components are related by the level of methylation—a methyl or hydrogen substitution in two R groups on the 2-amino-hexose residue (I). In gentamicin C1a, methyl groups are missing, whereas both in C1 and C2, a methyl group is present at the $6'$ position; gentamicin C1 is N-methylated at this position, while C1a and C2 have free amines. The C2 component consists of two stereoisomers [13]. The ratio of the gentamicin components varies depending on the drug's manufacturing method, the fermentation conditions, and the purification procedure [14,15].

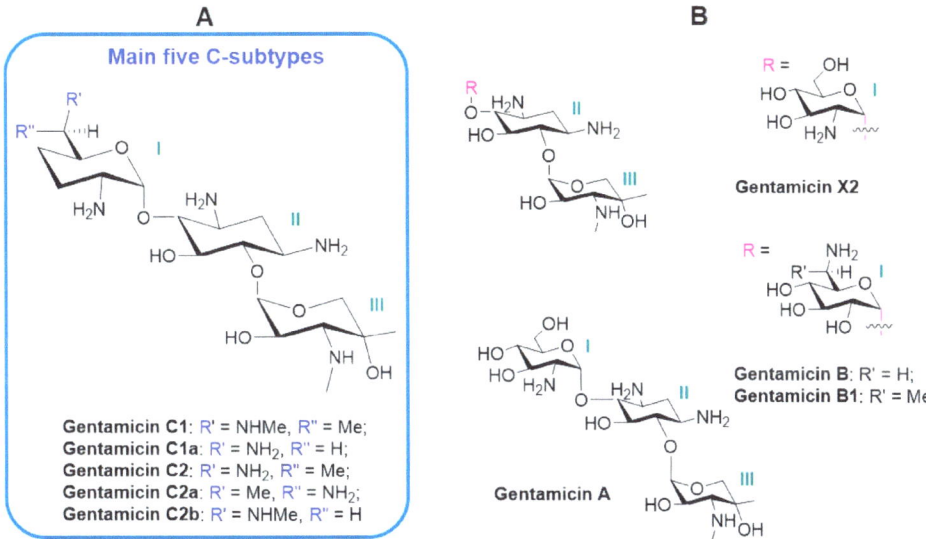

Figure 2. Structures of Gentamicin derivatives: (**A**): main C-subtypes; (**B**): minor components.

The major components constitute 92–99% of the gentamicin complex. Other gentamicin derivatives (Figure 2B), as the minor components, are found in the range between 0.8 and 5.3% [15,16].

According to the European Medicine Agency (EMA), the gentamicin composition consists of 10–30% C1a, 25–45% C1, and 35–55% C2, C2a, and C2b [17,18]. The ratio of gentamicin components has been studied using several methods based on paired-ion, high-performance liquid chromatography (HPLC) [19,20] and coupled liquid chromatography–NMR to compare the composition of different batches from various sources [15].

The clinical mechanism of action of the mixture is unclear; it is unknown whether the broad spectrum of antimicrobial action is due to multiple components. In other terms, it is unclear whether each component works across a narrower range of bacterial strains or species than the entire mixture [21]. Numerous research groups worldwide are working on the characterization of the structure–activity relationships of gentamicin components, studying the activity of the difficult-to-separate components of the commercial gentamicin samples, and characterizing specially prepared single components [21,22]. The relative toxicity and activity of the individual components in the commercial gentamicin samples have been studied since the 1970s [16,17]. These studies suggest that gentamicin C2 is less nephrotoxic than the other gentamicin constituents [23]; gentamicin C1 and C1a are less ototoxic than C2 [24]. In more recent studies evaluating the ototoxicity, it was indicated that gentamicin C1a was less ototoxic than a commercial gentamicin mixture. The minimum inhibitory concentration (MIC_{50} and MIC_{90}) values of both the gentamicin complex and gentamicin C1a against clinical isolates of five bacterial species from *E. coli*, *K. pheumoniae*, *A. baumannii*, *P. aeruginosa*, and *S. aureus* were comparable; however, a two-fold increase in MIC_{50} was observed for the gentamicin C1a isomer compared to the gentamicin complex. However, these two compounds showed rather different in vitro activities against a larger portion of 61 isolates from *E. coli*, *K. pheumoniae*, *A. baumannii*, *P. aeruginosa*, and *S. aureus* [25].

Further research on the activity–toxicity relationship of the gentamicin components is necessary to draw concrete conclusions regarding the potential gains of isolating and applying individual gentamicin subtypes.

3. Pharmacology, Stability, and Administration of Gentamicin

Gentamicin belongs to the 4,6-disubstituted-2-deoxystreptamine class of aminoglycosides [26]. Clinically, gentamicin has been used as a sulfate salt. It contains five basic nitrogens and requires five sulfuric acid equivalents per mole of every gentamicin base [27].

The mechanism of action prevents the synthesis of bacterial proteins through electrostatic binding with negatively charged phospholipids' head groups. Afterwards, the antibiotic binds to the specific ribosomal proteins, resulting in the formation of inactive complexes that cause misreadings in mRNA [28,29]. Gentamicin is a cationic antibiotic with a narrow therapeutic index [30,31]. Its antibacterial activity can be influenced by the pH. A low pH is associated with a decrease in activity [30]. The pharmacological action of gentamicin is concentration-dependent [6].

The pharmacokinetics of gentamicin are comparable to those of other aminoglycosides. Gentamicin is a polar molecule and is poorly absorbed when taken orally (less than 1%); therefore, systemic use requires parenteral administration [31–33]. In certain infections, topical and local administration is needed [34]. The local delivery of antibiotics might reduce potential toxic side effects and be of particular use in infections that require the long-term, sustained release of antibiotics, like osteomyelitis [35].

It has been suggested that the standard intravenous gentamicin starting dose of 7 mg/kg based on total body weight appears to optimize the chance of reaching the exposure target after the first administration in both adults and children older than 1 month, including critically ill patients. However, despite numerous recent population pharmacokinetic studies, the optimal pharmacokinetic–pharmacodynamic target for efficacy is still unclear [36]. If patients suffer from renal failure, the dosage of gentamicin needs to be lowered [37].

Gentamicin binds to serum proteins very poorly; in most cases, the binding to serum proteins is under 15% [38]. In the cerebrospinal fluid of patients with uninflamed meninges, it is found in very low concentrations [37]. Gentamicin does not easily penetrate cells; instead, it is mostly distributed in the extracellular fluid [33]. Pinocytosis is the main mechanism of free gentamicin uptake [39]. Gentamicin does not undergo metabolism in the body, and, through glomerular filtration, unchanged gentamicin is quickly eliminated [33,40]. Since gentamicin has a short plasma half-life of around 2 h, frequent administration is needed [31]. The biodistribution of gentamicin causes its most common side effects—nephrotoxicity and ototoxicity [41,42]. The half-life in the renal cortex is estimated to be around 100 h [43]. The pharmacokinetics of gentamicin are dependent on the overall health status of the patient. Altered pharmacokinetic parameters like the volume of distribution, peak concentrations, and renal clearance are affected by conditions like sepsis, heart failure, peritonitis, and renal impairment [33,44].

Gentamicin sulfate sterile solutions should be kept between 2 and 8 °C. Gentamicin solutions have proven to be stable when kept at room temperature and in boiling aqueous buffers with pH values ranging from 2 to 14 [27,45]. Recommendations under the auspices of the International Society for Peritoneal Dialysis (ISPD) underlined that gentamicin is stable for 14 days at all temperatures [46]. A protocol used for microbe–epithelium cocultures states that gentamicin is stable at 4 °C for 1 month [47]. The good stability of gentamicin over a wide range of storage conditions makes it a promising candidate for encapsulation in novel drug delivery systems like nanoparticles.

4. Polymeric Nanoformulations of Gentamicin

In the last two decades, nanoformulations have emerged as one of the frontrunners for the encapsulation and delivery of a wide range of active agents, including antibiotics. Nanoformulations for enhanced drug delivery have provided formulation scientists with the opportunity to achieve a higher bioavailability and biocompatibility, a controlled release, and increased target selectivity [48]. Although the use of nanoformulations in terms of their toxicity and distribution in the body is still under investigation, the potential gains of this approach drive further research in this field [14].

In the case of antibiotics, the main hope for the use of nanoformulations is that they will lower the chance of the development of antimicrobial resistance and achieve the targeted delivery of antibiotics with the lowest effective dose to avoid unwanted side effects for the patient [49,50]. For more than two decades, various lipids, polymers, and other materials have been applied to create micro- and nanoformulations, including nanoparticles, nanofibers, nanocomposites, and others, for the delivery of a wide range of antibiotics [50]. Gentamicin is no exception. In addition to polymeric nanoformulations, gentamicin has been successfully encapsulated into liposomes [51–53] and mesoporous silica nanoparticles [54–56], as well as being tested for synergic effects in combination with metallic nanoparticles [57–59]. A detailed overview of all nanoformulation types for the delivery of gentamicin has been thoroughly evaluated in a recent review paper by Athauda et al. [14]. The use of lipid-based nanoparticles for the delivery of antibiotics and the treatment of infections has already been reviewed in detail by Ferreira et al. [60,61]. Therefore, this review will only focus on recent advances in polymeric formulations, in particular, poly (lactic-co-glycolic acid) (PLGA) and chitosan-based systems, their potential applications, and the main variables impacting the systems and their kinetics. The sustained release properties of gentamicin-loaded nanoformulations and the possibility of enhancing the bioavailability of gentamicin are of particular importance; therefore, these topics will be discussed in detail in further subsections.

4.1. Gentamicin-Loaded PLGA Nanoparticles

PLGA is a polyester copolymer composed of lactic acid (PLA) and glycolic acid (PGA) in varying ratios. It is biodegradable, biocompatible, non-toxic, approved for parenteral use by both FDA and EMA, and allows for a wide range of surface modifications [62]. An overview of gentamicin-loaded PLGA nanoparticles and their main parameters can be found in Table 1.

Table 1. Gentamicin-loaded PLGA nanoparticles.

PLGA Type	Surfactant	Formulation Method	Size (nm)	PDI	Zeta Potential (mV)	Particle Characterization Methods	EE (%)	Drug Loading	Drug Release (In Vitro)	Bacteria (In Vitro Tests)	Potential Application	Ref.
50:50 (13.7 kDa)	PVA (15 kDa)	w/o/w solvent evaporation	320	NA	−15.5 ± 0.2	DLS ELS SEM XRD DSC	13.12–58.76	3.24–7.35 #	28 days	NT	Intracellular pathogens	[63]
50:50 (13.7 kDa)	PVA (15 kDa)	w/o/w solvent evaporation	310 ± 2.00	NA	NT	DLS	NT	6.2 *	NT	NT	Intracellular pathogens	[64]
50:50 (12 kDa)	PVA	w/o/w s/o/w solvent evaporation	241.3–358.5	0.10–0.23	−0.4–2.3	DLS ELS	NT	6.4–22.4 *	Over 16 days	P. aeruginosa	Planktonic- and biofilm-based infections	[65]
85:15 (80 kDa)	PVA (31 kDa)	w/o/w solvent evaporation	219–391	0.21–0.38	−7.2–−1.1	DLS ELS AFM	2.7–52.4	0.06–10.28%	35 days	S. aureus S. epidermidis	Osteomyelitis	[66]
50:50 (7–17 kDa)	PVA (85–124 kDa)	w/o/w solvent evaporation	280 ± 12.04	0.15 ± 0.01	−4.9 ± 0.84	DLS ELS SEM TEM	NT	60%	216 h	P. aeruginosa S. aureus	Surgical site infections	[67]
50:50 (7–17 kDa)	PVA	w/o/w solvent evaporation	227	0.162	−1.67	DLS ELS SEM	NT	135 *	120 h	K. pneumoniae	Intracellular pathogens	[68]
PLGA-PEG (70 kDa)	PVA (85–124 kDa)	s/o/w solvent evaporation	140.0–919.3	0.104–1.230	−5.54–0.36	DLS ELS TEM	43.97–64.61	2.9–7.9%	10 h	P. mirabilis E. coli P. aeruginosa S. aureus	Intracellular pathogens	[11]
75:25 (4–15 kDa)	PVA (89–98 kDa)	w/o/w solvent evaporation	32–2400	NA	NT	DLS SEM	NT	NT	10 h	E. coli	Wound treatment	[69]

#—μg gentamicin/mg particles; *—μg gentamicin/mg polymer; NA—not available; NT—not tested; PVA—poly (vinyl alcohol); PDI—polydispersity index; DLS—dynamic light scattering; ELS—electrophoretic light scattering; AFM—atomic force microscopy; TEM—transmission electron microscopy; SEM—scanning electron microscopy; DSC—differential scanning calorimetry; XRD—X-ray diffraction analysis.

Since gentamicin is highly hydrophilic, its penetration into cells might be hindered and the clearance of the drug is fast [11,31]. Hence, higher doses should be administered more frequently. In the case of gentamicin, the chance of developing side effects increases accordingly [31]. Low cellular penetration is especially associated with intracellular infections [64]. The encapsulation of gentamicin in polymeric nanoparticles like PLGA and chitosan could offer a solution to the problems caused by the high water-solubility of gentamicin. Drug-loaded nanoparticles have an improved bioavailability and permanence time at the site of infection, in addition to offering a sustained release and protection of premature degradation [11]. Polymers offer a wide variability of parameters, like molecular weight and the ratio between monomers, which can be applied to develop nanoformulations with optimal drug release properties.

In comparison to other polymers, like chitosan and alginate, PLGA nanoparticles can have controlled release properties without a chemical modification [67]. The sustained release of gentamicin from PLGA nanoparticles may be the most important advantage compared to using a free drug. The ratio between PLA and PGA is crucial to the hydrophobicity of the formulation [70]. A higher lactic acid content increases the hydrophobicity of the system and prolongs the release of drugs [64,70]. In addition, a sustained release of the drug can also be achieved by using a polymer with a higher molecular weight [71]. In case of chronic, long-lasting infections, a sustained release will determine the efficacy of the therapy. To date, PLGA 50:50 is the most commonly used PLA:PGA ratio in nanoformulations due to its favorable physiochemical properties and release kinetics [72].

The small molecular weight and the high water-solubility of gentamicin make it challenging to encapsulate it into nanocarriers [11]. One key advantage of using PLGA as a nanocarrier is its ability to encapsulate both hydrophobic and hydrophilic substances. However, different formulation methods need to be applied. For a hydrophilic drug (like gentamicin) encapsulation, multiple emulsions are needed so that the aqueous core containing the drug is coated by a polymer shell [65]. Therefore, the majority of published methods use the double emulsion w/o/w solvent evaporation method, with only a few authors reporting on the use of the s/o/w method [11,65]. A schematic illustration of the solvent evaporation method can be found in Figure 3.

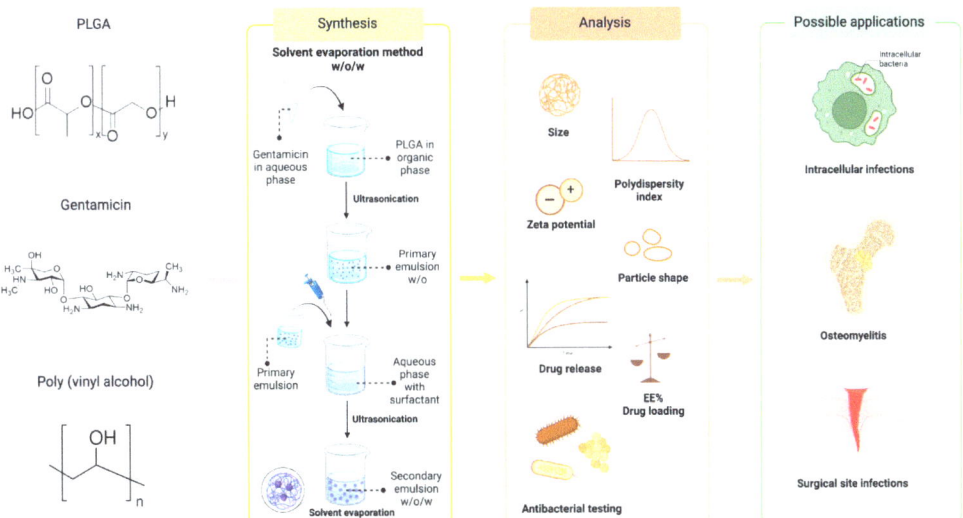

Figure 3. Synthesis, common characterization methods, and possible applications of gentamicin-loaded PLGA nanoparticles. Created with BioRender.com (accessed on 21 March 2024).

Cao et al. provide an in-depth overview of the influence of various parameters in the w/o/w method on the morphology and physiochemical properties of PLGA particles [73]. In short, the study determined that PLGA concentration and the colostrum emulsification speed are the most influential factors impacting the size of the particles. Lower PLGA concentration levels (10–20 mg/mL) produce particles with a narrow size distribution; however, the shape of the nanoparticles can be rather uneven. A higher PLGA concentration (30–40 mg/mL) allows for the formation of particles with round shapes, although the size distribution of the particles in this case is significantly larger. Up to a certain concentration, an increase in the PLGA concentration increases the drug loading. A higher polymer concentration leads to a higher viscosity and the particles solidify faster. As a consequence, less of the drug can escape from the particles, and the encapsulation efficiency (EE%) and drug loading (DL%) increase [73]. Regarding DL%, the second emulsification step is just as important. Higher emulsification speeds lead to the increased volatilization of solvents like DCM or chloroform, restricting the escape of drugs from particles [73].

Another factor significantly impacting the performance of the formulation method is the pH of the external aqueous phase. Increasing the pH of the external aqueous phase from 5 to 7.4 can increase the EE% up to three times [65]. This phenomenon is based on the deprotonation of the amino groups in the gentamicin molecule, making the molecule less hydrophilic [65].

Poly (vinyl alcohol) (PVA) is the most commonly used surfactant in PLGA-gentamicin nanoformulations. With increasing concentrations of PVA, it is possible to decrease the particle size as well as the polydispersity index (PDI) [66]. A study by Sun et al. suggests that a higher concentration of PVA (9%, 12%) is associated with a more uniform, spherical particle shape [69]. In addition, the hydrophilic nature of PVA could be responsible for the porous surface structures of nanoparticles due to the diffusion processes [69]. The pore size decreases with a higher PLGA concentration [69].

It has been determined that the size of nanoparticles will heavily impact their fate in biological systems. Nanocarriers under 100 nm are prone to endocytosis, while carriers larger than 500 nm will face phagocytosis [74]. The endocytosis of nanoparticles could be more efficient than the pinocytosis of free gentamicin, leading to an increase in the efficiency of the therapy [75]. In practice, most gentamicin-loaded PLGA nanoparticles range between 200 nm and 400 nm (see Table 1). PLGA nanoparticles are internalized using both pinocytosis- and clathrin-mediated endocytosis [76]. After internalization, the PLGA nanoparticles escape the lysosomes and enter the cytoplasm approximately 10 min after incubation [77,78]. It has been suggested that the naturally negative/anionic surface charge of PLGA nanoparticles (due to the carboxylic acid end groups) reverses to cationic with the low pH of endo-lysosomes (pH $\approx$ 4) [78]. The surface cationization allows for nanoparticles to escape into the cytosol, where the encapsulated drug is released [78]. Moreover, the sustained release of the drug is achievable intracellularly. Since the PLGA nanoparticles are only cationic in the endosomal compartment, and therefore do not cause lysosomal destruction, they could be less toxic in comparison to cationic lipids and cationic polymers [78].

The disadvantages of unmodified PLGA use are the lack of specific targeting properties and response to environmental stimuli, as well as vulnerability to aggregates during freeze-drying [79].

Since, without surface modifications, PLGA has no active targeting properties, it has to rely on passive targeting after intravenous administration. Passive targeting will be more effective against conditions that exhibit enhanced permeability and retention effects, such as cancers and inflammatory processes [80]. If no surface modifications to PLGA nanocarriers are applied, opsonization by macrophages usually occurs at high rates [65]. Due to the previously mentioned reasons and the chance of the development of antibacterial resistance, nanoformulations with gentamicin are most often applied for topical or local delivery.

However, in the case of systemic application, it is possible to apply surface modifications to PLGA to avoid clearance by phagocytes, limit opsonization, and prolong circulation time. The surface of PLGA is most often modified using polyethylene glycol (PEG), different lipids, and target-specific agents, like antibodies and bisphosphonates [81]. To the best of our knowledge, only one publication to date has explored the use of PLGA-PEG for the encapsulation of gentamicin [11].

Three main targets for PLGA–gentamicin nanoparticles can be differentiated—surgical site infections, osteomyelitis, and intracellular infections.

In the case of osteomyelitis, poor vascularization around bone tissues makes drug delivery to the site of infection very difficult [82]. For both surgical site infections and osteomyelitis, which are commonly caused by *Staphylococcus aureus, Pseudomonas aeruginosa*, and *Escherichia coli*, as well as more resistant strains like *Methicillin-resistant Staphylococcus aureus*, up to 6 weeks of the sustained delivery of gentamicin might be needed to eliminate the infections and their biofilms [66,83,84]. Although non-biodegradable bone cements, like poly (methyl methacrylate) (PMMA), possess several advantages for osteomyelitis treatment, the need for a second surgical intervention to remove them hinders their wider use [85,86]. Biodegradable PLGA-based nanocarrier administration via injection at the site of infection is a great alternative [66].

Another group of infections targeted by gentamicin-loaded PLGA nanoparticles are intracellular infections. Intracellular infections act as a reservoir of bacteria and lead to chronic conditions that can also be lethal. Targeting intracellular infections is much harder due to the poor cellular penetration of gentamicin [64,68]. To overcome this challenge, it is possible to turn to nanoformulations, which, in general, are often taken up by macrophages via phagocytosis. This strategy allows for the passive targeting of intracellular infections and enhances the efficacy of the therapy [68]. To date, gentamicin-loaded PLGA nanoparticles have been effectively explored against two intracellular infections—*Klebsiella pneumoniae* and *Brucella melitensis* [64,68]. Not only can gentamicin-loaded PLGA nanoparticles be taken up by infected macrophages, but they also reduce bacterial viability without inducing an inflammatory or apoptotic response on the macrophages [68].

The current evidence of the antibacterial effectiveness of PLGA nanoparticles loaded with gentamicin compared to the use of a free drug is mixed. Empty PLGA nanoparticles do not possess antibacterial properties; therefore, their effect is dependent on the drug content and the drug release mechanisms [65,69]. Some in vitro tests against *P. aeruginosa*, *S. aureus*, and *E. coli* have shown that the MIC and MBC levels of nanoparticles compared to a free drug are equal or one dilution higher [11,65]. Lower effective concentrations of nanoparticles compared to the free drug have been reported against *S. aureus* [11,67]. However, when Jiang et al. tested the use of gentamicin-loaded nanoparticles against *K. pneumoniae* in vitro, the MIC and MBC values for the nanoparticles were significantly higher than those of a free drug [68]. The MIC/MBC values of nanoparticles lowered when tested after a longer period (up to 120 h), while, for the free gentamicin, the values stayed the same. This observation suggests that simple in vitro antibacterial tests might not be suitable for testing nanoparticles with sustained release. Instead, nanoformulations should be tested in more complex physiological environments in vivo for a longer period of time. It was further proven in vivo that gentamicin-loaded nanoparticles were more effective, providing longer protective effects against the infection than the free form of the drug due to the sustained release of the gentamicin from nanoparticles [68]. An increased effectiveness in vivo was also observed with *P. aeruginosa* infection [65]. In addition, in terms of antibiofilm activity, the sustained release of gentamicin proves an advantage over a single dose of free gentamicin [65].

To alleviate the application of prepared nanoparticles and to further modify the release profile of the drugs, it is possible to incorporate the nanoparticles in various other drug delivery forms. For local application, gentamicin-loaded PLGA nanoparticles have been incorporated into transdermal patches and pullulan films [67,87,88].

In sum, the main advantages provided by PLGA nanoparticles are the sustained release of gentamicin for up to 35 days and an enhanced possibility of targeting intracellular infections and infections needing long-term treatment, leading to an increase in their bioavailability. The challenges regarding PLGA–gentamicin nanoparticles are that they require further process optimization to obtain reproducible results, in addition to a quite limited EE%. More studies on the antibacterial efficiency of these nanoparticles using in vivo tests are needed. Gentamicin-loaded PLGA nanoparticles with various surface modifications are an underexplored research field, with future potential for more targeted treatments of infections.

4.2. Gentamicin-Loaded Chitosan Nanoparticles

Chitosan is a natural, linear polysaccharide with wide use in the biomedical industry due to its physiochemical properties, biocompatibility, biodegradability, and antibacterial and antifungal activity [89,90]. It is composed of β-1,4 glucose amine and β-1,4-N-acetyl glucose amine units [91]. The antimicrobial properties of chitosan are explained by the electrostatic interaction between the positive charge of chitosan and the negatively charged bacterial cell walls [92,93]. Without the polycationic nature, the antibacterial properties of chitosan are reduced [93]. In addition, other factors, like molecular weight, positive charge density, and pH, can influence the antibacterial properties of chitosan [93,94]. The antimicrobial properties of chitosan make it a desirable polymer for nanoparticle formation and the encapsulation of antibiotics. Gentamicin-loaded chitosan nanoparticles have largely been explored only in the last 5 years. An overview of gentamicin-loaded chitosan nanoparticles and their main parameters can be found in Table 2.

Table 2. Gentamicin-loaded chitosan nanoparticles.

Chitosan Type	Crosslinker	Drugs	Formulation Method	Size (nm)	PDI	Zeta Potential (mV)	Particle Characterization Methods	EE (%)	Drug Loading (%)	Bacteria (In Vitro Tests)	Potential Application	Ref.
150 kDa, deacetylation degree 85.6%	TPP	Gentamicin	Ionic gelation	779.37 ± 51.79	NT	1.9 ± 0.5	DLS ELS	78.06 ± 2.13	63.10 ± 1.54	NT	Intracellular pathogens	[95]
80 kDa, deacetylation degree 95%	TPP	Gentamicin + salicylic acid	Ionic gelation	148–345	0.234–0.428	32.45–42.43	DLS ELS TEM SEM FTIR XRD	61.70–87.20	13.56–26.64	NT	Reduction in toxicity	[96]
140 kDa, deacetylation degree 85%	TPP	Gentamicin	Ionic gelation	100	NT	28	DLS ELS SEM	72	22	B. abortus B. melitensis	Intracellular pathogens	[75]
304 kDa, deacetylation degree >84%	-	Gentamicin + proanthocyanidin	Hydrogen bonding	242.9–277.4	0.344–0.391	34.5–38.5	DLS ELS SEM FTIR TGA	94	NT	E. coli S. aureus P. aeruginosa	Enhanced antimicrobial activity	[97]
Low molecular weight, deacetylation ≥ 75%	TPP	Gentamicin	Ionic gelation	151–212	0.21–0.29	37.2–51.1	DLS ELS TEM SEM DSC	36.6–42.7	NT	NT	Wound healing	[98]
NA	TPP	Gentamicin + ascorbic acid	Ionic gelation	278	NT	30.01	DLS ELS TEM FTIR	89	22	S. aureus P. aeruginosa	Reduction in toxicity	[99]

NA—not available; NT—not tested; TPP—sodium tripolyphosphate; DLS—dynamic light scattering; ELS—electrophoretic light scattering; TEM—transmission electron microscopy; SEM—scanning electron microscopy; TGA—thermogravimetric analysis; DSC—differential scanning calorimetry; FTIR—Fourier-transform infrared spectroscopy; XRD—X-ray diffraction analysis.

Both physical and chemical crosslinking can be applied to form chitosan nanoparticles [100]. The ionic gelation method, which is a type of physical crosslinking, has been most widely used to form gentamicin-loaded nanoparticles due to the simplicity and mild conditions of the method [96,99]. Sodium tripolyphosphate (TPP), in most cases, is used as a cross-linker. TPP is a non-toxic agent with negatively charged phosphate groups; therefore, it can react with the positively charged amino groups of chitosan, leading to gelling [101,102].

The cellular uptake of chitosan nanoparticles is dependent on their attachment to the negatively charged cell membranes due to electrostatic interactions. The chitosan nanoparticles are then transported via endocytosis, with subsequent release in subcellular compartments like lysosomes [103]. The "proton sponge effect" promotes chitosan nanoparticle escape from endosomes, meaning that the amino groups are more protonated in the acidic pH of endosomes. Subsequently, water and chloride ions enter the endosomes to balance out the osmotic imbalance. The volume increase ruptures the endosomes, allowing the nanoparticles to enter cytoplasm [104]. The same mechanism is also responsible for lysosome rupture [103]. In terms of their possible application, the use of gentamicin-loaded chitosan nanoparticles against intracellular bacteria and biofilms has been examined, as well as explored their potential as wound healing agents [75,95,98,105].

Regarding their antibacterial activity, gentamicin-loaded chitosan nanoparticles have shown promising results. Gentamicin-loaded chitosan nanoparticles have shown equal or better antibacterial properties compared to gentamicin in a free drug form [75,97,99,105]. The authors suggest that the higher antibacterial efficiency is observed due to the sustained release of gentamicin [75]. When tested in combination with other agents, like ascorbic acid, the dual-therapy chitosan particles show enhanced antibacterial activity and possible synergy between the components [99].

A disadvantage of using chitosan to encapsulate gentamicin is the positive charge of both molecules, which leads to electrostatic repulsion and, therefore, lower drug loading [95]. In addition, gentamicin release from the nanoparticles is rather short in comparison to that of gentamicin-loaded PLGA nanoparticles, with authors reporting drug release lasting up to 1 week and, in most cases, only around 3 days [75,95–97,99,105]. The release profile of chitosan nanoparticles could prohibit their potential use in hard-to-combat infections that require several weeks of treatment.

In recent years, novel publications can be found on chitosan nanoparticles that combine gentamicin with other active agents, like ascorbic acid, salicylic acid, and proanthocyanidin, to minimize the side effects of gentamicin and enhance the antibacterial activity, with promising results [96,97,99]. As strong antioxidants, these molecules could minimize the toxicity to cells created by reactive oxygen species (ROS) [99].

To further maximize the advantages of both polymeric and lipid drug delivery systems, combined hybrid nanoparticles are currently being researched. In the case of chitosan, Qiu et al. developed novel phosphatidylcholine–chitosan nanoparticles and coated the particles with gentamicin to enhance the drug delivery to biofilms and intracellular pathogens, with promising results [105].

4.3. The Release of Gentamicin from Polymeric Nanoparticles

The in vitro release study is crucial in evaluating drug delivery systems' safety, effectiveness, and quality when utilizing nanoparticles. However, despite its importance, no universally recognized standards or regulations currently govern this type of testing [106,107].

Various mechanisms are employed to assess the release of drugs from nanoparticles depending on the drug's physical and chemical properties and the matrix. These mechanisms include diffusion, erosion, swelling, and osmosis [108–112]. The effectiveness of drug release from biodegradable polymeric microspheres is determined by various factors, including drug loading efficiency, solubility, biodegradability, diffusion, and microsphere size [113].

As highlighted by the literature, gentamicin release studies involving the quantification of gentamicin face several challenges. Firstly, gentamicin is a complex mixture of five structurally distinct components (see Section 2). Secondly, gentamicin lacks chromophore groups, which means that it cannot absorb UV light and can be indirectly determined through chemical derivatization methods with o-phthaldialdehyde, phenyl isocyanate, 9-fluorenylmethyl chloroformate, 1-fluoro-2,4-dinitrobenzene, and others, which are time-consuming and produce unstable derivatives [114,115]. Most of the literature on gentamicin release from PLGA and chitosan mentions derivatization with o-phthaldialdehyde or ninhydrin [11,30,63,65–67]. The obtained fluorescent product can be determined through multiple methods. One of the most popular is the more rapid and cost-effective UV/VIS method. Alternatively, the most reliable method is high-performance liquid chromatography (HPLC), which enables UV, fluorescence, electrochemical, or MS detection [114,115].

The drug release profiles of nanoparticle-based formulations can be obtained through three methods: dialysis membrane, sample and separate methods, and the continuous-flow method [106,116,117]. For gentamicin-loaded PLGA and chitosan nanoparticles, the most commonly used methods are the first two.

One of the major challenges in comparing research findings in the field of gentamicin release is the absence of standardization in experimental methods. This leads to variations in the type of membranes used, stirring speed (50–200 rpm), medium (NaCl or PBS with pH 6.4–7.4), temperature (37 °C or 32 °C), and volume (500–900 mL) [11,30,63,65–67,69]. Even when the same techniques, such as UV/VIS, are employed, different wavelengths are often used to detect fluorescence or absorbance [11,30,69]. Fluorescence has been measured at 360/460 nm [63,65,68]. UV absorbance has been detected at 332 nm [66], 334 nm [75], 335 nm [67], and 400 nm [11]. Due to the variability in drug release profiles (Higuchi, first or zero order), it can be challenging to compare the published results and draw meaningful conclusions. This can lead to different interpretations of the drug release times and concentrations [69,113,118].

5. Hydrophobization of the Gentamicin Molecule

To increase the efficacy of antimicrobial drug activity against various infectious diseases, it is necessary to increase antimicrobial activity in the intracellular environment or prolong the presence of the antibiotic to produce a therapeutic effect. Gentamicin sulfate is a polar antimicrobial drug and, due to its hydrophilic nature, penetration into infected cells is limited. Moreover, as gentamicin shows a concentration-dependent bactericidal activity and post-antibiotic effect, it requires regular and high doses, which lead to increases in side effects [31]. Nanotechnology has developed a promising approach for the treatment of intracellular infections by providing the intracellular targeting and sustained release of encapsulated drugs inside the infected cells [119]. Initially, hydrophilic gentamicin sulfate was encapsulated in PLGA particles, and its encapsulation efficiency was achieved at 19.2% at 9.2 µg/mg of the polymer. However, drug release tests revealed that most of the gentamicin was released within the first hour. This can be explained by the possible absorption of gentamicin on the surface of PLGA particles [63]. Therefore, a highly efficient drug encapsulation strategy is required. The hydrophobic ion pairing of gentamicin with anionic surfactants without losing antimicrobial activity serves well for this purpose [120]. This method is well known to convert polar drugs into non-polar complexes and improve their encapsulation efficiency. For this purpose, active substances such as docusate sodium salt (AOT), sodium dodecyl sulfate, sodium oleate, and sodium deoxycholate sulfate are used [121]. Docusate sodium salt is one of the most promising anionic surfactants for gentamicin. The chemical structure of gentamicin and AOT are presented in Figure 4.

The ionic complex of the Gent–AOT ratio is 1:5, and the stoichiometric complexation of the five ionizable amino groups of gentamicin is neutralized with the AOT sulfate group. The lipophilic alkyl chains of AOT make this complex soluble in organic solvents [122]. The obtained complexes form particles with a size of 1000 nm [123], followed by further encapsulation of the hydrophobic Gent–AOT complex in a biodegradable water-insoluble polymer (PLGA), making it possible to obtain nanoparticles with a size of 200–300 nm [122–124]. This strategy allows for a gentamicin encapsulation efficacy close to quantitative yields and up to 60 μg/mg of the PLGA polymer compared to instances where sulfate is used as an ion pairing agent [125]. In addition, encapsulated gentamicin is released from PLGA particles much more slowly in drug release tests due to the hydrophobic gentamicin AOT complex. It was observed that only 10% of gentamicin was released during the first hour, but an almost linear sustained release of the drug over 10 weeks was observed later [122]. Other biodegradable polymers are also used for the encapsulation of hydrophobic Gent–AOT, for example, poly (ε-caprolactone) and poly (D,L-lactic acid) [126], polyvinyl alcohol [122], poly (aspartic acid) [127] or poly (methyl vinyl ether-co-maleic anhydride) [128]. The variation in surfactants is another tool to construct a drug delivery system, as the interactions of the gentamicin complex with the AOT that was entrapped into PLGA are known to provide a more efficient drug delivery than occurs in the absence of AOT [31].

The antibacterial properties of nanoparticles that contain Gent–AOT are superior. However, the toxicity of Gent–AOT should also be considered, and more research is needed to evaluate gentamicin nanoformulations [124,125].

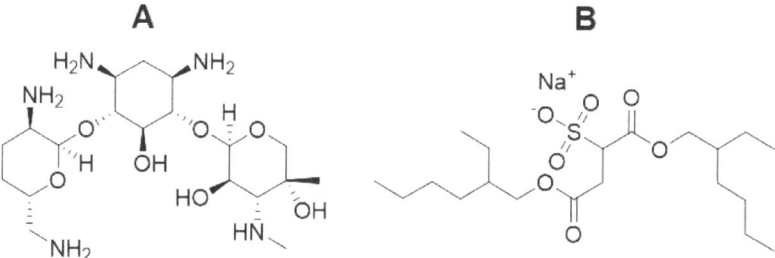

Figure 4. Structures of (A): gentamicin; (B): docusate sodium salt (AOT).

6. Gentamicin Combinations with Other Antibiotics

Early studies started investigating the synergic effects of gentamicin, together with other antibiotics, like β-lactams, in the 1970s, reporting better outcomes for the combination approach [129–131]. Currently, gentamicin is co-prescribed with a range of penicillins (amoxicillin, ampicillin, and benzylpenicillin) for the treatment of serious infections like sepsis, bacterial pneumonia, and peritoneal abscess [8]. The World Health Organization recommends gentamicin + azithromycin dual treatment for gonococcal infections in case treatment with cephalosporins fails, although this is a conditional recommendation with very low-quality evidence [132]. In the last decade, several studies have searched for new potential synergic combinations. Synergy has been observed when combining gentamicin with azithromycin [133,134], mitomycin C [135], fosfomycin [136,137], ciprofloxacin [136], daptomycin [138], and cefepime [139].

Recent tests on gentamicin in combination with other antibiotics have largely focused on its antibacterial activity against *P. aeruginosa* [134–136,139] and *Enterococci* species [137,138]. In addition, the combinational approach has also been tested against uncomplicated gonorrhea [133] and *E. coli* strains [136]. The synergic effects of combinations against biofilms of both *E. coli* (fosfomycin/gentamicin [136]) and *P. aeruginosa* (ciprofloxacin/gentamicin [136] and cefepime/gentamicin [139]) may be particularly important. A fosfomycin/gentamicin combination even retained its synergic effects against a gentamicin-resistant strain of *E. coli* [136].

The mechanisms behind the synergic effects of the two antibacterial agents are still largely unknown and underexplored. It has been suggested that the synergy of the azithromycin/gentamicin combination might be due to the suppression of trans-translation by gentamicin, enhancing the efficacy of azithromycin [134]. In addition, a bacterolytic effect of gentamicin has been hypothesized to explain the efficacy of the fosfomycin/gentamicin combination against a gentamicin-resistant strain [136]. Due to the high clinical significance, understanding the mechanism behind the synergic effects responsible for action against biofilms is critical.

Reports have been presented on the increased development of resistance after using the gentamicin combination compared to monotherapy [140]. Furthermore, the increased toxicity, especially the nephrotoxicity, of this approach is particularly concerning [29,140–142]. For example, a study of patients with gonorrhea revealed a strong adverse gastrointestinal effect rate in patients, which would likely limit the application of the azithromycin/gentamicin combination in clinical practice [133].

Further studies, including randomized controlled trials, should be executed to evaluate the risks and benefits of gentamicin + other antibiotic approaches. A search for alternative antibacterial agents, which have safer profiles and a lower likelihood of the development of resistance, like substances derived or isolated from natural products, is needed.

7. Gentamicin Combinations with Polyphenols

The used combination should lower the effective dose of antibiotic, as well as minimize the potential side-effects of the treatment [2,143]. These criteria could potentially be met by natural products like individual phytochemicals or herbal extracts.

Polyphenols are one of the largest groups of natural bioactive substances and are present in a very wide variety of plants [144]. Polyphenols possess not only antimicrobial but also antioxidant and anti-inflammatory properties [144,145]. Even though the effective concentrations of polyphenols often are much higher than those of antibiotics, their overall properties and potential for synergism make them attractive candidates for the combination approach [146].

A wide range of polyphenols, mainly flavonoids, have been tested together with gentamicin in the last 20 years. For the most part, more flavonoid aglycones than glycosides have been tested. Aglycones are known to have more potent biological activity than their respective glycosides [147]. An overview of studies with positive conclusions regarding synergy is found in Table 3. Polyphenols that, to date, have not shown any synergistic effects together with gentamicin have not been included in Table 3.

Table 3. Synergy between gentamicin and individual polyphenols.

Polyphenol	Bacteria	Bacterial Strain Type	Antibacterial Effect on Gentamicin	FICI	Synergy/Partial Synergy	Ref.
Caffeic acid	P. aeruginosa	Clinical isolates	MIC reduced from 625 µg/mL to 24.61 µg/mL	NA	Synergy	[148]
Epigallocatechin gallate	A. baumannii	Reference	MIC reduced from 27 µg/mL to 4 µg/mL	0.65	Partial synergy	[146]
	S. aureus	Clinical isolates	MIC reduced from 32 µg/mL to 6.4 µg/mL	0.325	Synergy	[149]
	E. coli	Clinical isolates	MIC reduced from 32 µg/mL to 6.4 µg/mL	0.325	Synergy	[149]
Daidzein	A. baumannii	Reference	MIC reduced from 27 µg/mL to 8 µg/mL	0.42	Synergy	[146]
Galangin	S. aureus (methicillin-resistant)	Clinical isolates/reference	Reduced MIC	0.18–0.25	Synergy	[150]
Gallic acid	S. aureus	Clinical isolates	MIC reduced from 49.21 µg/mL to 2.44 µg/mL	NA	Synergy	[148]
Genistein	A. baumannii	Reference	MIC reduced from 27 µg/mL to 4 µg/mL	0.4	Synergy	[146]
5-Hydroxy-3,7,4′-trimethoxyflavone	S. aureus	Clinical isolates	Reduced MIC	NA	Synergy	[151]
	E. coli	Clinical isolates	Reduced MIC	NA	Synergy	[151]
Kaempferol 7-O-β-D-(6″-O-cumaroyl)-glucopyranoside	S. aureus	Reference	MIC reduced from 16 µg/mL to 4 µg/mL	NA	Synergy	[3]
	E. coli	Reference	MIC reduced from 16 µg/mL to 8 µg/mL	NA	Synergy	[3]

Table 3. Cont.

Polyphenol	Bacteria	Bacterial Strain Type	Antibacterial Effect on Gentamicin	FICI	Synergy/Partial Synergy	Ref.
Luteolin	S. aureus	Reference	MIC reduced 4-fold	0.258	Synergy	[143]
	E. coli	Reference	Reduced MIC	0.504	Additive	[143]
Nordihydroguaiaretic acid	S. aureus (methicillin-sensitive)	Clinical isolates	Several-fold MIC reduction	<0.5	Synergy	[152]
	S. aureus (methicillin-resistant)	Clinical isolates	Several-fold MIC reduction	<0.5	Synergy	[152]
Quercetin	P. aeruginosa	Clinical isolates	MIC reduced from 128 µg/mL to 32 µg/mL	0.28–0.53	Synergy/Partial synergy	[153]
	P. aeruginosa	Clinical isolates/reference	Reduced MIC	0.375–0.75	Synergy/Partial synergy	[2]
	P. mirabilis	Clinical isolates	Restored antibacterial activity	NA	Synergy	[154]
Plumbagin	P. aeruginosa	Reference	Reduced MIC	0.152–0.485	Synergy	[155]
Pyrogallol	S. aureus	Clinical isolates	MIC reduced from 49.21 µg/mL to 2.44 µg/mL	NA	Synergy	[148]
Rutin	P. aeruginosa	Reference	MIC reduced from 10 µg/mL to 2.5 µg/mL	0.5	Synergy	[156]
Sophoraflavanone B	S. aureus (methicillin-resistant)	Clinical isolates/reference	MIC reduced 8- to 32-fold	0.25–0.375	Synergy	[157]
Vitexin	P. aeruginosa	Reference	Reduced MIC	0.078	Synergy	[158]

NA—not available; FICI—fractional inhibitory concentration index; MIC—minimum inhibitory concentration.

Three main mechanisms of polyphenol and gentamicin synergy can be distinguished. First, polyphenols inhibit the bacterial wall biosynthesis, allowing gentamicin to reenter the cells and leading to increased sensitivity [146,152,153]. Second, polyphenols can inhibit different bacterial efflux pumps; for example, AbeM and AdeABC [146,153]. Since these efflux pumps can be responsible for the development of resistance, their inhibition could increase bacterial sensitivity against antibiotics [146]. Third, polyphenols can inhibit quorum sensing, consequently regulating the bacterial population density [2,155,158]. Quorum sensing plays a significant role in biofilm production, hindering optimal drug delivery to pathogens. The inhibition of quorum sensing disrupts the biofilm structure, allowing gentamicin to reach and kill the pathogens [2,153,155].

Overall, most of the research focused on members of the ESKAPE group of pathogens, providing potential future alternatives to current approaches. To date, the lowest amount of evidence of synergy was found for E. coli, with only two papers finding synergy or additive effects using reference strains [3,143], and the rest reporting no or minimal effect [146,148,154,159].

In terms of the tested bacterial strains, it is advisable to use not only commercially available reference strains but also clinical isolates, since different strains may exhibit different synergic effects due to their diverse genetic and resistance mechanisms [2]. The synergic activity of polyphenols with gentamicin against reference strains does not always translate to clinical isolates [143].

In addition to the synergic effects, polyphenols have also been investigated to minimize the toxic effects of oxidative stress subsequent to the use of gentamicin [143,159].

8. Gentamicin Combinations with Natural Products

Another approach to enhance the antibacterial properties of gentamicin is to test multicomponent natural products like herbal extracts. Herbal extracts contain up to hundreds of bioactive substances and, therefore, could simultaneously act on multiple targets and enhance each other's antibacterial activity [160]. In addition, the use of multi-component products could lower the chances of antibacterial resistance development [161]. An overview of studies with positive conclusions regarding the synergy between natural products and gentamicin is found in Table 4. Natural products that, to date, have not shown any synergistic effects together with gentamicin are not included in Table 4.

Most positive outcomes regarding the synergy between natural products and gentamicin were obtained using bacterial reference strains, raising the question of whether the same observation could be seen using clinical isolates. If using medicinal plant extracts, the preparation method of the extract is crucial to the chemical composition of the extract. Furthermore, the wide variability in the chemical profiles and concentrations of bioactive substances in plants has to be kept in mind. Therefore, studies on the potential synergy between herbal extracts and antibiotics should also provide results on the chemical composition of the extract.

A concrete conclusion regarding the mechanisms responsible for the synergic activity of natural products together with antibiotics cannot be obtained [161–164]. Some authors have suggested that synergic effects could be observed due to changes in the efflux system, damage to cell membranes, and the inhibition of protein synthesis. Further research is needed to clearly understand the mechanisms [161,162,164]. A study using propolis revealed that the concentration of natural products is also crucial to the synergic activity [161]. Higher concentrations of propolis and antibiotics lead to a surprising loss of synergy [161]. This finding accentuates the important role of the ratio of components to produce synergic activity [161].

Table 4. Synergy between gentamicin and natural products.

Natural Product	Bacteria	Bacterial Strain Type	Antibacterial Effect on Gentamicin	FICI	Synergy/Partial Synergy	Ref.
Aniba rosaeodora essential oil	*B. cereus*	Reference	MIC reduction from 0.50 µg/mL to 0.12 µg/mL	0.30	Synergy	[40]
	B. subtilis	Reference	MIC reduction from 0.25 µg/mL to 0.06 µg/mL	0.34	Synergy	[40]
	S. aureus	Reference	MIC reduction from 0.50 µg/mL to 0.12 µg/mL and from 0.06 µg/mL to 0.01 µg/mL	0.30	Synergy	[40]
	E. coli	Reference	MIC reduction from 0.50 µg/mL to 0.12 µg/mL	0.35	Synergy	[40]
	A. baumannii	Reference	MIC reduction from 4.00 µg/mL to 0.24 µg/mL	0.11	Synergy	[40]
	S. marcescens	Reference	MIC reduction from 0.50 µg/mL to 0.12 µg/mL	0.30	Synergy	[40]
	Y. enterocolitica	Reference	MIC reduction from 0.25 µg/mL to 0.01 µg/mL	0.11	Synergy	[40]
Clinopodium vulgare L. extracts	*B. subtilis*	Clinical isolates	Reduction in MIC	0.395–0.44	Synergy	[164]
Daphne genkwa extract	*S. aureus* (methicillin-resistant)	Reference	Reduction in MIC	0.750	Partial synergy	[165]
Magnolia officinalis extract	*S. aureus* (methicillin-resistant)	Reference	Reduction in MIC	0.750	Partial synergy	[165]
Kaempferia parviflora extracts	*K. pneumoniae*	Clinical isolates	Reduction in MIC	0.141–0.625	Synergy/Partial synergy	[162]
	P. aeruginosa	Clinical isolates	Reduction in MIC	0.133–0.625	Synergy/Partial synergy	[162]
	A. baumannii	Clinical isolates	Reduction in MIC	0.133–0.563	Synergy/Partial synergy	[162]
Mentha piperita L. essential oil	*B. cereus*	Reference	MIC reduction from 2.00 µg/mL to 0.06 µg/mL	0.08	Synergy	[163]
	B. subtilis	Reference	MIC reduction from 0.50 µg/mL to 0.01 µg/mL	0.07	Synergy	[163]
	S. aureus	Reference	MIC reduction from 2.0 µg/mL to 0.06 µg/mL; from 0.5 µg/mL to 0.06 µg/mL; from 8.0 µg/mL to 2.0 µg/mL	0.103–0.3	Synergy	[163]
	E. faecalis	Reference	MIC reduction from 8.0 µg/mL to 1.0 µg/mL	0.32	Synergy	[163]
	E. coli	Reference	MIC reduction from 1.0 µg/mL to 0.03 µg/mL	0.43	Synergy	[163]
	K. pneumoniae	Reference	MIC reduction from 32.0 µg/mL to 1.0 µg/mL	0.43	Synergy	[163]
	A. baumannii	Reference	MIC reduction from 8.00 µg/mL to 0.5 µg/mL	0.46	Synergy	[163]
	P. aeruginosa	Reference	MIC reduction from 2.00 µg/mL to 0.06 µg/mL	0.08	Synergy	[163]

Table 4. Cont.

Natural Product	Bacteria	Bacterial Strain Type	Antibacterial Effect on Gentamicin	FICI	Synergy/Partial Synergy	Ref.
Pelargonium graveolens essential oil	B. cereus	Reference	MIC reduction from 0.50 µg/mL to 0.125 µg/mL	0.30	Synergy	[40]
	B. subtilis	Reference	MIC reduction from 0.25 µg/mL to 0.06 µg/mL	0.34	Synergy	[40]
	S. aureus	Reference	MIC reduction from 0.50 µg/mL to 0.01 µg/mL and from 0.12 to 0.04 µg/mL	0.28–0.35	Synergy	[40]
	E. coli	Reference	MIC reduction from 0.50 µg/mL to 0.12 µg/mL	0.30	Synergy	[40]
	A. baumannii	Reference	MIC reduction from 4.00 µg/mL to 0.24 µg/mL	0.11	Synergy	[40]
	S. marcescens	Reference	MIC reduction from 0.50 µg/mL to 0.12 µg/mL	0.45	Synergy	[40]
	Y. enterocolitica	Reference	MIC reduction from 0.25 µg/mL to 0.03 µg/mL	0.22	Synergy	[40]
Propolis	B. subtilis	Reference	MIC reduction from 1.25 µg/mL to 0.05 µg/mL	NA	Synergy	[161]
	B. cereus	Reference	MIC reduction from 1.25 µg/mL to 0.05 µg/mL	NA	Synergy	[161]
	B. megaterium	Reference	MIC reduction from 0.25 µg/mL to 0.01 µg/mL	NA	Synergy	[161]
	S. aureus (methicillin sensitive)	Reference	MIC reduction from 1.5 µg/mL to 0.5 µg/mL	NA	Synergy	[161]
	S. aureus (methicillin-resistant)	Reference	MIC reduction from >1.5 µg/mL to 0.5 µg/mL	NA	Synergy	[161]
	E. coli	Reference	MIC reduction from >1.5 µg/mL to 0.5 µg/mL	NA	Synergy	[161]

NA—not available; FICI—fractional inhibitory concentration index; MIC—minimum inhibitory concentration.

9. Conclusions and Future Perspectives

Even after 60 years on the market, gentamicin plays an important role in combating serious infections, especially those originating from the nosocomial ESKAPE pathogens. Several strategies, including encapsulation in nanoformulations, hydrophobization of the molecule, and combinations with various agents, have been investigated to enhance both the activity and drug delivery of gentamicin. Current evidence indicates that polymeric nanoformulations, especially PLGA nanoparticles, could provide a sustained release of gentamicin and offer higher bioavailability. Hydrophobization of the gentamicin molecule can significantly increase the encapsulation efficiency in nanoparticles and enhance the antibacterial properties of the system. Nevertheless, the currently used in vitro drug release methods lack standardization, hindering adequate comparison between studies. Further research on the toxicology of these nanoformulations is needed. Research on the synergic effects between gentamicin and polyphenols is an exciting research direction. Testing on a wider range of clinical isolates, not only reference strains of bacteria, will allow us to see if the results of synergy can be translated to clinical practice. The possible encapsulation of gentamicin–polyphenol combinations in drug delivery systems should be further investigated. As gentamicin is applied to treat hard-to-reach infections like osteomyelitis, target-specific surface modifications of drug delivery systems hold great potential for future research.

Author Contributions: Conceptualization, A.B. (Ance Bārzdiņa) and A.B. (Agnese Brangule); writing—original draft preparation, A.B. (Ance Bārzdiņa), A.B. (Agnese Brangule), A.P., A.S. and K.P.; writing—review and editing, A.B. (Ance Bārzdiņa), A.B. (Agnese Brangule), A.P., A.S., K.P. and D.B.; visualization, A.B. (Ance Bārzdiņa), A.P. and K.P.; supervision, A.B. (Agnese Brangule) and D.B.; project administration, A.B. (Agnese Brangule). All authors have read and agreed to the published version of the manuscript.

Funding: This project has received funding from the European Union's Horizon 2020 research and innovation program under the grant agreement No. 857287 (BBCE—Baltic Biomaterials Centre of Excellence).

Institutional Review Board Statement: Not applicable.

Informed Consent Statement: Not applicable.

Data Availability Statement: Not applicable.

Acknowledgments: The authors acknowledge the access to the infrastructure and expertise of the BBCE—Baltic Biomaterials Centre of Excellence (European Union's Horizon 2020 research and innovation programme under the grant agreement No. 857287) and the SPRINGBOARD project (European Union's Horizon 2020 research and innovation programme under grant agreement No. 951883).

Conflicts of Interest: The authors declare no conflicts of interest.

References

1. Chen, J.W.; Lau, Y.Y.; Krishnan, T.; Chan, K.G.; Chang, C.Y. Recent Advances in Molecular Diagnosis of Pseudomonas aeruginosa Infection by State-of-the-Art Genotyping Techniques. *Front. Microbiol.* **2018**, *9*, 1104. [CrossRef]
2. Vipin, C.; Saptami, K.; Fida, F.; Mujeeburahiman, M.; Rao, S.S.; Athmika; Arun, A.B.; Rekha, P.D. Potential synergistic activity of quercetin with antibiotics against multidrug-resistant clinical strains of *Pseudomonas aeruginosa*. *PLoS ONE* **2020**, *15*, e0241304. [CrossRef] [PubMed]
3. Cruz, B.G.; dos Santos, H.S.; Bandeira, P.N.; Rodrigues, T.H.S.; Matos, M.G.C.; Nascimento, M.F.; de Carvalho, G.G.C.; Braz-Filho, R.; Teixeira, A.M.R.; Tintino, S.R.; et al. Evaluation of antibacterial and enhancement of antibiotic action by the flavonoid kaempferol 7-O-β-D-(6″-O-cumaroyl)-glucopyranoside isolated from *Croton piauhiensis* müll. *Microb. Pathog.* **2020**, *143*, 104144. [CrossRef] [PubMed]
4. Santajit, S.; Indrawattana, N. Mechanisms of Antimicrobial Resistance in ESKAPE Pathogens. *Biomed. Res. Int.* **2016**, *2016*, 2475067. [CrossRef] [PubMed]
5. Tacconelli, E.; Carrara, E.; Savoldi, A.; Harbarth, S.; Mendelson, M.; Monnet, D.L.; Pulcini, C.; Kahlmeter, G.; Kluytmans, J.; Carmeli, Y.; et al. Discovery, research, and development of new antibiotics: The WHO priority list of antibiotic-resistant bacteria and tuberculosis. *Lancet Infect. Dis.* **2018**, *18*, 318–327. [CrossRef]
6. Chen, C.; Chen, Y.; Wu, P.; Chen, B. Update on new medicinal applications of gentamicin: Evidence-based review. *J. Formos. Med. Assoc.* **2014**, *113*, 72–82. [CrossRef]
7. Alapi, M.E.; Fisher, J. *Analogue-Based Drug Discovery*; Fischer, J., Ganellin, C.R., Eds.; Wiley-VCH Verlag GmbH & Co.: Weinheim, Germany; KgaA: Weinheim, Germany, 2006; p. 507. ISBN 9783527607495.
8. WHO Electronic Essential Medicines List. Gentamicin. Model List of Essential Medicines. Available online: https://list.essentialmeds.org/medicines/229 (accessed on 19 February 2024).
9. Gentamicin sulfate. In *Merative Micromedex® DRUGDEX® (Electronic Version)*; Merative Healthcare Solutions/EBSCO Information Services: Greenwood Village, CO, USA; Cambridge, MA, USA. Available online: https://www.dynamed.com/drug-monograph/gentamicin-sulfate (accessed on 16 March 2024).
10. Elsevier Drug Information. Drug Monograph. Gentamicin. In *ClinicalKey*; Elsevier: Amsterdam, The Netherlands, 2024. Available online: https://www.clinicalkey.com/#!/content/drug_monograph/6-s2.0-275 (accessed on 16 March 2024).
11. Dorati, R.; DeTrizio, A.; Spalla, M.; Migliavacca, R.; Pagani, L.; Pisani, S.; Chiesa, E.; Conti, B.; Modena, T.; Genta, I. Gentamicin Sulfate PEG-PLGA/PLGA-H Nanoparticles: Screening Design and Antimicrobial Effect Evaluation toward Clinic Bacterial Isolates. *Nanomaterials* **2018**, *8*, 37. [CrossRef]
12. Weinstein, M.J.; Luedemann, G.M.; Oden, E.M.; Wagman, G.H.; Rosselet, J.P.; Marquez, J.A.; Coniglio, C.T.; Charney, W.; Herzog, H.L.; Black, J. Gentamicin, a new antibiotic complex from micromonospora. *J. Med. Chem.* **1963**, *6*, 463–464. [CrossRef] [PubMed]
13. Isoherranen, N.; Lavy, E.; Soback, S. Pharmacokinetics of gentamicin C_1, C_{1a}, and C_2 in beagles after a single intravenous dose. *Antimicrob. Agents Chemother.* **2000**, *44*, 1443–1447. [CrossRef]
14. Athauda, I.D.; Shetty, M.G.; Pai, P.; Hegde, M.; Gurumurthy, S.C.; Babitha, K.S. Enhanced Bactericidal Effects and Drug Delivery with Gentamicin-Conjugated Nanoparticles. *J. Clust. Sci.* **2023**, *35*, 371–390. [CrossRef]
15. Deubner, R.; Schollmayer, C.; Wienen, F.; Holzgrabe, U. Assignment of the major and minor components of gentamicin for evaluation of batches. *Magn. Reson. Chem.* **2003**, *41*, 589–598. [CrossRef]
16. Friesen, W.J.; Johnson, B.; Sierra, J.; Zhuo, J.; Vazirani, P.; Xue, X.; Tomizawa, Y.; Baiazitov, R.; Morrill, C.; Ren, H.; et al. The minor gentamicin complex component, X2, is a potent premature stop codon readthrough molecule with therapeutic potential. *PLoS ONE* **2018**, *13*, e0206158. [CrossRef] [PubMed]
17. O'Sullivan, M.E.; Song, Y.; Greenhouse, R.; Lin, R.; Perez, A.; Atkinson, P.J.; MacDonald, J.P.; Siddiqui, Z.; Lagasca, D.; Comstock, K.; et al. Dissociating antibacterial from ototoxic effects of gentamicin C-subtypes. *Proc. Natl. Acad. Sci. USA* **2020**, *117*, 32423–32432. [CrossRef] [PubMed]

18. Eren, E.; Parkin, J.; Adelanwa, A.; Cheneke, B.; Movileanu, L.; Khalid, S.; van den Berg, B. Toward understanding the outer membrane uptake of small molecules by *Pseudomonas aeruginosa*. *J. Biol. Chem.* **2013**, *288*, 12042–12053. [CrossRef] [PubMed]
19. Claes, P.J.; Busson, R.; Vanderhaeghe, H. Determination of the component ratio of commercial gentamicins by high-performance liquid chromatography using pre-column derivatization. *J. Chromatogr. A* **1984**, *298*, 445–457. [CrossRef] [PubMed]
20. Kohlhepp, S.J.; Loveless, M.O.; Kohnen, P.W.; Houghton, D.C.; Bennett, W.M.; Gilbert, D.N. Nephrotoxicity of the Constituents of the Gentamicin Complex. *J. Infect. Dis.* **1984**, *149*, 605–614. [CrossRef] [PubMed]
21. Jana, S.; Rajasekaran, P.; Haldimann, K.; Vasella, A.; Böttger, E.C.; Hobbie, S.N.; Crich, D. Synthesis of Gentamicins C1, C2, and C2a and Antiribosomal and Antibacterial Activity of Gentamicins B1, C1, C1a, C2, C2a, C2b, and X2. *ACS Infect. Dis.* **2023**, *9*, 1622–1633. [CrossRef] [PubMed]
22. Gu, Y.; Ni, X.; Ren, J.; Gao, H.; Wang, D.; Xia, H. Biosynthesis of Epimers C2 and C2a in the Gentamicin C Complex. *ChemBioChem* **2015**, *16*, 1933–1942. [CrossRef] [PubMed]
23. Sandoval, R.M.; Reilly, J.P.; Running, W.; Campos, S.B.; Santos, J.R.; Phillips, C.L.; Molitoris, B.A. A Non-Nephrotoxic Gentamicin Congener That Retains Antimicrobial Efficacy. *J. Am. Soc. Nephrol.* **2006**, *17*, 2697–2705. [CrossRef]
24. Kobayashi, M.; Sone, M.; Umemura, M.; Nabeshima, T.; Nakashima, T.; Hellström, S. Comparisons of cochleotoxicity among three gentamicin compounds following intratympanic application. *Acta Otolaryngol.* **2008**, *128*, 245–249. [CrossRef]
25. Ishikawa, M.; García-Mateo, N.; Čusak, A.; López-Hernández, I.; Fernández-Martínez, M.; Müller, M.; Rüttiger, L.; Singer, W.; Löwenheim, H.; Kosec, G.; et al. Lower ototoxicity and absence of hidden hearing loss point to gentamicin C1a and apramycin as promising antibiotics for clinical use. *Sci. Rep.* **2019**, *9*, 2410. [CrossRef]
26. Recht, M.I.; Puglisi, J.D. Aminoglycoside resistance with homogeneous and heterogeneous populations of antibiotic-resistant ribosomes. *Antimicrob. Agents Chemother.* **2001**, *45*, 2414–2419. [CrossRef]
27. Rosenkrantz, B.E.; Greco, J.R.; Hoogerheide, J.G.; Oden, E.M. Gentamicin Sulfate. In *Analytical Profiles of Drug Substances*; Florey, K., Ed.; Academic Press: Cambridge, MA, USA, 1981; Volume 9, pp. 295–340. [CrossRef]
28. Tangy, F.; Moukkadem, M.; Vindimian, E.; Capmau, M.L.; Le Goffic, F. Mechanism of action of gentamicin components. Characteristics of their binding to *Escherichia coli* ribosomes. *Eur. J. Biochem.* **1985**, *147*, 381–386. [CrossRef]
29. Beganovic, M.; Luther, M.K.; Rice, L.B.; Arias, C.A.; Rybak, M.J.; LaPlante, K.L. A Review of Combination Antimicrobial Therapy for *Enterococcus faecalis* Bloodstream Infections and Infective Endocarditis. *Clin. Infect. Dis.* **2018**, *67*, 303–309. [CrossRef]
30. Prior, S.; Gamazo, C.; Irache, J.M.; Merkle, H.P.; Gander, B. Gentamicin encapsulation in PLA/PLGA microspheres in view of treating Brucella infections. *Int. J. Pharm.* **2000**, *196*, 115–125. [CrossRef] [PubMed]
31. Duran, S.; Anwar, J.; Moin, S.T. Interaction of gentamicin and gentamicin-AOT with poly-(lactide-co-glycolate) in a drug delivery system—Density functional theory calculations and molecular dynamics simulation. *Biophys. Chem.* **2023**, *294*, 106958. [CrossRef] [PubMed]
32. Crcek, M.; Zdovc, J.; Kerec Kos, M. A review of population pharmacokinetic models of gentamicin in paediatric patients. *J. Clin. Pharm. Ther.* **2019**, *44*, 659–674. [CrossRef] [PubMed]
33. Craig, W.A. Optimizing aminoglycoside use. *Crit. Care Clin.* **2011**, *27*, 107–121. [CrossRef]
34. Pisani, S.; Dorati, R.; Chiesa, E.; Genta, I.; Modena, T.; Bruni, G.; Grisoli, P.; Conti, B. Release Profile of Gentamicin Sulfate from Polylactide-co-Polycaprolactone Electrospun Nanofiber Matrices. *Pharmaceutics* **2019**, *11*, 161. [CrossRef]
35. Wassif, R.K.; Elkayal, M.; Shamma, R.N.; Elkheshen, S.A. Recent advances in the local antibiotics delivery systems for management of osteomyelitis. *Drug Deliv.* **2021**, *28*, 2392–2414. [CrossRef]
36. Hodiamont, C.J.; van den Broek, A.K.; de Vroom, S.L.; Prins, J.M.; Mathôt, R.A.A.; van Hest, R.M. Clinical Pharmacokinetics of Gentamicin in Various Patient Populations and Consequences for Optimal Dosing for Gram-Negative Infections: An Updated Review. *Clin. Pharmacokinet.* **2022**, *61*, 1075–1094. [CrossRef] [PubMed]
37. Scholar, E. Gentamicin. In *xPharm: The Comprehensive Pharmacology Reference*; Enna, S.J., Bylund, D.B., Eds.; Elsevier: New York, NY, USA, 2007; pp. 1–6. [CrossRef]
38. Bailey, D.N.; Briggs, J.R. Gentamicin and Tobramycin Binding to Human Serum In Vitro. *J. Anal. Toxicol.* **2004**, *28*, 187–189. [CrossRef] [PubMed]
39. Drevets, D.A.; Canono, B.P.; Leenen, P.J.; Campbell, P.A. Gentamicin kills intracellular Listeria monocytogenes. *Infect. Immun.* **1994**, *62*, 2222–2228. [CrossRef] [PubMed]
40. Rosato, A.; Piarulli, M.; Corbo, F.; Muraglia, M.; Carone, A.; Vitali, M.E.; Vitali, C. In vitro synergistic antibacterial action of certain combinations of gentamicin and essential oils. *Curr. Med. Chem.* **2010**, *17*, 3289–3295. [CrossRef] [PubMed]
41. Lopez-Novoa, J.M.; Quiros, Y.; Vicente, L.; Morales, A.I.; Lopez-Hernandez, F.J. New insights into the mechanism of aminoglycoside nephrotoxicity: An integrative point of view. *Kidney Int.* **2011**, *79*, 33–45. [CrossRef] [PubMed]
42. Fu, X.; Wan, P.; Li, P.; Wang, J.; Guo, S.; Zhang, Y.; An, Y.; Ye, C.; Liu, Z.; Gao, J.; et al. Mechanism and Prevention of Ototoxicity Induced by Aminoglycosides. *Front. Cell Neurosci.* **2021**, *15*, 692762. [CrossRef] [PubMed]
43. Dorati, R.; DeTrizio, A.; Genta, I.; Grisoli, P.; Merelli, A.; Tomasi, C.; Conti, B. An experimental design approach to the preparation of pegylated polylactide-co-glicolide gentamicin loaded microparticles for local antibiotic delivery. *Mater. Sci. Eng. C* **2016**, *58*, 909–917. [CrossRef]
44. Abbasi, M.Y.; Chaijamorn, W.; Wiwattanawongsa, K.; Charoensareerat, T.; Doungngern, T. Recommendations of Gentamicin Dose Based on Different Pharmacokinetic/Pharmacodynamic Targets for Intensive Care Adult Patients: A Redefining Approach. *Clin. Pharmacol.* **2023**, *15*, 67–76. [CrossRef]

45. Cepec, E.; Trček, J. Antimicrobial Resistance of Acetobacter and Komagataeibacter Species Originating from Vinegars. *Int. J. Environ. Res. Public. Health* **2022**, *19*, 463. [CrossRef]
46. Li, P.K.T.; Szeto, C.C.; Piraino, B.; de Arteaga, J.; Fan, S.; Figueiredo, A.E.; Fish, D.N.; Goffin, E.; Kim, Y.L.; Salzer, W.; et al. ISPD Peritonitis Recommendations: 2016 Update on Prevention and Treatment. *Perit. Dial. Int.* **2016**, *36*, 481–508. [CrossRef]
47. Puschhof, J.; Pleguezuelos-Manzano, C.; Martinez-Silgado, A.; Akkerman, N.; Saftien, A.; Boot, C.; de Waal, A.; Beumer, J.; Dutta, D.; Heo, I.; et al. Intestinal organoid cocultures with microbes. *Nat. Protoc.* **2021**, *16*, 4633–4649. [CrossRef] [PubMed]
48. Patra, J.K.; Das, G.; Fraceto, L.F.; Campos, E.V.R.; Rodriguez-Torres, M.D.P.; Acosta-Torres, L.S.; Diaz-Torres, L.A.; Grillo, R.; Swamy, M.K.; Sharma, S.; et al. Nano based drug delivery systems: Recent developments and future prospects. *J. Nanobiotechnol.* **2018**, *16*, 71. [CrossRef] [PubMed]
49. Adeniji, O.O.; Nontongana, N.; Okoh, J.C.; Okoh, A.I. The Potential of Antibiotics and Nanomaterial Combinations as Therapeutic Strategies in the Management of Multidrug-Resistant Infections: A Review. *Int. J. Mol. Sci.* **2022**, *23*, 15038. [CrossRef] [PubMed]
50. Mamun, M.M.; Sorinolu, A.J.; Munir, M.; Vejerano, E.P. Nanoantibiotics: Functions and Properties at the Nanoscale to Combat Antibiotic Resistance. *Front. Chem.* **2021**, *9*, 687660. [CrossRef] [PubMed]
51. Alhariri, M.; Majrashi, M.A.; Bahkali, A.H.; Almajed, F.S.; Azghani, A.O.; Khiyami, M.A.; Alyamani, E.J.; Aljohani, S.M.; Halwani, M.A. Efficacy of neutral and negatively charged liposome-loaded gentamicin on planktonic bacteria and biofilm communities. *Int. J. Nanomed.* **2017**, *12*, 6949–6961. [CrossRef] [PubMed]
52. Jia, Y.; Joly, H.; Omri, A. Liposomes as a carrier for gentamicin delivery: Development and evaluation of the physicochemical properties. *Int. J. Pharm.* **2008**, *359*, 254–263. [CrossRef]
53. Rukholm, G.; Mugabe, C.; Azghani, A.O.; Omri, A. Antibacterial activity of liposomal gentamicin against *Pseudomonas aeruginosa*: A time–kill study. *Int. J. Antimicrob. Agents* **2006**, *27*, 247–252. [CrossRef]
54. Mosselhy, D.A.; Ge, Y.; Gasik, M.; Nordström, K.; Natri, O.; Hannula, S.-P. Silica-Gentamicin Nanohybrids: Synthesis and Antimicrobial Action. *Materials* **2016**, *9*, 170. [CrossRef]
55. Perni, S.; Martini-Gilching, K.; Prokopovich, P. Controlling release kinetics of gentamicin from silica nano-carriers. *Colloids Surf. A: Physicochem. Eng. Asp.* **2018**, *541*, 212–221. [CrossRef]
56. Purcar, V.; Rădițoiu, V.; Nichita, C.; Bălan, A.; Rădițoiu, A.; Căprărescu, S.; Raduly, F.M.; Manea, R.; Şomoghi, R.; Nicolae, C.A.; et al. Preparation and Characterization of Silica Nanoparticles and of Silica-Gentamicin Nanostructured Solution Obtained by Microwave-Assisted Synthesis. *Materials* **2021**, *14*, 2086. [CrossRef]
57. Katva, S.; Das, S.; Moti, H.S.; Jyoti, A.; Kaushik, S. Antibacterial Synergy of Silver Nanoparticles with Gentamicin and Chloramphenicol against *Enterococcus faecalis*. *Pharmacogn. Mag.* **2018**, *13*, S828–S833. [CrossRef] [PubMed]
58. Birla, S.S.; Tiwari, V.V.; Gade, A.K.; Ingle, A.P.; Yadav, A.P.; Rai, M.K. Fabrication of silver nanoparticles by Phoma glomerata and its combined effect against *Escherichia coli*, *Pseudomonas aeruginosa* and *Staphylococcus aureus*. *Lett. Appl. Microbiol.* **2009**, *48*, 173–179. [CrossRef]
59. Feizi, S.; Cooksley, C.M.; Nepal, R.; Psaltis, A.J.; Wormald, P.-J.; Vreugde, S. Silver nanoparticles as a bioadjuvant of antibiotics against biofilm-mediated infections with methicillin-resistant *Staphylococcus aureus* and *Pseudomonas aeruginosa* in chronic rhinosinusitis patients. *Pathology* **2022**, *54*, 453–459. [CrossRef] [PubMed]
60. Ferreira, M.; Aguiar, S.; Bettencourt, A.; Gaspar, M.M. Lipid-based nanosystems for targeting bone implant-associated infections: Current approaches and future endeavors. *Drug Deliv. Transl. Res.* **2021**, *11*, 72–85. [CrossRef]
61. Ferreira, M.; Ogren, M.; Dias, J.N.R.; Silva, M.; Gil, S.; Tavares, L.; Aires-da-Silva, F.; Gaspar, M.M.; Aguiar, S.I. Liposomes as Antibiotic Delivery Systems: A Promising Nanotechnological Strategy against Antimicrobial Resistance. *Molecules* **2021**, *26*, 2047. [CrossRef]
62. Danhier, F.; Ansorena, E.; Silva, J.M.; Coco, R.; Le Breton, A.; Préat, V. PLGA-based nanoparticles: An overview of biomedical applications. *J. Control. Release* **2012**, *161*, 505–522. [CrossRef]
63. Lecaroz, C.; Gamazo, C.; Renedo, M.J.; Blanco-Prieto, M.J. Biodegradable micro- and nanoparticles as long-term delivery vehicles for gentamicin. *J. Microencapsul.* **2006**, *23*, 782–792. [CrossRef]
64. Lecaroz, M.C.; Blanco-Prieto, M.J.; Campanero, M.A.; Salman, H.; Gamazo, C. Poly(D,L-lactide-coglycolide) particles containing gentamicin: Pharmacokinetics and pharmacodynamics in Brucella melitensis-infected mice. *Antimicrob. Agents Chemother.* **2007**, *51*, 1185–1190. [CrossRef]
65. Abdelghany, S.M.; Quinn, D.J.; Ingram, R.J.; Gilmore, B.F.; Donnelly, R.F.; Taggart, C.C.; Scott, C.J. Gentamicin-loaded nanoparticles show improved antimicrobial effects towards *Pseudomonas aeruginosa* infection. *Int. J. Nanomed.* **2012**, *7*, 4053–4063. [CrossRef]
66. Posadowska, U.; Brzychczy-Włoch, M.; Pamuła, E. Gentamicin loaded PLGA nanoparticles as local drug delivery system for the osteomyelitis treatment. *Acta Bioeng. Biomech.* **2015**, *17*, 41–48. [CrossRef]
67. Dhal, C.; Mishra, R. Formulation development and in vitro evaluation of gentamicin sulfate-loaded PLGA nanoparticles based film for the treatment of surgical site infection by Box–Behnken design. *Drug Dev. Ind. Pharm.* **2019**, *45*, 805–818. [CrossRef] [PubMed]
68. Jiang, L.; Greene, M.K.; Insua, J.L.; Pessoa, J.S.; Small, D.M.; Smyth, P.; McCann, A.P.; Cogo, F.; Bengoechea, J.A.; Taggart, C.C.; et al. Clearance of intracellular *Klebsiella pneumoniae* infection using gentamicin-loaded nanoparticles. *J. Control. Release* **2018**, *279*, 316–325. [CrossRef]

69. Sun, Y.; Bhattacharjee, A.; Reynolds, M.; Li, Y.V. Synthesis and characterizations of gentamicin-loaded poly-lactic-co-glycolic (PLGA) nanoparticles. *J. Nanoparticle Res.* **2021**, *23*, 155. [CrossRef]
70. Rezvantalab, S.; Drude, N.I.; Moraveji, M.K.; Güvener, N.; Koons, E.K.; Shi, Y.; Lammers, T.; Kiessling, F. PLGA-Based Nanoparticles in Cancer Treatment. *Front. Pharmacol.* **2018**, *9*, 1260. [CrossRef] [PubMed]
71. Xu, Y.; Kim, C.-S.; Saylor, D.M.; Koo, D. Polymer degradation and drug delivery in PLGA-based drug–polymer applications: A review of experiments and theories. *J. Biomed. Mater. Res. B Appl. Biomater.* **2017**, *105*, 1692–1716. [CrossRef]
72. Lü, J.M.; Wang, X.; Marin-Muller, C.; Wang, H.; Lin, P.H.; Yao, Q.; Chen, C. Current advances in research and clinical applications of PLGA-based nanotechnology. *Expert. Rev. Mol. Diagn.* **2009**, *9*, 325–341. [CrossRef]
73. Cao, X.; Dai, L.; Sun, S.; Ma, R.; Liu, X. Preparation and performance of porous hydroxyapatite/poly(lactic-co-glycolic acid) drug-loaded microsphere scaffolds for gentamicin sulfate delivery. *J. Mater. Sci.* **2021**, *56*, 15278–15298. [CrossRef]
74. Sivaraman, B.; Ramamurthi, A. Multifunctional nanoparticles for doxycycline delivery towards localized elastic matrix stabilization and regenerative repair. *Acta Biomater.* **2013**, *9*, 6511–6525. [CrossRef] [PubMed]
75. Razei, A.; Cheraghali, A.M.; Saadati, M.; Fasihi Ramandi, M.; Panahi, Y.; Hajizade, A.; Siadat, S.D.; Behrouzi, A. Gentamicin-Loaded Chitosan Nanoparticles Improve Its Therapeutic Effects on Brucella-Infected J774A.1 Murine Cells. *Galen. Med. J.* **2019**, *8*, e1296. [CrossRef]
76. Shakya, A.K.; Al-Sulaibi, M.; Naik, R.R.; Nsairat, H.; Suboh, S.; Abulaila, A. Review on PLGA Polymer Based Nanoparticles with Antimicrobial Properties and Their Application in Various Medical Conditions or Infections. *Polymers* **2023**, *15*, 3597. [CrossRef]
77. Vasir, J.K.; Labhasetwar, V. Biodegradable nanoparticles for cytosolic delivery of therapeutics. *Adv. Drug Deliv. Rev.* **2007**, *59*, 718–728. [CrossRef] [PubMed]
78. Panyam, J.; Zhou, W.-Z.; Prabha, S.; Sahoo, S.K.; Labhasetwar, V. Rapid endo-lysosomal escape of poly(DL-lactide-coglycolide) nanoparticles: Implications for drug and gene delivery. *FASEB J.* **2002**, *16*, 1217–1226. [CrossRef] [PubMed]
79. Kosinski, A.M.; Brugnano, J.L.; Seal, B.L.; Knight, F.C.; Panitch, A. Synthesis and characterization of a poly (lactic-co-glycolic acid) core + poly (N-isopropylacrylamide) shell nanoparticle system. *Biomatter* **2012**, *2*, 195–201. [CrossRef] [PubMed]
80. Acharya, S.; Sahoo, S.K. PLGA nanoparticles containing various anticancer agents and tumour delivery by EPR effect. *Adv. Drug Deliv. Rev.* **2011**, *63*, 170–183. [CrossRef]
81. El-Hammadi, M.M.; Arias, J.L. Recent Advances in the Surface Functionalization of PLGA-Based Nanomedicines. *Nanomaterials* **2022**, *12*, 354. [CrossRef] [PubMed]
82. Nandi, S.K.; Bandyopadhyay, S.; Das, P.; Samanta, I.; Mukherjee, P.; Roy, S.; Kundu, B. Understanding osteomyelitis and its treatment through local drug delivery system. *Biotechnol. Adv.* **2016**, *34*, 1305–1317. [CrossRef] [PubMed]
83. Owens, C.D.; Stoessel, K. Surgical site infections: Epidemiology, microbiology and prevention. *J. Hosp. Infect.* **2008**, *70*, 3–10. [CrossRef]
84. Worku, S.; Abebe, T.; Alemu, A.; Seyoum, B.; Swedberg, G.; Abdissa, A.; Mihret, A.; Beyene, G.T. Bacterial profile of surgical site infection and antimicrobial resistance patterns in Ethiopia: A multicentre prospective cross-sectional study. *Ann. Clin. Microbiol. Antimicrob.* **2023**, *22*, 96. [CrossRef]
85. Liu, Y.; Li, X.; Liang, A. Current research progress of local drug delivery systems based on biodegradable polymers in treating chronic osteomyelitis. *Front. Bioeng. Biotechnol.* **2022**, *10*, 1042128. [CrossRef]
86. Flores, C.; Degoutin, S.; Chai, F.; Raoul, G.; Hornez, J.-C.; Martel, B.; Siepmann, J.; Ferri, J.; Blanchemain, N. Gentamicin-loaded poly(lactic-co-glycolic acid) microparticles for the prevention of maxillofacial and orthopedic implant infections. *Mater. Sci. Engineering C* **2016**, *64*, 108–116. [CrossRef]
87. Akhtar, B.; Muhammad, F.; Aslam, B.; Saleemi, M.K.; Sharif, A. Biodegradable nanoparticle based transdermal patches for gentamicin delivery: Formulation, characterization and pharmacokinetics in rabbits. *J. Drug Deliv. Sci. Technol.* **2020**, *57*, 101680. [CrossRef]
88. Dhal, C.; Mishra, R. In vitro and in vivo evaluation of gentamicin sulphate-loaded PLGA nanoparticle-based film for the treatment of surgical site infection. *Drug Deliv. Transl. Res.* **2020**, *10*, 1032–1043. [CrossRef]
89. Aranaz, I.; Alcántara, A.R.; Civera, M.C.; Arias, C.; Elorza, B.; Heras Caballero, A.; Acosta, N. Chitosan: An Overview of Its Properties and Applications. *Polymers* **2021**, *13*, 3256. [CrossRef]
90. Kou, S.; Peters, L.; Mucalo, M. Chitosan: A review of molecular structure, bioactivities and interactions with the human body and micro-organisms. *Carbohydr. Polym.* **2022**, *282*, 119132. [CrossRef] [PubMed]
91. El-Alfy, E.A.; El-Bisi, M.K.; Taha, G.M.; Ibrahim, H.M. Preparation of biocompatible chitosan nanoparticles loaded by tetracycline, gentamycin and ciprofloxacin as novel drug delivery system for improvement the antibacterial properties of cellulose based fabrics. *Int. J. Biol. Macromol.* **2020**, *161*, 1247–1260. [CrossRef]
92. Yan, D.; Li, Y.; Liu, Y.; Li, N.; Zhang, X.; Yan, C. Antimicrobial Properties of Chitosan and Chitosan Derivatives in the Treatment of Enteric Infections. *Molecules* **2021**, *26*, 7136. [CrossRef]
93. Yilmaz Atay, H. Antibacterial Activity of Chitosan-Based Systems. In *Functional Chitosan: Drug Delivery and Biomedical Applications*; Jana, S., Jana, S., Eds.; Springer: Singapore, 2019; pp. 457–489.
94. Chandrasekaran, M.; Kim, K.D.; Chun, S.C. Antibacterial Activity of Chitosan Nanoparticles: A Review. *Processes* **2020**, *8*, 1173. [CrossRef]
95. Lu, E.; Franzblau, S.; Onyuksel, H.; Popescu, C. Preparation of aminoglycoside-loaded chitosan nanoparticles using dextran sulphate as a counterion. *J. Microencapsul.* **2009**, *26*, 346–354. [CrossRef] [PubMed]

96. Ji, J.; Hao, S.; Wu, D.; Huang, R.; Xu, Y. Preparation, characterization and in vitro release of chitosan nanoparticles loaded with gentamicin and salicylic acid. *Carbohydr. Polym.* **2011**, *85*, 803–808. [CrossRef]
97. Alfaro-Viquez, E.; Esquivel-Alvarado, D.; Madrigal-Carballo, S.; Krueger, C.G.; Reed, J.D. Antimicrobial proanthocyanidin-chitosan composite nanoparticles loaded with gentamicin. *Int. J. Biol. Macromol.* **2020**, *162*, 1500–1508. [CrossRef]
98. Asgarirad, H.; Ebrahimnejad, P.; Mahjoub, M.A.; Jalalian, M.; Morad, H.; Ataee, R.; Hosseini, S.S.; Farmoudeh, A. A promising technology for wound healing; in-vitro and in-vivo evaluation of chitosan nano-biocomposite films containing gentamicin. *J. Microencapsul.* **2021**, *38*, 100–107. [CrossRef]
99. Abdel-Hakeem, M.A.; Abdel Maksoud, A.I.; Aladhadh, M.A.; Almuryif, K.A.; Elsanhoty, R.M.; Elebeedy, D. Gentamicin-Ascorbic Acid Encapsulated in Chitosan Nanoparticles Improved In Vitro Antimicrobial Activity and Minimized Cytotoxicity. *Antibiotics* **2022**, *11*, 1530. [CrossRef]
100. Jafernik, K.; Ładniak, A.; Blicharska, E.; Czarnek, K.; Ekiert, H.; Wiącek, A.E.; Szopa, A. Chitosan-Based Nanoparticles as Effective Drug Delivery Systems—A review. *Molecules* **2023**, *28*, 1963. [CrossRef] [PubMed]
101. Abdelgawad, A.M.; Hudson, S.M. Chitosan nanoparticles: Polyphosphates cross-linking and protein delivery properties. *Int. J. Biol. Macromol.* **2019**, *136*, 133–142. [CrossRef]
102. Pan, C.; Qian, J.; Zhao, C.; Yang, H.; Zhao, X.; Guo, H. Study on the relationship between crosslinking degree and properties of TPP crosslinked chitosan nanoparticles. *Carbohydr. Polym.* **2020**, *241*, 116349. [CrossRef] [PubMed]
103. Aibani, N.; Rai, R.; Patel, P.; Cuddihy, G.; Wasan, E.K. Chitosan Nanoparticles at the Biological Interface: Implications for Drug Delivery. *Pharmaceutics* **2021**, *13*, 1686. [CrossRef]
104. Cao, Y.; Tan, Y.F.; Wong, Y.S.; Liew, M.W.J.; Venkatraman, S. Recent Advances in Chitosan-Based Carriers for Gene Delivery. *Mar. Drugs* **2019**, *17*, 381. [CrossRef] [PubMed]
105. Qiu, Y.; Xu, D.; Sui, G.; Wang, D.; Wu, M.; Han, L.; Mu, H.; Duan, J. Gentamicin decorated phosphatidylcholine-chitosan nanoparticles against biofilms and intracellular bacteria. *Int. J. Biol. Macromol.* **2020**, *156*, 640–647. [CrossRef] [PubMed]
106. Weng, J.; Tong, H.H.Y.; Chow, S.F. In Vitro Release Study of the Polymeric Drug Nanoparticles: Development and Validation of a Novel Method. *Pharmaceutics* **2020**, *12*, 732. [CrossRef]
107. Gao, J.; Karp, J.M.; Langer, R.; Joshi, N. The Future of Drug Delivery. *Chem. Mater.* **2023**, *35*, 359–363. [CrossRef]
108. Kapoor, D.N.; Bhatia, A.; Kaur, R.; Sharma, R.; Kaur, G.; Dhawan, S. PLGA: A unique polymer for drug delivery. *Ther. Deliv.* **2015**, *6*, 41–58. [CrossRef] [PubMed]
109. Herdiana, Y.; Wathoni, N.; Shamsuddin, S.; Muchtaridi, M. Drug release study of the chitosan-based nanoparticles. *Heliyon* **2022**, *8*, e08674. [CrossRef] [PubMed]
110. Fredenberg, S.; Wahlgren, M.; Reslow, M.; Axelsson, A. The mechanisms of drug release in poly(lactic-co-glycolic acid)-based drug delivery systems—A review. *Int. J. Pharm.* **2011**, *415*, 34–52. [CrossRef] [PubMed]
111. Hines, D.J.; Kaplan, D.L. Poly(lactic-co-glycolic) acid-controlled-release systems: Experimental and modeling insights. *Crit. Rev. Ther. Drug Carrier Syst.* **2013**, *30*, 257–276. [CrossRef] [PubMed]
112. Chavan, Y.R.; Tambe, S.M.; Jain, D.D.; Khairnar, S.V.; Amin, P.D. Redefining the importance of polylactide-co-glycolide acid (PLGA) in drug delivery. *Ann. Pharm. Fr.* **2022**, *80*, 603–616. [CrossRef] [PubMed]
113. Trang, T.T.T.; Mariatti, M.; Badrul, H.Y.; Masakazu, K.; Nguyen, X.T.T.; Zuratul, A.A.H. Drug Release Profile Study of Gentamicin Encapsulated Poly (lactic Acid) Microspheres for Drug Delivery. *Mater. Today Proc.* **2019**, *17*, 836–845. [CrossRef]
114. Ivković, B.; Milutinović, I.; Čudina, O.; Marković, B. A new simple liquid chromatographic assay for gentamicin in presence of methylparaben and propylparaben. *Acta Chromatogr.* **2023**, *35*, 81–87. [CrossRef]
115. Ismail, A.F.H.; Mohamed, F.; Rosli, L.M.M.; Shafri, M.A.M.; Haris, M.S.; Adina, A.B. Spectrophotometric Determination of Gentamicin Loaded PLGA Microparticles and Method Validation via Ninhydrin-Gentamicin Complex as a Rapid Quantification Approach. *J. Appl. Pharm. Sci.* **2016**, *6*, 007–014. [CrossRef]
116. D'Souza, S. A Review of In Vitro Drug Release Test Methods for Nano-Sized Dosage Forms. *Adv. Pharm.* **2014**, *2014*, 304757. [CrossRef]
117. D'Souza, S.S.; DeLuca, P.P. Methods to Assess in Vitro Drug Release from Injectable Polymeric Particulate Systems. *Pharm. Res.* **2006**, *23*, 460–474. [CrossRef]
118. Gosau, M.; Müller, B.W. Release of gentamicin sulphate from biodegradable PLGA-implants produced by hot melt extrusion. *Pharmazie* **2010**, *65*, 487–492. [CrossRef] [PubMed]
119. Hetta, H.F.; Ramadan, Y.N.; Al-Harbi, A.I.; Ahmed, E.A.; Battah, B.; Abd Ellah, N.H.; Zanetti, S.; Donadu, M.G. Nanotechnology as a Promising Approach to Combat Multidrug Resistant Bacteria: A Comprehensive Review and Future Perspectives. *Biomedicines* **2023**, *11*, 413. [CrossRef] [PubMed]
120. Imbuluzqueta, E.; Gamazo, C.; Lana, H.; Campanero, M.; Salas, D.; Gil, A.G.; Elizondo, E.; Ventosa, N.; Veciana, J.; Blanco-Prieto, M.J. Hydrophobic gentamicin-loaded nanoparticles are effective against *Brucella melitensis* infection in mice. *Antimicrob. Agents Chemother.* **2013**, *57*, 3326–3333. [CrossRef] [PubMed]
121. Kwiecień, K.; Brzychczy-Włoch, M.; Pamuła, E. Antibiotics modified by hydrophobic ion-pairing—A solution world's problems with resistant bacteria? *Sustain. Mater. Technol.* **2023**, *37*, e00662. [CrossRef]
122. Imbuluzqueta, E.; Elizondo, E.; Gamazo, C.; Moreno-Calvo, E.; Veciana, J.; Ventosa, N.; Blanco-Prieto, M.J. Novel bioactive hydrophobic gentamicin carriers for the treatment of intracellular bacterial infections. *Acta Biomater.* **2011**, *7*, 1599–1608. [CrossRef] [PubMed]

123. Imbuluzqueta, E.; Lemaire, S.; Gamazo, C.; Elizondo, E.; Ventosa, N.; Veciana, J.; Van Bambeke, F.; Blanco-Prieto, M.J. Cellular pharmacokinetics and intracellular activity against *Listeria monocytogenes* and *Staphylococcus aureus* of chemically modified and nanoencapsulated gentamicin. *J. Antimicrob. Chemother.* **2012**, *67*, 2158–2164. [CrossRef] [PubMed]
124. Pudełko, I.; Moskwik, A.; Kwiecień, K.; Kriegseis, S.; Krok-Borkowicz, M.; Schickle, K.; Ochońska, D.; Dobrzyński, P.; Brzychczy-Włoch, M.; Gonzalez-Julian, J.; et al. Porous Zirconia Scaffolds Functionalized with Calcium Phosphate Layers and PLGA Nanoparticles Loaded with Hydrophobic Gentamicin. *Int. J. Mol. Sci.* **2023**, *24*, 8400. [CrossRef] [PubMed]
125. Kwiecień, K.; Pudełko, I.; Knap, K.; Reczyńska-Kolman, K.; Krok-Borkowicz, M.; Ochońska, D.; Brzychczy-Włoch, M.; Pamuła, E. Insight in Superiority of the Hydrophobized Gentamycin in Terms of Antibiotics Delivery to Bone Tissue. *Int. J. Mol. Sci.* **2022**, *23*, 12077. [CrossRef]
126. Rotman, S.G.; Thompson, K.; Grijpma, D.W.; Richards, R.G.; Moriarty, T.F.; Eglin, D.; Guillaume, O. Development of bone seeker–functionalised microspheres as a targeted local antibiotic delivery system for bone infections. *J. Orthop. Translat* **2020**, *21*, 136–145. [CrossRef] [PubMed]
127. Rotman, S.G.; Moriarty, T.F.; Nottelet, B.; Grijpma, D.W.; Eglin, D.; Guillaume, O. Poly(Aspartic Acid) Functionalized Poly(ε-Caprolactone) Microspheres with Enhanced Hydroxyapatite Affinity as Bone Targeting Antibiotic Carriers. *Pharmaceutics* **2020**, *12*, 885. [CrossRef]
128. Elizondo, E.; Sala, S.; Imbuluzqueta, E.; González, D.; Blanco-Prieto, M.J.; Gamazo, C.; Ventosa, N.; Veciana, J. High loading of gentamicin in bioadhesive PVM/MA nanostructured microparticles using compressed carbon-dioxide. *Pharm. Res.* **2011**, *28*, 309–321. [CrossRef] [PubMed]
129. Sande, M.A.; Courtney, K.B. Nafcillin-gentamicin synergism in experimental staphylococcal endocarditis. *J. Lab. Clin. Med.* **1976**, *88*, 118–124. [PubMed]
130. Andriole, V.T. Antibiotic synergy in experimental infection with Pseudomonas. II. The effect of carbenicillin, cephalothin, or cephanone combined with tobramycin or gentamicin. *J. Infect. Dis.* **1974**, *129*, 124–133. [CrossRef] [PubMed]
131. Archer, G.; Fekety, F.R., Jr. Experimental Endocarditis Due to *Pseudomonas aeruginosa*. II. Therapy with Carbenicillin and Gentamicin. *J. Infect. Dis.* **1977**, *136*, 327–335. [CrossRef] [PubMed]
132. World Health Organization. WHO Guidelines for the Treatment of Neisseria Gonorrhoeae. Available online: https://www.who.int/publications/i/item/9789241549691 (accessed on 19 February 2024).
133. Kirkcaldy, R.D.; Weinstock, H.S.; Moore, P.C.; Philip, S.S.; Wiesenfeld, H.C.; Papp, J.R.; Kerndt, P.R.; Johnson, S.; Ghanem, K.G.; Hook, E.W., III; et al. The Efficacy and Safety of Gentamicin Plus Azithromycin and Gemifloxacin Plus Azithromycin as Treatment of Uncomplicated Gonorrhea. *Clin. Infect. Dis.* **2014**, *59*, 1083–1091. [CrossRef] [PubMed]
134. Ren, H.; Liu, Y.; Zhou, J.; Long, Y.; Liu, C.; Xia, B.; Shi, J.; Fan, Z.; Liang, Y.; Chen, S.; et al. Combination of Azithromycin and Gentamicin for Efficient Treatment of *Pseudomonas aeruginosa* Infections. *J. Infect. Dis.* **2019**, *220*, 1667–1678. [CrossRef] [PubMed]
135. Svedholm, E.; Bruce, B.; Parcell, B.J.; Coote, P.J. Repurposing Mitomycin C in Combination with Pentamidine or Gentamicin to Treat Infections with Multi-Drug-Resistant (MDR) *Pseudomonas aeruginosa*. *Antibiotics* **2024**, *13*, 177. [CrossRef]
136. Wang, L.; Di Luca, M.; Tkhilaishvili, T.; Trampuz, A.; Gonzalez Moreno, M. Synergistic Activity of Fosfomycin, Ciprofloxacin, and Gentamicin against *Escherichia coli* and *Pseudomonas aeruginosa* Biofilms. *Front. Microbiol.* **2019**, *10*, 2522. [CrossRef]
137. Oliva, A.; Tafin, U.F.; Maiolo, E.M.; Jeddari, S.; Bétrisey, B.; Trampuz, A. Activities of Fosfomycin and Rifampin on Planktonic and Adherent *Enterococcus faecalis* Strains in an Experimental Foreign-Body Infection Model. *Antimicrob. Agents Chemother.* **2014**, *58*, 1284–1293. [CrossRef]
138. Luther, M.K.; Arvanitis, M.; Mylonakis, E.; LaPlante, K.L. Activity of Daptomycin or Linezolid in Combination with Rifampin or Gentamicin against Biofilm-Forming *Enterococcus faecalis* or *E. faecium* in an In Vitro Pharmacodynamic Model Using Simulated Endocardial Vegetations and an In Vivo Survival Assay Using Galleria mellonella Larvae. *Antimicrob. Agents Chemother.* **2014**, *58*, 4612–4620. [CrossRef]
139. Usman, M.; Marcus, A.; Fatima, A.; Aslam, B.; Zaid, M.; Khattak, M.; Bashir, S.; Masood, S.; Rafaque, Z.; Dasti, J.I. Synergistic Effects of Gentamicin, Cefepime, and Ciprofloxacin on Biofilm of *Pseudomonas aeruginosa*. *Infect. Drug Resist.* **2023**, *16*, 5887–5898. [CrossRef] [PubMed]
140. Tamma, P.D.; Cosgrove, S.E.; Maragakis, L.L. Combination Therapy for Treatment of Infections with Gram-Negative Bacteria. *Clin. Microbiol. Rev.* **2012**, *25*, 450–470. [CrossRef] [PubMed]
141. Fernández-Hidalgo, N.; Almirante, B.; Gavaldà, J.; Gurgui, M.; Peña, C.; de Alarcón, A.; Ruiz, J.; Vilacosta, I.; Montejo, M.; Vallejo, N.; et al. Ampicillin Plus Ceftriaxone Is as Effective as Ampicillin Plus Gentamicin for Treating *Enterococcus faecalis* Infective Endocarditis. *Clin. Infect. Dis.* **2013**, *56*, 1261–1268. [CrossRef] [PubMed]
142. Pericas, J.M.; Cervera, C.; del Rio, A.; Moreno, A.; Garcia de la Maria, C.; Almela, M.; Falces, C.; Ninot, S.; Castañeda, X.; Armero, Y.; et al. Changes in the treatment of *Enterococcus faecalis* infective endocarditis in Spain in the last 15 years: From ampicillin plus gentamicin to ampicillin plus ceftriaxone. *Clin. Microbiol. Infect.* **2014**, *20*, O1075–O1083. [CrossRef] [PubMed]
143. Bustos, P.S.; Deza-Ponzio, R.; Páez, P.L.; Cabrera, J.L.; Virgolini, M.B.; Ortega, M.G. Flavonoids as protective agents against oxidative stress induced by gentamicin in systemic circulation. Potent protective activity and microbial synergism of luteolin. *Food Chem. Toxicol.* **2018**, *118*, 294–302. [CrossRef] [PubMed]
144. Rana, A.; Samtiya, M.; Dhewa, T.; Mishra, V.; Aluko, R.E. Health benefits of polyphenols: A concise review. *J. Food Biochem.* **2022**, *46*, e14264. [CrossRef] [PubMed]
145. Daglia, M. Polyphenols as antimicrobial agents. *Curr. Opin. Biotechnol.* **2012**, *23*, 174–181. [CrossRef] [PubMed]

146. Buchmann, D.; Schultze, N.; Borchardt, J.; Böttcher, I.; Schaufler, K.; Guenther, S. Synergistic antimicrobial activities of epigallocatechin gallate, myricetin, daidzein, gallic acid, epicatechin, 3-hydroxy-6-methoxyflavone and genistein combined with antibiotics against ESKAPE pathogens. *J. Appl. Microbiol.* **2022**, *132*, 949–963. [CrossRef] [PubMed]
147. Xiao, J. Dietary flavonoid aglycones and their glycosides: Which show better biological significance? *Crit. Rev. Food Sci. Nutr.* **2017**, *57*, 1874–1905. [CrossRef]
148. Lima, V.N.; Oliveira-Tintino, C.D.M.; Santos, E.S.; Morais, L.P.; Tintino, S.R.; Freitas, T.S.; Geraldo, Y.S.; Pereira, R.L.S.; Cruz, R.P.; Menezes, I.R.A.; et al. Antimicrobial and enhancement of the antibiotic activity by phenolic compounds: Gallic acid, caffeic acid and pyrogallol. *Microb. Pathog.* **2016**, *99*, 56–61. [CrossRef]
149. Parvez, M.A.K.; Saha, K.; Rahman, J.; Munmun, R.A.; Rahman, M.A.; Dey, S.K.; Rahman, M.S.; Islam, S.; Shariare, M.H. Antibacterial activities of green tea crude extracts and synergistic effects of epigallocatechingallate (EGCG) with gentamicin against MDR pathogens. *Heliyon* **2019**, *5*, e02126. [CrossRef] [PubMed]
150. Lee, Y.S.; Kang, O.H.; Choi, J.G.; Oh, Y.C.; Chae, H.S.; Kim, J.H.; Park, H.; Sohn, D.H.; Wang, Z.T.; Kwon, D.Y. Synergistic effects of the combination of galangin with gentamicin against methicillin-resistant *Staphylococcus aureus*. *J. Microbiol.* **2008**, *46*, 283–288. [CrossRef] [PubMed]
151. Macedo, I.; Silva, J.; Silva, P.; Cruz, B.; Vale, J.; Santos, H.; Bandeira, P.; Souza, E.; Xavier, R.; Coutinho, H.; et al. Structural and Microbiological Characterization of 5-Hydroxy-3,7,4′-Trimethoxyflavone: A Flavonoid Isolated from Vitex gardneriana Schauer Leaves. *Microb. Drug Resist.* **2019**, *25*, 434–438. [CrossRef] [PubMed]
152. Cunningham-Oakes, E.; Soren, O.; Moussa, C.; Rathor, G.; Liu, Y.; Coates, A.; Hu, Y. Nordihydroguaiaretic acid enhances the activities of aminoglycosides against methicillin- sensitive and resistant *Staphylococcus aureus* in vitro and in vivo. *Front. Microbiol.* **2015**, *6*, 1195. [CrossRef] [PubMed]
153. Luo, S.; Kang, X.; Luo, X.; Li, C.; Wang, G. Study on the inhibitory effect of quercetin combined with gentamicin on the formation of *Pseudomonas aeruginosa* and its bioenvelope. *Microb. Pathog.* **2023**, *182*, 106274. [CrossRef]
154. Elssaig, E.; Alnour, T.; Ahmed, E.; Ullah, M.; Abu-Duhier, F. Antimicrobial synergistic effects of dietary flavonoids rutin and quercetin in combination with antibiotics gentamicin and ceftriaxone against *E. coli* (MDR) and *P. mirabilis* (XDR) strains isolated from human infections: Implications for food–medicine interactions. *Ital. J. Food Sci.* **2022**, *34*, 34–42. [CrossRef]
155. Gupta, P.; Sarkar, A.; Sandhu, P.; Daware, A.; Das, M.C.; Akhter, Y.; Bhattacharjee, S. Potentiation of antibiotic against *Pseudomonas aeruginosa* biofilm: A study with plumbagin and gentamicin. *J. Appl. Microbiol.* **2017**, *123*, 246–261. [CrossRef]
156. Sathiya Deepika, M.; Thangam, R.; Sakthidhasan, P.; Arun, S.; Sivasubramanian, S.; Thirumurugan, R. Combined effect of a natural flavonoid rutin from *Citrus sinensis* and conventional antibiotic gentamicin on *Pseudomonas aeruginosa* biofilm formation. *Food Control* **2018**, *90*, 282–294. [CrossRef]
157. Mun, S.H.; Kang, O.H.; Joung, D.K.; Kim, S.B.; Seo, Y.S.; Choi, J.G.; Lee, Y.S.; Cha, S.W.; Ahn, Y.S.; Han, S.H.; et al. Combination Therapy of Sophoraflavanone B against MRSA: In Vitro Synergy Testing. *Evid. Based Complement. Alternat Med.* **2013**, *2013*, 823794. [CrossRef]
158. Das, M.C.; Sandhu, P.; Gupta, P.; Rudrapaul, P.; De, U.C.; Tribedi, P.; Akhter, Y.; Bhattacharjee, S. Attenuation of *Pseudomonas aeruginosa* biofilm formation by Vitexin: A combinatorial study with azithromycin and gentamicin. *Sci. Rep.* **2016**, *6*, 23347. [CrossRef]
159. Bustos, P.S.; Deza-Ponzio, R.; Páez, P.L.; Albesa, I.; Cabrera, J.L.; Virgolini, M.B.; Ortega, M.G. Protective effect of quercetin in gentamicin-induced oxidative stress in vitro and in vivo in blood cells. Effect on gentamicin antimicrobial activity. *Environ. Toxicol. Pharmacol.* **2016**, *48*, 253–264. [CrossRef] [PubMed]
160. Caesar, L.K.; Cech, N.B. Synergy and antagonism in natural product extracts: When 1 + 1 does not equal 2. *Nat. Prod. Rep.* **2019**, *36*, 869–888. [CrossRef] [PubMed]
161. Freitas, A.S.; Cunha, A.; Oliveira, R.; Almeida-Aguiar, C. Propolis antibacterial and antioxidant synergisms with gentamicin and honey. *J. Appl. Microbiol.* **2022**, *132*, 2733–2745. [CrossRef] [PubMed]
162. Sookkhee, S.; Sakonwasun, C.; Mungkornasawakul, P.; Khamnoi, P.; Wikan, N.; Nimlamool, W. Synergistic Effects of Some Methoxyflavones Extracted from Rhizome of *Kaempferia parviflora* Combined with Gentamicin against Carbapenem-Resistant Strains of *Klebsiella pneumoniae*, *Pseudomonas aeruginosa*, and *Acinetobacter baumannii*. *Plants* **2022**, *11*, 3128. [CrossRef] [PubMed]
163. Rosato, A.; Carocci, A.; Catalano, A.; Clodoveo, M.L.; Franchini, C.; Corbo, F.; Carbonara, G.G.; Carrieri, A.; Fracchiolla, G. Elucidation of the synergistic action of *Mentha piperita* essential oil with common antimicrobials. *PLoS ONE* **2018**, *13*, e0200902. [CrossRef] [PubMed]
164. Stefanovic, O.; Stankovic, M.; Čomić, L. In vitro antibacterial efficacy of *Clinopodium vulgare* L. extracts and their synergistic interaction with antibiotics. *J. Med. Plant Res.* **2011**, *5*, 4074–4079.
165. Kuok, C.F.; Hoi, S.O.; Hoi, C.F.; Chan, C.H.; Fong, I.H.; Ngok, C.K.; Meng, L.R.; Fong, P. Synergistic antibacterial effects of herbal extracts and antibiotics on methicillin-resistant *Staphylococcus aureus*: A computational and experimental study. *Exp. Biol. Med.* **2017**, *242*, 731–743. [CrossRef]

Disclaimer/Publisher's Note: The statements, opinions and data contained in all publications are solely those of the individual author(s) and contributor(s) and not of MDPI and/or the editor(s). MDPI and/or the editor(s) disclaim responsibility for any injury to people or property resulting from any ideas, methods, instructions or products referred to in the content.

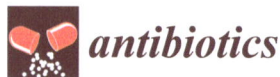 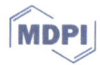

Article

Chlorhexidine-Containing Electrospun Polymeric Nanofibers for Dental Applications: An *In Vitro* Study

Luana Dutra de Carvalho [1], Bernardo Urbanetto Peres [2], Ya Shen [3], Markus Haapasalo [3], Hazuki Maezono [4], Adriana P. Manso [1], Frank Ko [5], John Jackson [6,*] and Ricardo M. Carvalho [2]

[1] Department of Oral Health Sciences, Division of Restorative Dentistry, Faculty of Dentistry, University of British Columbia, 2199 Wesbrook Mall, Vancouver, BC V6T 1Z3, Canada; luanadc@dentistry.ubc.ca (L.D.d.C.); amanso@dentistry.ubc.ca (A.P.M.)

[2] Department of Oral Biological and Medical Sciences, Division of Biomaterials, Faculty of Dentistry, University of British Columbia, 2199 Wesbrook Mall, Vancouver, BC V6T 1Z3, Canada; buperes@gmail.com (B.U.P.); rickmc@dentistry.ubc.ca (R.M.C.)

[3] Department of Oral Health Sciences, Division of Endodontics, Faculty of Dentistry, University of British Columbia, 2199 Wesbrook Mall, Vancouver, BC V6T 1Z3, Canada; yashen@dentistry.ubc.ca (Y.S.); markush@dentistry.ubc.ca (M.H.)

[4] Department of Restorative Dentistry and Endodontology, Graduate School of Dentistry, Osaka Dental University, Osaka 565-0871, Japan; maezono.hazuki.dent@osaka-u.ac.jp

[5] Department of Materials Engineering, Faculty of Applied Sciences, University of British Columbia, 309-6350 Stores Road, Vancouver, BC V6T 1Z4, Canada; frank.ko@ubc.ca

[6] Faculty of Pharmaceutical Sciences, University of British Columbia, 2405 East Mall, Vancouver, BC V6T 1Z3, Canada

* Correspondence: jackson@mail.ubc.ca

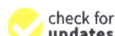

Citation: de Carvalho, L.D.; Peres, B.U.; Shen, Y.; Haapasalo, M.; Maezono, H.; Manso, A.P.; Ko, F.; Jackson, J.; Carvalho, R.M. Chlorhexidine-Containing Electrospun Polymeric Nanofibers for Dental Applications: An *In Vitro* Study. *Antibiotics* **2023**, *12*, 1414. https:// doi.org/10.3390/antibiotics12091414

Academic Editor: Anisha D'Souza

Received: 1 August 2023
Revised: 29 August 2023
Accepted: 1 September 2023
Published: 6 September 2023

Copyright: © 2023 by the authors. Licensee MDPI, Basel, Switzerland. This article is an open access article distributed under the terms and conditions of the Creative Commons Attribution (CC BY) license (https:// creativecommons.org/licenses/by/ 4.0/).

Abstract: Chlorhexidine is the most commonly used anti-infective drug in dentistry. To treat infected void areas, a drug-loaded material that swells to fill the void and releases the drug slowly is needed. This study investigated the encapsulation and release of chlorhexidine from cellulose acetate nanofibers for use as an antibacterial treatment for dental bacterial infections by oral bacteria *Streptococcus mutans* and *Enterococcus faecalis*. This study used a commercial electrospinning machine to finely control the manufacture of thin, flexible, chlorhexidine-loaded cellulose acetate nanofiber mats with very-small-diameter fibers (measured using SEM). Water absorption was measured gravimetrically, drug release was analyzed by absorbance at 254 nm, and antibiotic effects were measured by halo analysis in agar. Slow electrospinning at lower voltage (14 kV), short target distance (14 cm), slow traverse and rotation, and syringe injection speeds with controlled humidity and temperature allowed for the manufacture of strong, thin films with evenly cross-meshed, uniform low-diameter nanofibers (640 nm) that were flexible and absorbed over 600% in water. Chlorhexidine was encapsulated efficiently and released in a controlled manner. All formulations killed both bacteria and may be used to fill infected voids by swelling for intimate contact with surfaces and hold the drug in the swollen matrix for effective bacterial killing in dental settings.

Keywords: nanofiber; controlled release preparation; chlorhexidine; anti-bacterial

1. Introduction

Electrospun nanofibers are finding uses as effective drug-delivery biomaterials. The nanoscale properties of these fibers offer the advantage of creating fiber mats with flexibility for good handling and a considerable increase in contact surface area. This allows for improved adhesion to tissues, making these mats attractive for numerous applications in health sciences [1].

Electrospinning is the most popular method for nanofiber production due to the ease of equipment handling and the versatility of the composition of polymeric solutions [2]. The potential application of nanofibers in various fields of dentistry has been investigated, very often as drug release systems, using a wide variety of polymers and drugs [3–8].

Souza et al. [8] review anti-infective nanofiber technology that describes all the work conducted with numerous antibiotics, including tetracycline, ciprofloxacin, metronidazole, minocycline and doxycycline, for dental applications. Depending on the polymers employed for nanofiber production, the release can be controlled by different mechanisms (diffusion or diffusion with the degradation of the matrix) [9]. Certain dental applications require an antibiotic delivery system to be highly flexible, swell in aqueous media, and be easily squeezed into voids, such as root canal channels or caries decay sites [8]. For nanofiber systems, this might be achieved with more hydrophilic, cellulose-based polymers electrospun with small-diameter fibers to maximize flexibility and surface area for rapid wetting/swelling. This water absorption would be limited by void space and not create any significant hydrodynamic pressure.

Chlorhexidine is one of the most commonly prescribed antiseptic agents in dental fields. It has long-lasting antibacterial activity compared to other similar agents, with broad-spectrum action, and it has been shown to reduce plaque, gingival inflammation and bleeding [10–12]. Despite a recent systematic review that highlighted the resistance of some microorganisms to chlorhexidine, chlorhexidine rinses favor the resolution of microbial dysbiosis by lowering community diversity and promoting widespread reductions in bacterial genera [13]. Its use is considered a powerful co-adjuvant to mechanical oral hygiene [14]. Several studies have proposed its use as an enzyme inhibitor to reduce collagen degradation [15–19]. Although chlorhexidine may combat collagen degradation and provide benefits to dentin [20], it may present some adverse effects when used in mouthwashes with concentrations higher than 0.2%, which may limit its use in the required extended residence time of the agent in the oral setting [12]. Generally, chlorhexidine application in a cavity is in liquid or gel form, making it difficult to control the amount of agent remaining in the cavity. In these application forms, the chlorhexidine available is restricted to that in contact with the exposed area, and a depot reservoir to supply additional chlorhexidine for long-term action is not presently available. Moreover, any other bioactive agent to be applied would need a separate procedure.

Cellulose acetate is a biocompatible polymer conducive to electrospinning into flexible mats [21–27]. The material has uses in dentistry as a composite membrane [28] or in the form of electrospun membranes [26,27]. Antibiotic-loaded cellulose acetate electrospun membranes were shown to be effective treatments for diabetic wound treatment [29], underlining the long-term compatibility of the material with sensitive tissues. The objective of this study was to investigate the encapsulation and release of chlorhexidine from cellulose acetate nanofibers for use as an antibacterial treatment for dental bacterial infections by oral bacteria *Streptococcus mutans* and *Enterococcus faecalis*. Because such fibers would likely release the chlorhexidine rapidly, a titanium binding agent was incorporated into the CA fiber mats to slow the release of the drug.

2. Results

2.1. Morphological Characterization

SEM images showed randomly oriented fibers in all groups. The mean fiber diameter (±standard deviation) of all groups is presented in Table 1.

Table 1. Mean fiber diameter (nm) present in the different mats.

CA-PEO	CA-TTE	CA-CHX 0.3	CA-CHX 1.2	CA-PEO POST-SPIN
588 (±57)	600 (±54)	569 (±76)	613 (±122)	584 (±62)

CA-PEO: Cellulose acetate and Polyethylene oxide; CA-TTE: Cellulose acetate, Polyethylene oxide and Titanium triethanolamine linker; CA-CHX 0.3: Cellulose acetate, Polyethylene oxide, Titanium triethanolamine linker and Chlorhexidine diacetate powder at wt% 0.3; CA-CHX 1.2: Cellulose acetate, Polyethylene oxide, Titanium triethanolamine linker and Chlorhexidine diacetate powder at wt% 1.2; CA-PEO POST-SPIN: Cellulose acetate and Polyethylene oxide immersed in 5% (w/v) Chlorhexidine digluconate aqueous solution binded via the Titanium triethanolamine.

One-way ANOVA analysis showed that the different formulations of the fibers produced did not result in different fiber diameters ($p > 0.05$). Figures 1–5 show nanofibers from the five experimental groups under three magnifications each.

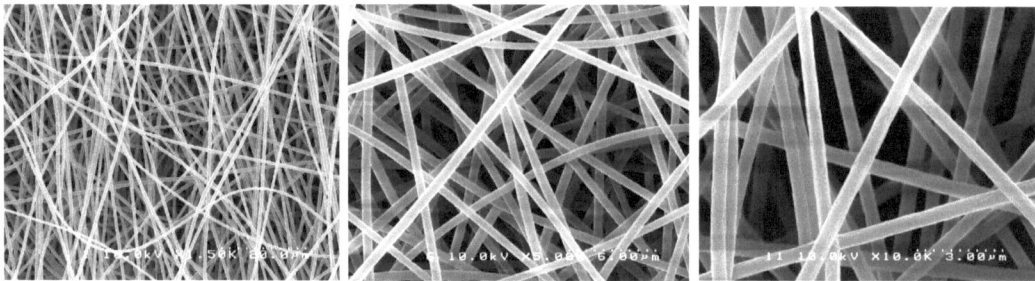

Figure 1. SEM photomicrographs of CA-PEO mats under different magnifications.

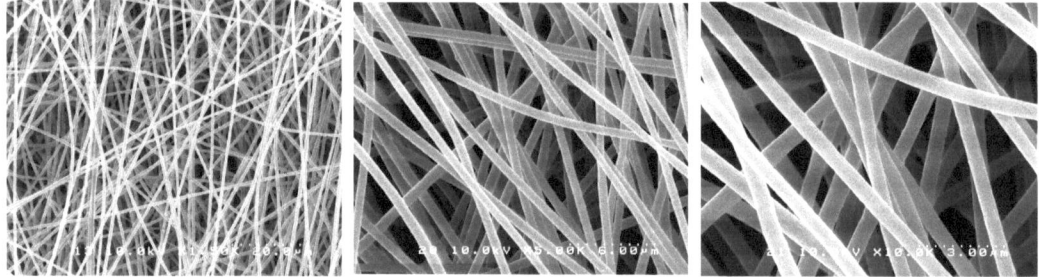

Figure 2. SEM photomicrographs of CA-TTE mats under different magnifications.

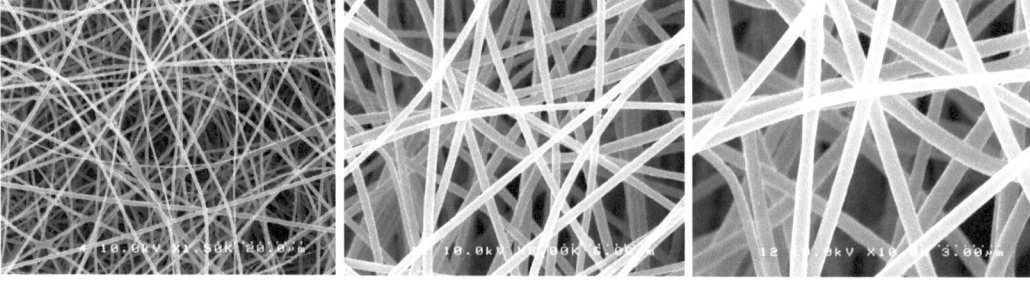

Figure 3. SEM photomicrographs of CA-CHX 0.3 mats under different magnifications.

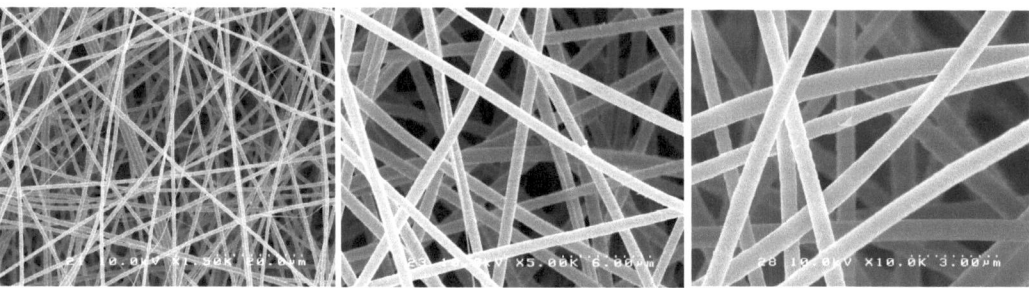

Figure 4. SEM photomicrographs of CA-CHX 1.2 mats under different magnifications.

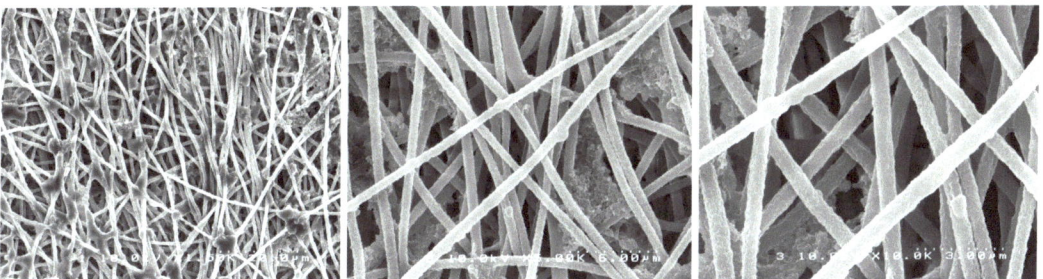

Figure 5. SEM photomicrographs of CA-PEO with post-spin treatment mats under different magnifications.

2.2. Nanofiber Mat Water Absorption

All nanofiber mats absorbed water rapidly, reaching levels of approximately 600% within 5 min followed by minor increases in water absorption over the next two hours. There was little difference in water absorption between fiber mats, but the chlorhexidine-soaked mats showed slightly higher absorption levels that were significant at the two- and three-hour time points ($p < 0.05$) (Figure 6).

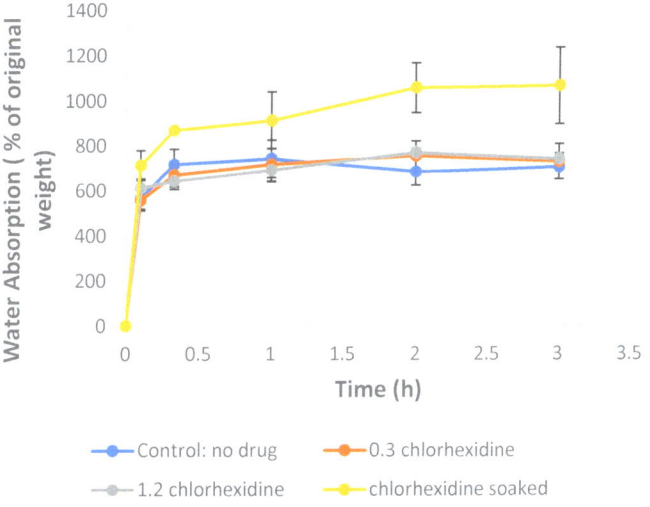

Figure 6. Water absorption of chlorhexidine-loaded cellulose acetate nanofiber mats (0.3 and 1.2 indicate the loading % of chlorhexidine in cellulose acetate).

2.3. Drug Release

Chlorhexidine release from the different mats was characterized by a burst phase over the first 2 h, followed by a slow release over the rest of the experiment (Figure 7). The mats containing 1.2 wt% chlorhexidine showed statically higher increased release when compared to the other groups in the first 2 h. However, the release from the group where the fibers received the post-spin treatment was higher over time, showing the ability to still release a certain amount of CHX after the three months (last data), which is significantly higher when compared to the other groups ($p < 0.05$).

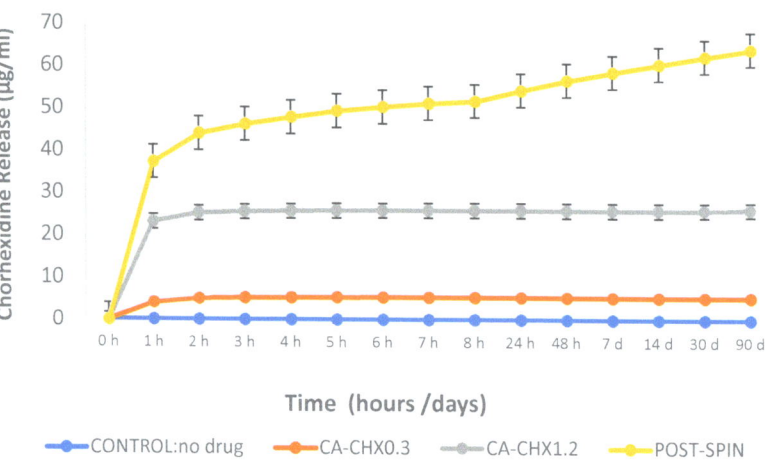

Figure 7. Release of chlorhexidine (μg/mL) from the nanofiber mats.

2.4. Antibacterial Assay

The antibacterial assay showed that inhibition halos were formed against *S. mutans* and *E. faecalis* in all mats containing chlorhexidine (Figures 8–10). The mats with 1.2 wt% of the drug and the one treated after the spinning process showed statistically higher inhibition than both the positive control (chlorhexidine solution at 300 μg/mL) and the mats with 0.3 wt% of the drug ($p < 0.05$). In general, the inhibition was higher against *S. mutans* than *E. faecalis* for all groups containing CHX. The initial concentration calculated for *S. mutans* was 5.0×10^8 CFU/mL, and for *E. faecalis*, it was 1.2×10^8 CFU/mL. A comparison of the size of the diameter of the halos are represented graphically (Figures 8 and 9) and through images (Figure 10A,B).

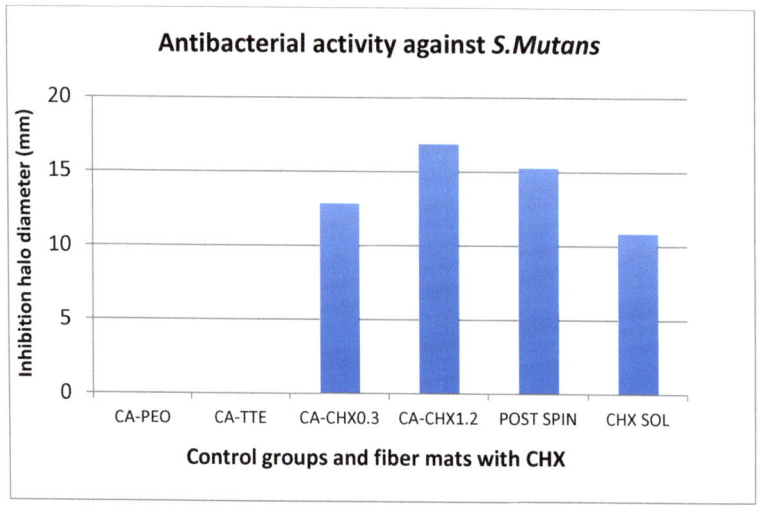

Figure 8. Comparison of the size of the inhibition halos against *S. mutans* formed around the different fiber mats and controls.

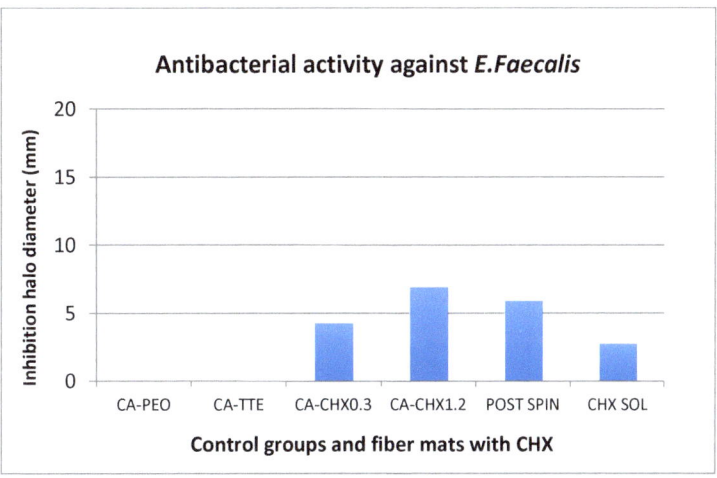

Figure 9. Comparison of the size of the inhibition halos against *E. faecalis* formed around the different fiber mats and controls.

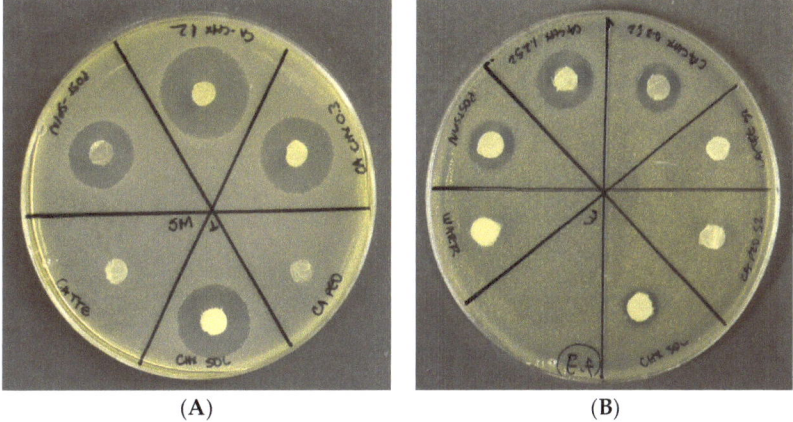

Figure 10. The inhibition halos observed when the experimental mats were applied against *S. mutans* (**A**) and *E. faecalis* (**B**).

2.5. Minimum Bactericidal Concentration

The concentration of chlorhexidine solution to prevent the dental biofilm bacteria growth was detected with solutions at 270 µg/mL and 27 µg/mL. The MBC value was determined to be 2.7 µg/mL against the plaque bacteria.

3. Discussion

Cellulose and derivates are polymers often used for nanofiber production through the electrospinning process [21,22]. A great number of publications have suggested the use of cellulose acetate nanofibers for biomedical applications [23–25] and often specifically for dental applications [26,27]. Furthermore, depending on the application, it can be blended with other polymers to control drug diffusion and release and is a suitable matrix for the incorporation of antimicrobial compounds [24,25,30,31]. Cellulose acetate has been described as a suitable biomaterial for obtaining a prolonged drug release from cast films [32], suggesting the potential for similar properties from nanofiber mats. The strategy of incorporating a drug into the fibers may be achieved in a number of ways: by evenly distributing or dissolving the active agent in the polymer solution before electrospinning, by confining the active agent in the core of the fiber through coaxial electrospinning, by encapsulating the active agent in nanostructures before dispersing them in the electrospinning solution, by post-treatment of the fiber after electrospinning to convert a precursor to its active form, or the attachment of the active agent onto the fiber surface [33]. In most studies to date, the active agents are blended into the polymer solutions before electrospinning [34]. This technique is simple and able to accommodate a large range of active agents, and the resultant fibers tend to release the active agents in a burst fashion (essential for the initial bacterial killing) followed by a slower release to top up and maintain the bactericidal concentration.

For this investigation, we used a similar method to Chen et al. [35] who encapsulated chlorhexidine into cellulose acetate nanofibers with an average diameter of 950 nm. The use of a commercial electrospinning machine in this study allowed for much finer control of spinning conditions than the lab-assembled systems used by others. We found that using high polymer concentrations in DMF (6%) with the control of chamber humidity and temperature and lower voltage (14 kV), shorter target distance (14 cm), and slower drum rotation with spinning over extended times (12 h) allowed for the production of much smaller-diameter nanofibers in very smooth easy-to-handle sheets. The optimal solution concentration choice was based on a pilot study where the concentrations of 3, 5, and 6 wt% of CA were tested with 0.2 or 0.3 wt% of PEO. The 6 wt% CA and 0.2 wt% PEO were very stable and with suitable viscosity, producing a mat with the best characteristics. It is known that fiber diameter has a direct impact on fiber properties and may eventually influence drug release profiles [34,36]. The task of transforming polymeric solutions into nanofibers is governed by factors related to the process itself, the environment, and factors related to the polymeric solution, such as the choice of solvent, viscosity, and polymer concentration. Although "nano" is normally meant to mean a size range under 100 nm, most of the publications have applied the term "nanofibers" for their fabrics, even in cases where the average diameters were 200–800 nm (submicron), obtained in major works where cellulose acetate fibers were produced by electrospinning, and also in our experiment. The fibers formed were uniform, well distributed, and free of beads, and the mats were easy to handle. The drug incorporation did not interfere with the fiber characteristics. In this study, by using a commercial electrospinning machine, fine control over all spinning parameters was allowed, and very slow overnight spinning was found to give optimal lower-diameter fibers formed into easy-to-handle mats. The manufacturing process was considered a great success, as following many trial-and-error pilot studies, the effective encapsulation of chlorhexidine in usable nanofiber mats was achieved. Furthermore, these mats allowed for the release of the drug and provided excellent antibacterial effects against two particularly problematic dental bacteria.

The antibacterial action of these nanofiber formulations of chlorhexidine was tested against common oral pathogens, frequently related to active carious lesions or dental infections. Dental biofilm may contain thousands of different bacteria, so it was interesting to assess a bactericidal concentration for a culture of these bacteria because a nanofiber formulation might encounter preexisting biofilm deposits on teeth rather than low-level infection with just one or two bacteria. In our studies, all plaque bacteria were killed using a chlorhexidine concentration of 27 μg/mL. The specific bacteria *S. mutants* and *E. faecalis* are particularly difficult to kill using chlorhexidine with high MBC values, often reported to be close to 100 μg/mL for both bacteria [35,37]. Certainly, then, any drug released from nanofibers should be able to maintain concentrations above this value for some time after placement to achieve the initial first killing of localized infections [8]. In this study, the nanofiber formulations released the drug into release media at levels reaching 5–25 μg/mL over 24 h, but this was into 20 mL release media. These mats measured 5 cm by 1 cm and when moist, this size of film was easily manipulated down into a wet ball so that inside a void, slow drug diffusion from the inside of such a mass might help maintain anti-infective concentrations at the interface with tissues where drug clearance mechanisms would normally reduce drug concentration. A particular limitation of this study is that no animal studies were possible to test the practical application of these nanofiber mats, so these projections of *in vivo* application and effective void concentrations are speculative.

The nanofiber mats containing either low (0.3 wt%) or high (1.2 wt%) loadings of chlorhexidine were able to effectively eliminate both bacteria in agar plate tests with a similar efficiency to chlorhexidine alone (Figures 8–10).

Since chlorhexidine remains the gold-standard antiseptic in dentistry, being able to act in several dental fields [14], many authors have tried to maintain the chlorhexidine release for long periods through many different strategies, including nanofiber technology [38–45]. In this study, it is assumed that the high levels of drug release after placement in a moist dental void setting would achieve bactericidal concentrations and the compressed swollen mat would retain the released drug in the matrix to maintain the high local concentration. This scenario is totally different from the use of chlorhexidine solution washing of tissue surfaces where the drug is clearly washed away from the target area rapidly.

This study, despite the limitations related to the use of the electrospinning method, which may generate fiber mats with slightly different characteristics among the samples and the simple method of drug incorporation, successfully provided the manufacture of biocompatible drug-loaded nanofiber mats that might allow for easy dry placement (forceps pushing fibers into void) so that the matrix would absorb enough water, fill the void, release chlorhexidine and ensure immediate contact with potentially infected tissue surfaces. The experiments described in this paper are considered fundamental studies to generate evidence for future research.

4. Materials and Methods

4.1. Nanofiber Mat Production

The fibers were produced from a solution containing cellulose acetate Mn ~ 50,000 (CA) and Polyethylene oxide Mw ~ 5,000,000 (PEO) (Sigma-Aldrich, St. Louis, MO, USA), the latter essential to provide the appropriate viscosity of the solution to allow for the formation of the fibers. The polymers were dissolved in N, N-Dimethylformamide (DMF, Fisher Scientific, Waltham, MA, USA), considered a suitable solvent for CA and chlorhexidine powder (CHX). First, the high-molecular-weight PEO (24 mg or 0.2 wt%) was dissolved in a beaker with 12 g of DMF and stirred at 350 rpm at 60 °C for 30 min. After the achievement of a clear solution, 720 mg (6 wt%) of the cellulose acetate powder was added, mixed with a metal spatula and left stirring for 45 min at 60 °C. For the control group 1 (CA-PEO), the clear solution was transferred to a 10 mL plastic syringe to fit in a Nanofiber Electrospinning Unit (NEU–Kato Tech, Kyoto, Japan) to start the electrospinning process. For the groups that received chlorhexidine, titanium triethanolamine was included in the formulation to potentially bind the drug and potentially slow the rate of drug release. A volume of 10 mL of the CA-PEO-DMF solutions was added to 0.1 mL (1 wt%) of Tyzor®TE (TTE) (80 wt% titanium triethanolamine in isopropanol), and different amounts of chlorhexidine diacetate were added according to each group (0.3 wt% or 1.2 wt%) and stirred for 10 min at 90 °C. The second control group received TTE but did not receive CHX. The electrospinning parameters were applied voltage of 14 kV; distance between the needle tip and the collector plate of 14 cm; target speed of 1.0 m/min; and traverse speed of 1 cm/min. The syringe pump speed was 0.065 mm/min. Temperature and humidity in the chamber were monitored. Air humidity was kept under 30%, controlled by a dryer unit, and temperature varied between 24 °C and 27 °C. The collector plate was covered with an aluminum foil, the fibers were produced over 12 h in a random mode, and no attempt to align them was made. The formed fiber mats were gently removed from the collector plate and stored in a sealed plastic bag away from heat and humidity until use.

The last experimental group was obtained with a post-spin treatment of the CA-PEO fiber mats with a chlorhexidine solution. The electrospun fiber mats obtained from 6 wt% CA and 0.2 wt% PEO were immersed for 1 h in 10 wt% titanium triethanolamine solution in isopropanol, which was obtained by dilution of the TTE solutions supplied by the manufacturer. The fiber meshes were cured in an oven at 110 °C for 10 min to bind TTE to CA. The fibers were then rinsed with water several times and dried. The resulting fibers were placed in 5% (w/v) chlorhexidine digluconate aqueous solution for 1 h and cured at 90 °C for 30 min to immobilize the CHX via the titanate linkers. The treated fibers were rinsed with water several times and dried under vacuum to constant weight.

Based on the composition/treatment of the mats, five experimental groups were formed (Table 2). Triplicate fiber mats were produced for each group.

Table 2. Polymers, solvents, and drugs added to the solutions of the experimental groups.

Groups	Composition				
	CA	PEO	TTE	DMF	CHX
CA-PEO	0.78 g	0.025 g	-	12 g	-
CA-PEO-TTE	0.78 g	0.025 g	0.12 g	12 g	-
CA-PEO-TTE-CHX 0.3	0.78 g	0.025 g	0.12 g	12 g	0.038 g
CA-PEO-TTE-CHX 1.2	0.78 g	0.026 g	0.13 g	12 g	0.15 g
CA-PEO-POST-SPIN	0.78 g	0.025 g	-	12 g	Post-spin treatment

CA: Cellulose acetate; PEO: Polyethylene oxide; TTE: Titanium triethanolamine linker; DMF: N,N-Dimethylformamide; CHX: Chlorhexidine diacetate powder.

4.2. Nanofiber Water Absorption Studies

Twenty mg sections of each nanofiber mat were placed on Millipore vacuum filter membranes. These mat sections had been pre-weighed both dry and after wetting followed by vacuum removal of excess water. The mats and filter combination were wetted and left for various times in a Petri dish. The filter and mats were removed from water and tilted with forceps to remove excess water and then vacuum treated for three seconds to remove any obvious remaining excess water. The filter and swollen mats were then weighed before returning to the water. The percentage of water absorption was then simply calculated by the ratio of dry weight to wet weight.

4.3. Morphological Characterization of Nanofibers

The nanofibers' morphological characteristics were initially observed under an optical microscope during the electrospinning process (Nikon Eclipse LV100 Optical Microscope, Tokyo, Japan). Samples were collected on a glass slide placed next to the revolving drum to confirm the production of the fibers. A scanning electron microscope (SEM S-238ON, Hitachi, Tokyo, Japan) was used to evaluate the final electrospun mats with an acceleration voltage of 10 kV. The mats were analyzed to evaluate the structure of the fibers. Randomly selected areas of each mat were cut into 5×5 mm squares and mounted on stubs with carbon tape ($n = 3$). The stubs were then coated with platinum/palladium (Pt/Pd) with an ion sputter coater (Hitachi E-1030 Ion Sputter Coater, Hitachi, Tokyo, Japan). Random images were taken from the selected pieces of each mat. Average fiber diameter was calculated based on 15 random measurements from pictures taken at the same magnification, using image software (ImageJ version 1.54, NIH, Stapelton, NY, USA).

4.4. Chlorhexidine Release Profile

In order to analyze the chlorhexidine released from the fiber mats, samples obtained from each fiber mat (5×1 cm) were immersed in vials with 20 mL of distilled water, which were capped and kept in a mixer machine at 100 rpm. The drug release analysis was performed by removing aliquots of the drug-containing solution from each vial, in specific periods (1 h, 2 h, 3 h, 4 h, 5 h, 6 h, 7 h, 8 h, 24 h, 48 h, 7 d, 14 d, 30 d, and 90 d). After each sampling, the media were replaced with 20 mL of freshwater. Chlorhexidine release was analyzed using UV-visible spectrophotometer (UV-1800, Shimadzu, Kyoto, Japan) with the wavelength for chlorhexidine detection at 254 nm. Chlorhexidine release was presented as µg/mL not a percentage of the total, as it was not possible to determine the total amount of encapsulated drug in the formulations.

4.5. Antibacterial Assay

Streptococcus mutans (NTCC# 10449) and *Enterococcus faecalis* (181) were the dental bacteria used in this study. These bacteria are commonly found in dental biofilms or root canal infections [30]. The preparation of bacterial suspension was conducted with the removal of 20 mL of *S. mutans* from the stock (frozen at $-80\,°C$) of the UBC Endodontics Lab. Bacteria were cultured overnight in 5 mL of brain–heart infusion broth (BHI), at 37 °C in aerobic conditions. After that, 20–50 µL of the overnight culture was put into 8 mL of BHI to obtain another overnight growth solution. On the other hand, the preparation of *E. faecalis* was conducted by the removal of one colony from the stock on BHI agar and placement on a new agar plate in an incubator at 37 °C under aerobic conditions. After the overnight growth, 5–10 colonies were removed from the plate and added to 8 mL of BHI at 37 °C, in aerobic conditions. For the test execution, 500 µL of each diluted bacterial solution (100×) was plated on the new BHI agar plate and left to dry at room temperature. Discs with a 6 mm diameter of the fiber mats were positioned over the smeared bacteria and incubated overnight at 37 °C. Filter paper with water and the CA mats with no drugs were used as the negative control, and filter paper immersed in chlorhexidine solution (concentration 300 µg/mL) was used as the positive control. The fiber mats with different concentrations of chlorhexidine had their antibacterial action tested based on the inhibition halos formed around the discs. After the incubation period, inhibition halos were measured. The experiments were performed in triplicate.

4.6. Minimum Bactericidal Concentration

To determine the minimum bactericidal concentration of chlorhexidine solution (the concentration that reduces bacterial numbers to below an assay detection limit) on a mixed plaque sample, the bacterial suspension was prepared (mix of human plaque plus BHI) with an optical density of 0.1 at 405 nm for a colony-forming unit concentration of approximately 1×10^7 cfu/mL. This was diluted to 1×10^5 cfu and mixed with chlorhexidine at 270, 27, 2.7, 0.27, and 0.027 µg/mL (final concentration). Then, 20 µL of each solution was plated on BHI agar plate (triplicates) to be incubated in aerobic conditions at 37 °C for three days. The minimum concentration of chlorhexidine to prevent the multispecies bacterial growth was determined in the plates where no bacterial colonies were observed.

4.7. Statistical Analysis

Differences in the average fiber diameters, drug release at each period, and inhibition halo diameters were compared using one-way ANOVA for each experiment ($\alpha \leq 0.05$), with the normality test conducted using Shapiro–Wilk test and post hoc Tukey's test to detect significant pairwise comparisons between groups ($p \leq 0.05$). Sigma Plot software version 14.5 (Systat Software, San Jose, CA, USA) was used for statistical analysis.

5. Conclusions

The chlorhexidine-loaded cellulose acetate nanofiber mats developed in this study may offer dentists an improved treatment method over chlorhexidine rinsing of surfaces. Chlorhexidine was encapsulated efficiently and released in a controlled manner. The mats were successful in eliminating *S. mutans* and *E. faecalis*, which are two particularly difficult-to-kill dental bacteria and would swell into a soft gel-like matrix that might enable intimate contact with dental surface for extended periods of time.

Author Contributions: Conceptualization, R.M.C. and A.P.M.; methodology, A.P.M., F.K., R.M.C. and A.P.M.; investigation, L.D.d.C., B.U.P., H.M., J.J., M.H. and Y.S.; writing—original draft preparation, L.D.d.C.; writing—review and editing, J.J., R.M.C. and A.P.M. supervision, R.M.C. project administration, R.M.C. All authors have read and agreed to the published version of the manuscript.

Funding: This research received no external funding.

Institutional Review Board Statement: Not applicable.

Informed Consent Statement: Not applicable.

Data Availability Statement: Not applicable.

Acknowledgments: The authors gratefully acknowledge the support given by the National Council of Scientific and Technological Development (CNPq) and the Ministry of Science, Technology and Innovation, Brazil.

Conflicts of Interest: The authors declare no conflict of interest.

References

1. Leung, V.; Ko, F. Biomedical Applications of Nanofibers. *Polym. Adv. Technol.* **2011**, *22*, 350–365. [CrossRef]
2. Petrik, S. Industrial Production Technology for Nanofibers. In *Nanofibers—Production, Properties and Functional Applications*; Lin, T., Ed.; InTech: Houston, TX, USA, 2011; ISBN 978-953-307-420-7.
3. Lee, J.B.; Park, H.N.; Ko, W.-K.; Bae, M.S.; Heo, D.N.; Yang, D.H.; Kwon, I.K. Poly(L-Lactic Acid)/Hydroxyapatite Nanocylinders as Nanofibrous Structure for Bone Tissue Engineering Scaffolds. *J. Biomed. Nanotechnol.* **2013**, *9*, 424–429. [CrossRef] [PubMed]
4. Albuquerque, M.T.P.; Valera, M.C.; Moreira, C.S.; Bresciani, E.; de Melo, R.M.; Bottino, M.C. Effects of Ciprofloxacin-Containing Scaffolds on Enterococcus Faecalis Biofilms. *J. Endod.* **2015**, *41*, 710–714. [CrossRef] [PubMed]
5. Bottino, M.C.; Kamocki, K.; Yassen, G.H.; Platt, J.A.; Vail, M.M.; Ehrlich, Y.; Spolnik, K.J.; Gregory, R.L. Bioactive Nanofibrous Scaffolds for Regenerative Endodontics. *J. Dent. Res.* **2013**, *92*, 963–969. [CrossRef] [PubMed]
6. Tonglairoum, P.; Ngawhirunpat, T.; Rojanarata, T.; Panomsuk, S.; Kaomongkolgit, R.; Opanasopit, P. Fabrication of Mucoadhesive Chitosan Coated Polyvinylpyrrolidone/Cyclodextrin/Clotrimazole Sandwich Patches for Oral Candidiasis. *Carbohydr. Polym.* **2015**, *132*, 173–179. [CrossRef]
7. Sill, T.J.; von Recum, H.A. Electrospinning: Applications in Drug Delivery and Tissue Engineering. *Biomaterials* **2008**, *29*, 1989–2006. [CrossRef]
8. Sousa, M.G.C.; Maximiano, M.R.; Costa, R.A.; Rezende, T.M.B.; Franco, O.L. Nanofibers as Drug-Delivery Systems for Infection Control in Dentistry. *Expert Opin. Drug Deliv.* **2020**, *17*, 919–930. [CrossRef]
9. Ambrosio, Z.M.H.; Marim, D.O.A.; Neto, P.C.N.; Robles, V.M.V.; Rolim, B.A. *Method and Nanofibres Produced by Electrospinning Containing Active Substances for Controlled Release Cosmetic Application*; World Intellectual Property Organization/WIPO: Geneva, Switzerland, 2014.
10. Brookes, Z.L.S.; Bescos, R.; Belfield, L.A.; Ali, K.; Roberts, A. Current Uses of Chlorhexidine for Management of Oral Disease: A Narrative Review. *J. Dent.* **2020**, *103*, 103497. [CrossRef]
11. Brookes, Z.L.S.; Belfield, L.A.; Ashworth, A.; Casas-Agustench, P.; Raja, M.; Pollard, A.J.; Bescos, R. Effects of Chlorhexidine Mouthwash on the Oral Microbiome. *J. Dent.* **2021**, *113*, 103768. [CrossRef]
12. Poppolo Deus, F.; Ouanounou, A. Chlorhexidine in Dentistry: Pharmacology, Uses, and Adverse Effects. *Int. Dent. J.* **2022**, *72*, 269–277. [CrossRef]
13. do Amaral, G.C.L.S.; Hassan, M.A.; Sloniak, M.C.; Pannuti, C.M.; Romito, G.A.; Villar, C.C. Effects of Antimicrobial Mouthwashes on the Human Oral Microbiome: Systematic Review of Controlled Clinical Trials. *Int. J. Dent. Hyg.* **2023**, *21*, 128–140. [CrossRef] [PubMed]
14. Varoni, E.; Tarce, M.; Lodi, G.; Carrassi, A. Chlorhexidine (CHX) in Dentistry: State of the Art. *Minerva Stomatol.* **2012**, *61*, 399–419. [PubMed]
15. Breschi, L.; Mazzoni, A.; Nato, F.; Carrilho, M.; Visintini, E.; Tjäderhane, L.; Ruggeri, A.; Tay, F.R.; Dorigo, E.D.S.; Pashley, D.H. Chlorhexidine Stabilizes the Adhesive Interface: A 2-Year in Vitro Study. *Dent. Mater.* **2010**, *26*, 320–325. [CrossRef] [PubMed]
16. Carrilho, M.R.O.; Carvalho, R.M.; de Goes, M.F.; di Hipólito, V.; Geraldeli, S.; Tay, F.R.; Pashley, D.H.; Tjäderhane, L. Chlorhexidine Preserves Dentin Bond in Vitro. *J. Dent. Res.* **2007**, *86*, 90–94. [CrossRef]
17. Ricci, H.A.; Sanabe, M.E.; de Souza Costa, C.A.; Pashley, D.H.; Hebling, J. Chlorhexidine Increases the Longevity of in Vivo Resin-Dentin Bonds. *Eur. J. Oral Sci.* **2010**, *118*, 411–416. [CrossRef]
18. Carvalho, R.M.; Manso, A.P.; Geraldeli, S.; Tay, F.R.; Pashley, D.H. Durability of Bonds and Clinical Success of Adhesive Restorations. *Dent. Mater.* **2012**, *28*, 72–86. [CrossRef]
19. Hebling, J.; Pashley, D.H.; Tjäderhane, L.; Tay, F.R. Chlorhexidine Arrests Subclinical Degradation of Dentin Hybrid Layers in Vivo. *J. Dent. Res.* **2005**, *84*, 741–746. [CrossRef]
20. Carrilho, M.R.; Carvalho, R.M.; Sousa, E.N.; Nicolau, J.; Breschi, L.; Mazzoni, A.; Tjäderhane, L.; Tay, F.R.; Agee, K.; Pashley, D.H. Substantivity of Chlorhexidine to Human Dentin. *Dent. Mater.* **2010**, *26*, 779–785. [CrossRef]
21. Ohkawa, K. Nanofibers of Cellulose and Its Derivatives Fabricated Using Direct Electrospinning. *Molecules* **2015**, *20*, 9139–9154. [CrossRef]
22. Christoforou, T.; Doumanidis, C. Biodegradable Cellulose Acetate Nanofiber Fabrication via Electrospinning. *J. Nanosci. Nanotechnol.* **2010**, *10*, 6226–6233. [CrossRef]

23. Khoshnevisan, K.; Maleki, H.; Samadian, H.; Shahsavari, S.; Sarrafzadeh, M.H.; Larijani, B.; Dorkoosh, F.A.; Haghpanah, V.; Khorramizadeh, M.R. Cellulose Acetate Electrospun Nanofibers for Drug Delivery Systems: Applications and Recent Advances. *Carbohydr. Polym.* **2018**, *198*, 131–141. [CrossRef] [PubMed]
24. Castillo-Ortega, M.M.; Montaño-Figueroa, A.G.; Rodríguez-Félix, D.E.; Munive, G.T.; Herrera-Franco, P.J. Amoxicillin Embedded in Cellulose Acetate-Poly (Vinyl Pyrrolidone) Fibers Prepared by Coaxial Electrospinning: Preparation and Characterization. *Mater. Lett.* **2012**, *76*, 250–254. [CrossRef]
25. Liu, X.; Lin, T.; Gao, Y.; Xu, Z.; Huang, C.; Yao, G.; Jiang, L.; Tang, Y.; Wang, X. Antimicrobial Electrospun Nanofibers of Cellulose Acetate and Polyester Urethane Composite for Wound Dressing. *J. Biomed. Mater. Res. Part B Appl. Biomater.* **2012**, *100*, 1556–1565. [CrossRef] [PubMed]
26. Boyd, S.A.; Su, B.; Sandy, J.R.; Ireland, A.J. Cellulose Nanofibre Mesh for Use in Dental Materials. *Coatings* **2012**, *2*, 120–137. [CrossRef]
27. Narang, R.S.; Narang, J.K. Nanomedicines for Dental Applications-Scope and Future Perspective. *Int. J. Pharm. Investig.* **2015**, *5*, 121. [CrossRef] [PubMed]
28. Al-Harbi, N.; Hussein, M.A.; Al-Hadeethi, Y.; Felimban, R.I.; Tayeb, H.H.; Bedaiwi, N.M.H.; Alosaimi, A.M.; Bekyarova, E.; Chen, M. Bioactive Hybrid Membrane-Based Cellulose Acetate/Bioactive Glass/Hydroxyapatite/Carbon Nanotubes Nanocomposite for Dental Applications. *J. Mech. Behav. Biomed. Mater.* **2023**, *141*, 105795. [CrossRef] [PubMed]
29. Samadian, H.; Zamiri, S.; Ehterami, A.; Farzamfar, S.; Vaez, A.; Khastar, H.; Alam, M.; Ai, A.; Derakhshankhah, H.; Allahyari, Z.; et al. Electrospun Cellulose Acetate/Gelatin Nanofibrous Wound Dressing Containing Berberine for Diabetic Foot Ulcer Healing: In Vitro and in Vivo Studies. *Sci. Rep.* **2020**, *10*, 8312. [CrossRef]
30. Ahrari, F.; Eslami, N.; Rajabi, O.; Ghazvini, K.; Barati, S. The Antimicrobial Sensitivity of Streptococcus Mutans and Streptococcus Sangius to Colloidal Solutions of Different Nanoparticles Applied as Mouthwashes. *Dent. Res. J.* **2015**, *12*, 44–49.
31. Sundararaj, S.C.; Al-Sabbagh, M.; Rabek, C.L.; Dziubla, T.D.; Thomas, M.V.; Puleo, D.A. Comparison of Sequential Drug Release in Vitro and in Vivo. *J. Biomed. Mater. Res. Part B Appl. Biomater.* **2016**, *104*, 1302–1310. [CrossRef] [PubMed]
32. Çetin, E.Ö.; Buduneli, N.; Atılhan, E.; Kırılmaz, L. In Vitro Studies on Controlled-Release Cellulose Acetate Films for Local Delivery of Chlorhexidine, Indomethacin, and Meloxicam. *J. Clin. Periodontol.* **2004**, *31*, 1117–1121. [CrossRef] [PubMed]
33. Gao, Y.; Bach Truong, Y.; Zhu, Y.; Louis Kyratzis, I. Electrospun Antibacterial Nanofibers: Production, Activity, and in Vivo Applications. *J. Appl. Polym. Sci.* **2014**, *131*, 40797. [CrossRef]
34. Sun, Y.; Cheng, S.; Lu, W.; Wang, Y.; Zhang, P.; Yao, Q. Electrospun Fibers and Their Application in Drug Controlled Release, Biological Dressings, Tissue Repair, and Enzyme Immobilization. *RSC Adv.* **2019**, *9*, 25712–25729. [CrossRef] [PubMed]
35. Chen, L.; Bromberg, L.; Hatton, T.A.; Rutledge, G.C. Electrospun Cellulose Acetate Fibers Containing Chlorhexidine as a Bactericide. *Polymer* **2008**, *49*, 1266–1275. [CrossRef]
36. Chou, S.-F.; Carson, D.; Woodrow, K.A. Current Strategies for Sustaining Drug Release from Electrospun Nanofibers. *J. Control. Release* **2015**, *220*, 584–591. [CrossRef] [PubMed]
37. Deng, D.M.; Hoogenkamp, M.A.; Exterkate, R.A.M.; Jiang, L.M.; van der Sluis, L.W.M.; ten Cate, J.M.; Crielaard, W. Influence of Streptococcus Mutans on Enterococcus Faecalis Biofilm Formation. *J. Endod.* **2009**, *35*, 1249–1252. [CrossRef]
38. Gonzales, J.R.; Harnack, L.; Schmitt-Corsitto, G.; Boedeker, R.H.; Chakraborty, T.; Domann, E.; Meyle, J. A Novel Approach to the Use of Subgingival Controlled-Release Chlorhexidine Delivery in Chronic Periodontitis: A Randomized Clinical Trial. *J. Periodontol.* **2011**, *82*, 1131–1139. [CrossRef]
39. Priyadarshini, B.M.; Selvan, S.T.; Lu, T.B.; Xie, H.; Neo, J.; Fawzy, A.S. Chlorhexidine Nanocapsule Drug Delivery Approach to the Resin-Dentin Interface. *J. Dent. Res.* **2016**, *95*, 1065–1072. [CrossRef]
40. Shen, C.; Zhang, N.-Z.; Anusavice, K.J. Fluoride and Chlorhexidine Release from Filled Resins. *J. Dent. Res.* **2010**, *89*, 1002–1006. [CrossRef]
41. Stanislawczuk, R.; Reis, A.; Malaquias, P.; Pereira, F.; Farago, P.V.; Meier, M.M.; Loguercio, A.D. Mechanical Properties and Modeling of Drug Release from Chlorhexidine-Containing Etch-and-Rinse Adhesives. *Dent. Mater.* **2014**, *30*, 392–399. [CrossRef]
42. Kwon, T.-Y.; Hong, S.-H.; Kim, Y.K.; Kim, K.-H. Antibacterial Effects of 4-META/MMA-TBB Resin Containing Chlorhexidine. *J. Biomed. Mater. Res. Part B Appl. Biomater.* **2010**, *92*, 561–567. [CrossRef]
43. Seneviratne, C.J.; Leung, K.C.-F.; Wong, C.-H.; Lee, S.-F.; Li, X.; Leung, P.C.; Lau, C.B.S.; Wat, E.; Jin, L. Nanoparticle-Encapsulated Chlorhexidine against Oral Bacterial Biofilms. *PLoS ONE* **2014**, *9*, e103234. [CrossRef] [PubMed]
44. Luo, D.; Zhang, X.; Shahid, S.; Cattell, M.J.; Gould, D.J.; Sukhorukov, G.B. Electrospun Poly(Lactic Acid) Fibers Containing Novel Chlorhexidine Particles with Sustained Antibacterial Activity. *Biomater. Sci.* **2016**, *5*, 111–119. [CrossRef] [PubMed]
45. Arnold, R.R.; Wei, H.H.; Simmons, E.; Tallury, P.; Barrow, D.A.; Kalachandra, S. Antimicrobial Activity and Local Release Characteristics of Chlorhexidine Diacetate Loaded within the Dental Copolymer Matrix, Ethylene Vinyl Acetate. *J. Biomed. Mater. Res. Part B Appl. Biomater.* **2008**, *86*, 506–513. [CrossRef] [PubMed]

Disclaimer/Publisher's Note: The statements, opinions and data contained in all publications are solely those of the individual author(s) and contributor(s) and not of MDPI and/or the editor(s). MDPI and/or the editor(s) disclaim responsibility for any injury to people or property resulting from any ideas, methods, instructions or products referred to in the content.

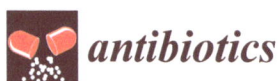

Article

Lyophilized Lipid Liquid Crystalline Nanoparticles as an Antimicrobial Delivery System

Muhammed Awad [1,2,3], Timothy J. Barnes [1] and Clive A. Prestidge [1,*]

[1] Centre for Pharmaceutical Innovation, Clinical and Health Sciences, University of South Australia, Adelaide 5000, Australia; muhammed.awad@mymail.unisa.edu (M.A.); tim.barnes@unisa.edu.au (T.J.B.)
[2] Basil Hetzel Institute for Translational Health Research, Woodville South 5011, Australia
[3] Pharmaceutical Analytical Chemistry, Faculty of Pharmacy, Azhar University, Assiut 71524, Egypt
* Correspondence: clive.prestidge@unisa.edu.au

Abstract: Lipid liquid crystalline nanoparticles (LCNPs) are unique nanocarriers that efficiently deliver antimicrobials through biological barriers. Yet, their wide application as an antimicrobial delivery system is hindered by their poor stability in aqueous dispersions. The production of dried LCNP powder via lyophilization is a promising approach to promote the stability of LCNPs. However, the impact of the process on the functionality of the loaded hydrophobic cargoes has not been reported yet. Herein, we investigated the potential of lyophilization to produce dispersible dry LCNPs loaded with a hydrophobic antimicrobial compound, gallium protoporphyrin (GaPP). The effect of lyophilization on the physicochemical characteristics and the antimicrobial activity of rehydrated GaPP-LCNPs was studied. The rehydrated GaPP-LCNPs retained the liquid crystalline structure and were monodisperse (PDI: 0.27 ± 0.02), with no significant change in nanoparticle concentration despite the minor increase in hydrodynamic diameter (193 ± 6.5 compared to 173 ± 4.2 prior to freeze-drying). Most importantly, the efficacy of the loaded GaPP as an antimicrobial agent and a photosensitizer was not affected as similar MIC values were obtained against *S. aureus* (0.125 µg/mL), with a singlet oxygen quantum yield of 0.72. These findings indicate the suitability of lyophilization to produce a dry form of LCNPs and pave the way for future studies to promote the application of LCNPs as an antimicrobial delivery system.

Keywords: antimicrobial; lyophilization; photodynamic therapy; lipid liquid crystalline; nanoparticles

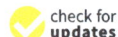

Citation: Awad, M.; Barnes, T.J.; Prestidge, C.A. Lyophilized Lipid Liquid Crystalline Nanoparticles as an Antimicrobial Delivery System. *Antibiotics* **2023**, *12*, 1405. https://doi.org/10.3390/antibiotics12091405

Academic Editor: Anisha D'Souza

Received: 15 August 2023
Revised: 31 August 2023
Accepted: 31 August 2023
Published: 4 September 2023

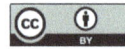

Copyright: © 2023 by the authors. Licensee MDPI, Basel, Switzerland. This article is an open access article distributed under the terms and conditions of the Creative Commons Attribution (CC BY) license (https://creativecommons.org/licenses/by/4.0/).

1. Introduction

The application of lipid-based nanomaterials as a delivery system for therapeutics is a promising approach that can tackle many clinical challenges and promote the efficacy of different therapeutics [1,2]. One promising class of nanomaterials that have shown great potential as a delivery system are lipid liquid crystalline nanoparticles (LCNPs) [3]. The crystalline structure of LCNPs with mesh-like lipid bilayer separated with inner water channels makes them ideal carriers for both hydrophilic and hydrophobic compounds, where hydrophobic molecules are entrapped in the lipid bilayer and hydrophilic compounds are trapped in the water channels [3]. In addition, LCNPs have been shown to efficiently permeate through biological barriers and promote the efficiency of antimicrobial agents [2,4,5]. Recently, we demonstrated that LCNP fabricated from glycerol monooleate (GMO) could promote the potential of gallium protoporphyrin (GaPP) as an antimicrobial against bacterial biofilms [6–8]. GaPP was successfully loaded in the LCNP lipid bilayer, which promoted its antibacterial and photodynamic activities through efficient solubilization and enhancing its delivery into bacterial biofilms [8]. The positive impact of LCNP on the antibacterial activity of GaPP is thought to enable its clinical application as a promising antimicrobial photosensitizer [7].

However, LCNP colloidal dispersions suffer poor long-term stability and cannot be stored at room temperature for extended periods [9], which limits their practical application.

The ester linkage in GMO (Figure 1) is prone to hydrolysis in aqueous solutions [3], which subsequently disrupts the crystalline structure of LCNPs and leads to aggregation of the loaded GaPP in aqueous solutions. Therefore, obtaining LCNPs in a dispersible dry powder is hypothesized to improve the stability and promote the practical application of GaPP-LCNPs [10,11].

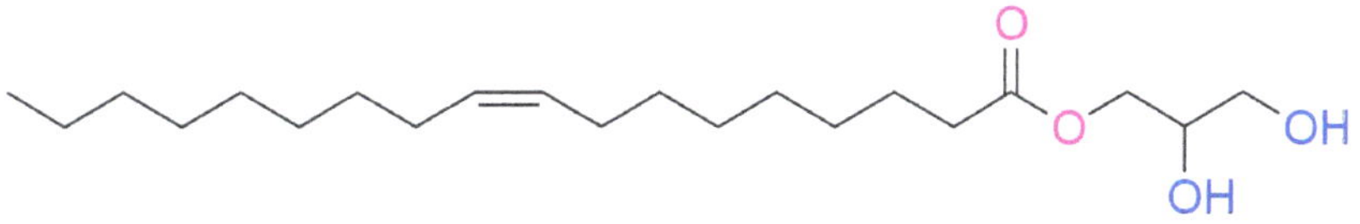

Figure 1. Chemical structure of glycerol monooleate.

Freeze-drying is a simple and more convenient technique to acquire dry powder formulations. Compared to spray drying [11–14], it can be used for heat-sensitive materials and small-volume samples, and it is easy to scale up [11]. During the freeze-drying process, stress is produced that can disrupt the integrity of nanoparticles; thus, cryoprotective agents are added to protect nanoparticles from freezing stress and improve their stability upon storage [11].

Disaccharides have been successfully used as cryoprotectants for biological samples and nanoformulations [15–18]. They are thought to protect the lipid bilayer from stress either by replacing water in the spaces between the hydrophilic groups in the lipid bilayer or by forming a protective amorphous matrix around it [19,20]. Trehalose is among the most renowned cryoprotectants that has been widely used in lyophilization of nanoparticles and biological samples [16,21]. The high safety profile and low molecular size of trehalose has prompted its utilization in this study as it is hypothesized it can enter the water channels of LCNPs and provide the necessary protection to the lipid bilayer [22].

A few studies have investigated lyophilization of LCNPs as a tool to promote its stability and shelf-life [9,22,23]. However, there is still a need to elucidate the effect of freeze-drying on the functionality of LCNPs as a delivery system for photodynamic applications. Hydrophobic photosensitizers such as GaPP tend to form dimers via π-π interactions, which lowers their photodynamic activity [1]. Thus, confirming the integrity of LCNPs' lipid bilayer and the uniform distribution of GaPP in LCNPs after rehydration is essential to validate the use of freeze-drying to obtain dispersible dry GaPP-LCNP formulation. To this end, we investigated the effect of freeze-drying using trehalose as cryoprotectant on the photodynamic activity of GaPP within LCNPs as a proof-of-concept study, which can pave the way for future implementation of GaPP-LCNPs as an antimicrobial agent and a photosensitizer.

2. Materials

Glycerol monooleate (Myverol 18–92 K, Kerry ingredients, product number: 4552180, composed of 95% unsaturated monoglycerides) was kindly donated by DKSH Performance Materials Australia. Gallium protoporphyrin was purchased from Frontier Scientific (Logan, UT, USA). Trehalose, Pluronic F127, propylene glycol, uric acid and methanol with HPLC gradient grade $\geq$ 99.9% were purchased from Sigma Aldrich (St. Louis, MO, USA). Tryptic soy broth (TSB) and agar were purchased from Oxoid Limited; cation-adjusted Muller–Hinton broth was obtained from BD Difco™ (Thermo Fisher Scientific Australia Pty Ltd., Scoresby, VIC, Australia). All the reagents used were of analytical reagent grade, and double-distilled MQ water was used for all experiments conducted.

Staphylococcus aureus Xen 29 bioluminescent strain derived from a parental strain from the American Type Culture Collection (ATCC) (part number: 119240) was kindly gifted by Prof. Allison Cowen. *S. aureus*-Xen29 possesses a stable copy of the *Photorhabdus luminescens* lux operon on the bacterial chromosome.

2.1. Fabrication of Liquid Crystalline Nanoparticle Dispersions

LCNPs loaded with GaPP were prepared as previously described with slight modifications. Briefly, aqueous dispersion of GaPP-LCNPs was prepared in a scintillation glass by mixing glycerol monooleate (15 mg) with 260 µL of propylene glycol and Pluronic F127 (3 mg) and the methanolic solution of GaPP (1.5 mM). Excess methanol was further added to bring the mixture to a homogenous methanolic solution. Following methanol evaporation under N_2 gas, the lipid film was reconstituted using an aqueous solution of 2% w/v trehalose to obtain a final volume of 5 mL. Blank LCNP samples were prepared similarly by omitting GaPP from the formulation.

2.2. Freeze-Drying and Redispersion

LCNP and GaPP-LCNP aqueous dispersions in scintillation glass vials were frozen at $-80\ ^\circ C$ for 24 h. The frozen samples were lyophilized in a Labconco® Dry Ice bench-top freeze dryer overnight. The dry cakes of LCNPs and GaPP-LCNPs were redispersed with MQ water for characterization.

2.3. Determination of Nanoparticle Diameter

The z-average diameter and polydispersity index (PDI) of the nanoparticle dispersions before and after the lyophilization process were determined using Zetasizer Nano ZS (Malvern, Worcestershire, UK). Both LCNP and GaPP-LCNP dispersions were diluted 1:100 in 1 mM KCL, with a refractive index of 1.48, at 25 $^\circ$C. The data reported were the average of three independent formulations.

2.4. Measuring LCNP Concentration

Nanoparticle tracking analysis technique was used to determine the concentrations of blank LCNPs and GaPP-loaded LCNPs before and after lyophilization using Nanosight NS300 (Malvern, Worcestershire, UK) equipped with a blue (405 nm) laser. The samples were diluted 1:100 in Milli-Q water and measured in triplicates at room temperature. The particle motion was recorded using an sCMOS camera, and the data were analyzed using an analysis software (NTA 3.4 Build 3.4.003).

2.5. Quantifying GaPP in LCNPs

The concentration of entrapped GaPP within LCNPs before and after the lyophilization process was determined using spectrofluorimetric assay as previously described [7]. The fluorescent signal of GaPP at 585 nm after excitation at 405 nm was examined to determine the concentration of GaPP using a Fluostar® Omega microplate reader. A calibration curve was plotted in the range between 0.3 and 3 µM with a correlation coefficient of 0.9998. GaPP-LCNP dispersions were centrifuged for 10 min at $31,120\times g$ to separate unentrapped GaPP from GaPP-loaded LCNPs. The supernatant containing GaPP-LCNPs was collected and dissolved in methanol to release GaPP from LCNPs. Aliquots of the released GaPP was further diluted in methanol and the concentration was determined from the corresponding calibration curve.

2.6. Cryogenic Transmission Electron Microscopy

The morphology of GaPP-LCNPs following freeze-drying was imaged using Glacios 200 kV Cryo-TEM (Thermo Fisher Scientific). A total of 5 µL aliquot of GaPP-LCNPs was applied to 300-mesh copper grids that were glow discharged for 30 s. A mixture of liquid ethane/propane was used for sample vitrification, and the samples were kept at $-180\ ^\circ$C during observation. Micrographs were recorded using a NANOSPRT15 camera (Thermo Fisher Scientific) operating a microscope at 120 kV under a bright field. All the reagents used were of analytical reagent grade to avoid any interference with imaging.

2.7. Small-Angle X-ray Scattering (SAXS)

The influence of trehalose on LCNP crystalline structure before and after freeze-drying was determined using small-angle X-ray scattering (SAXS). The measurements were conducted at the Australian Synchrotron (Melbourne, Australia) using a Bruker Nanostar system fitted with an X-ray source operating at 11 keV, 100 mA and Cu-Kα radiation with a wavelength of 1.27 Å. The sample-to-detector length was set to cover the q range (0.05 to 0.4) relevant for these samples, and the scattering pattern was collected using a Pilatus 1M detector.

2.8. Illumination Setup

The illumination setup used for light activation was composed of a blue LED lamp emitting light at 405 nm (M405L4) [7]. Using an aspheric condenser lens (Ø1″, f = 16 mm, NA = 0.79, ARC: 350–700 nm) attached to the LED lamp with an SM1 Lens Tube, 1.00″, the light beam was collimated to illuminate 1 cm² area. A T-Cube LED Driver (LEDD1B) was used to control the output power, which was monitored using a PM100USB power meter connected to a S302C thermal sensor head; all were purchased from Thorlabs (Newton, NJ, USA).

2.9. Determination of Singlet Oxygen Quantum Yield

The singlet oxygen quantum yield (Φ_Δ) following photoactivation of GaPP-LCNPs was determined indirectly using uric acid as a probe [6,24]. Briefly, uric acid (0.12 µM) dissolved in 0.001% v/v Tween 20 was mixed with GaPP-LCNPs (1.2 µM) in a 1 mL quartz cuvette, followed by light activation at an output power of 20 mW/cm². The declines in uric acid absorbance at 291 nm and GaPP-LCNPs at 405 nm were determined every 30 s for 5 min using an Evolution™ 201/220 UV-VIS spectrophotometer. The photodynamic activity was calculated using Equation (1) [6,24]:

$$PA = \frac{\Delta Abs_{(UA)} \times 10^5}{E \times t \times PS} \quad (1)$$

where PA is the photodynamic activity of GaPP; $\Delta Abs_{(UA)}$ is the delta absorbance of uric acid before and after illumination multiplied by a correction factor (10^5) for (t) time; E is the output power of blue light (mW/cm²); and PS is the absorbance of GaPP at an irradiation wavelength of 405 nm following illumination.

Following determination of the photodynamic activity, the singlet oxygen quantum yield was calculated using Equation (2) [6,24]:

$$\Phi_\Delta = \frac{\Phi_\Delta^S}{Y_\Delta^S} Y_\Delta \quad (2)$$

where Φ_Δ is the singlet oxygen quantum yield; Φ_Δ^S is the singlet oxygen quantum yield of the standard photosensitizer, Rose Bengal = 0.79 [25]; Y_Δ^S is the photodynamic activity of Rose Bengal determined using Equation (1); and Y_Δ is the photodynamic activity of GaPP.

2.10. Determination of Antibacterial Activity

The minimum inhibitory concentration (MIC) of GaPP-LCNPs against *S. aureus* Xen 29 before lyophilization and after rehydration was determined using the broth microdilution method as previously described [26]. Briefly, a single colony of *S. aureus* Xen 29 from a freshly streaked agar plate was suspended in TSB overnight. The culture of Xen 29 in TSB broth was adjusted to 0.5 McFarland, followed by 1:100 dilution in cation-adjusted Muller–Hinton broth (CaMHB). Two-fold dilutions of GaPP-LCNPs and blank LCNPs were prepared in CaMHB and mixed with bacterial suspension in 96-well plates (5 technical replicates per plate), and one row containing nanoparticles in CaMHB without bacterial cells served as a blank for the turbidity measurement. MIC was identified as the minimum concentration that inhibited bacterial growth, where no visible bacterial growth or turbidity was detected.

3. Results and Discussion

3.1. Physicochemical Characteristics of LCNP Dispersion and Rehydrated Powder

Herein, we investigated the potential of trehalose in the concentration range between 0.5 and 5% w/v as a cryoprotectant to produce dispersible powder of LCNPs and GaPP-LCNPs. At lower concentrations (0.5% and 1% w/v), sticky masses of LCNPs were formed. However, at higher concentrations (2% and 5% w/v) of trehalose, we obtained dry porous dispersible cakes of LCNPs and GaPP-LCNPs (Figure 2a,b). Upon rehydration, all LCNP blank formulations (0.5–5 w/v%) formed milky white dispersions that were characteristic for LCNPs with no sign of aggregates. On the other hand, sticky masses of GaPP-LCNPs at 0.5% and 1% w/v of trehalose could not be fully dispersed, with GaPP aggregates remaining on the container's wall (see Supplementary Figure S1). However, at higher trehalose concentrations, i.e., 2% and 5% w/v, the dry cakes were efficiently dispersed, forming uniform dispersions (Figure 2d), which implied trehalose conferred effective protection to GaPP-LCNPs at these concentrations that allowed the reformation of GaPP-LCNP dispersions.

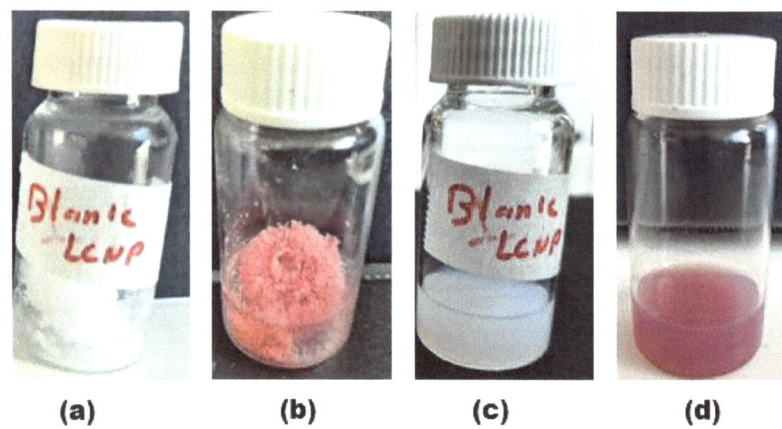

Figure 2. Illustrative images showing the physical appearance of blank LCNPs and GaPP-LCNP dry cakes cryoprotected with 2% w/v trehalose following freeze-drying (**a**,**b**), respectively, and the uniform dispersions (**c**,**d**) after rehydration.

The influence of incorporating trehalose on the hydrodynamic diameters of LCNPs with and without GaPP was investigated, and the diameters of the formulations were compared to the original dispersions without trehalose. In the concentration range between 0.5 and 2 w/v% trehalose, the nanoparticles had a z-average diameter < 200 nm with a polydispersity index (PDI) $\leq$ 0.2, similar to LCNPs prepared without trehalose [6,8]. However, at 5% w/v, the size of LCNPs increased to ~300 nm with a PDI $\geq$ 0.31 (Figure 3). This increase in size could be attributed to the entrapment of trehalose within the water channels of LCNPs.

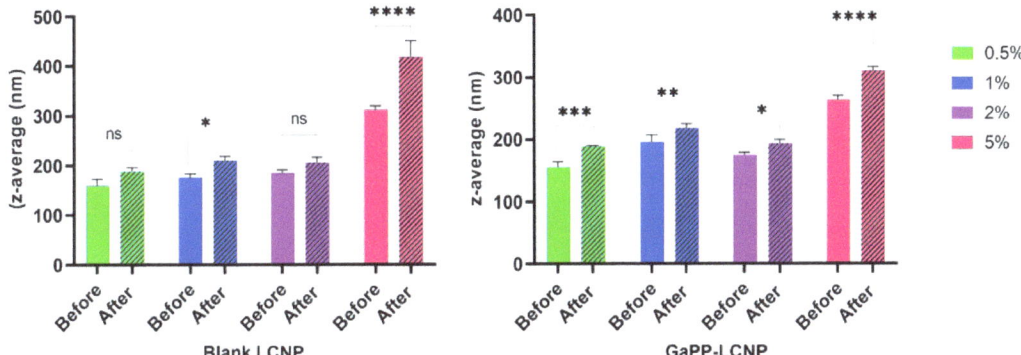

Figure 3. z-average diameter of blank LCNP and GaPP-LCNP dispersions containing trehalose in the concentration range between 0.5 and 5 w/v%. Date are presented as mean ± SD, n = 3; ns: non-significant; * p = 0.03, ** p = 0.006, *** p = 0.0001, and **** p < 0.0001. (Two-way ANOVA test followed by Sidak's multiple comparison test).

The rehydrated LCNPs were larger in size compared to the dispersions before lyophilization. The increase in hydrodynamic diameter was more pronounced in the formulations containing 5% w/v trehalose (p < 0.0001), where the recorded z-average dimeters were 418 ± 33 nm and 312 ± 7 nm for LCNPs and GaPP-LCNPs, respectively, with a PDI ≥ 0.3. On the other hand, formulations containing 2% w/v trehalose had z-average diameters of 206 ± 10.5 nm and 193 ± 6.5 nm for LCNPs and GaPP-LCNPs, respectively, with a PDI ~ 0.2 (see Supplementary Table S1). The better size distribution and smaller hydrodynamic diameter of ~200 nm, in addition to the formation of dispersible cakes, prompted the use of 2% w/v trehalose as a cryoprotectant for GaPP-LCNPs in subsequent investigations.

To further investigate the reproduction of LCNPs following rehydration, we determined LCNPs' concentration (number of nanoparticles/mL) and particle diameter using nanoparticle tracking analysis (NTA). Akin to the hydrodynamic diameter data, NTA showed an increase in the particles' diameter (Figure 4). However, no significant change in nanoparticle concentration was observed (Student's t-test p = 0.4). This indicated that most nanoparticles were redispersed upon rehydration [27], as shown in Table 1.

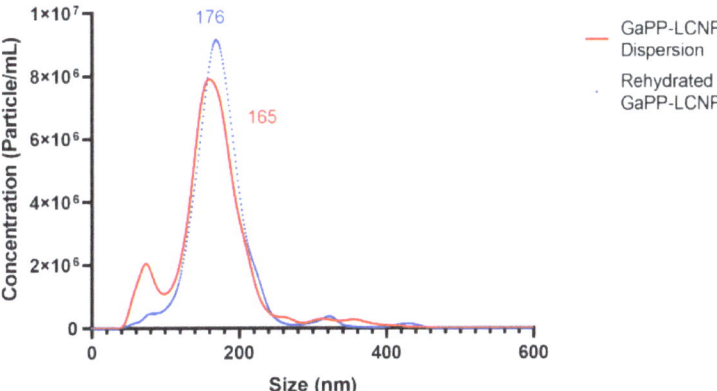

Figure 4. Mean particle diameter of GaPP-LCNPs with trehalose (2% w/v) before lyophilization (red) and after rehydration (blue). Data are presented as the average mean diameter obtained from NTA for 5 runs at 60 S each.

Table 1. Comparison of mean particle diameter and nanoparticle concentration between LCNPs and GaPP-LCNPs before and after lyophilization.

Sample	Original LCNPs		Reconstituted LCNPs	
	Mean Diameter	Concentration of Nanoparticles/mL	Mean Diameter	Concentration of Nanoparticles/mL
Blank LCNPs	154 ± 3.8	$7.8 \times 10^8 \pm 1.1 \times 10^8$	180 ± 5.1	$7.5 \times 10^8 \pm 3.6 \times 10^7$
GaPP-LCNPs	165 ± 4.2	$6.8 \times 10^8 \pm 4.9 \times 10^7$	176 ± 4.3	$6.5 \times 10^8 \pm 2.1 \times 10^7$

The increase in diameter following rehydration can be attributed to the merging of smaller colloidal particles to form larger LCNPs in the reconstitution step. The particle-size distribution curve before lyophilization (red) shows a mean particle diameter of 165 nm and a small peak indicating the presence of nanoparticles with a dimeter lower than 50 nm. However, the small peak disappears in the blue curve representing reconstituted particles with a higher mean diameter of 176 nm, which indicates the formation of larger LCNPs.

3.2. Effect of Freeze-Drying on the Crystalline Structure of LCNPs

Following the investigation of the effect of lyophilization on LCNP particle diameter, we determined its effect on the crystalline structure of LCNPs. Firstly, the morphology of GaPP-LCNPs following rehydration was investigated using Cryo-TEM. The images indicate that GaPP-LCNPs maintained the crystalline mesh-like structure of LCNP lipid bilayer following rehydration (Figure 5).

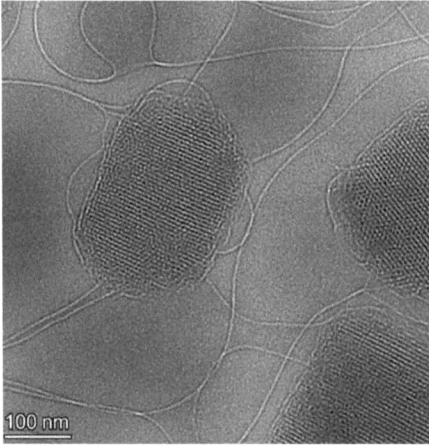

Figure 5. Cryo-TEM images of lyophilized GaPP-LCNPs following redispersion showing the cubic crystalline form of LCNPs with mesh-like lipid bilayer.

Moreover, we used SAXS to determine the influence of trehalose on LCNP crystalline structure. Before the addition of trehalose, LCNPs had an *Im3m* cubic structure at 25 °C, which agrees with previous reports [28–30]. There was no change in the crystalline structure upon the addition of trehalose at all tested concentrations (1, 2 and 5% w/v), where the SAXS profiles showed peaks at $\sqrt{2}$, $\sqrt{4}$, $\sqrt{6}$ and $\sqrt{8}$ that were indicative for primitive cubic *Im3m* phase [31], with a lattice parameter of 121.7 Å compared to 126.5 Å in the absence of sugar. The non-significant effect of trehalose on the internal structure of LCNPs was supported by the scattering peaks observed at the same q-values (Figure 6).

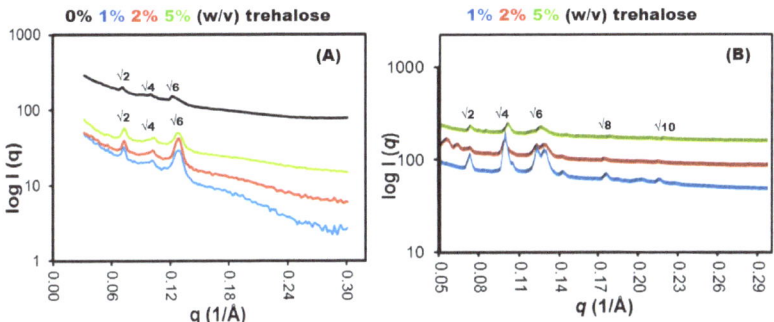

Figure 6. SAXS profiles of LCNPs at 25 °C. (**A**) LCNP before freeze-drying showing q peaks at $\sqrt{2}$, $\sqrt{4}$ and $\sqrt{6}$, indicative for Im3m phase. A value of 0% indicates LCNP without trehalose, while 1%, 2% and 5% *w/v* indicate different trehalose concentrations being tested. (**B**) Represents LCNP regaining the Im3m crystalline structure showing q peaks at $\sqrt{2}$, $\sqrt{4}$ and $\sqrt{6}$.

After redispersion in MQ water, LCNPs regained their *Im3m* crystalline form as demonstrated from the q peaks at $\sqrt{2}$, $\sqrt{4}$, $\sqrt{6}$ and $\sqrt{8}$, with a lattice parameter of 119 Å. The negligible change in lattice parameter and the reformation of the crystalline structure confirm the protective nature of trehalose during lyophilization. Furthermore, these results imply that trehalose did not occupy the space between the polar head groups of the monooleate lipid bilayer as previously reported with liposomes [19,32]; rather, it formed a glassy amorphous matrix around the lipid bilayer. In addition to the retained integrity of LCNPs, the reproduced nanoparticles efficiently entrapped GaPP molecules following the redispersion process, with GaPP entrapment efficiencies of 98.2 ± 3.2% and 99.2 ± 4.2% before and after lyophilization, respectively. It is noteworthy that the efficient entrapment of GaPP within LCNPs was observed when 2 and 5% *w/v* trehalose were used, while a reduction of >15% in the entrapment efficiency was reported at lower trehalose concentrations due to the incomplete redispersion of the formed sticky masses.

3.3. Effect of Lyophilization on the Antimicrobial and Photodynamic Activities of GaPP

The main aim of this study was to promote the stability and shelf-life of GaPP-LCNPs to advance their clinical application. Thus, it was fundamental to probe the activity of GaPP-LCNPs before and after lyophilization. Since GaPP is a metalloporphyrin complex, it can form molecular clusters inside the lipid bilayer through the magnetic properties of metal ions [33]. However, we previously demonstrated that through properly adjusting GaPP to lipid molar ratio, GaPP was uniformly distributed in its monomer form, which improved both the photodynamic and antimicrobial activities of GaPP [6,8]. Therefore, we quantified the singlet oxygen quantum yield (Φ_Δ) of GaPP-LCNPs using Equations (1) and (2). Interestingly, the calculated singlet oxygen value after the addition of 2% *w/v* trehalose was similar to the obtained value with the original formulation (PA = 105 ± 0.85 and Φ_Δ = 0.72). These results confirm the suggested protective mechanism of trehalose by forming a protective matrix without disturbing the integrity of the lipid bilayer.

Following testing the photodynamic activity of GaPP-LCNPs, we investigated the effect of trehalose on the antimicrobial activity of GaPP as an iron mimetic agent. Trehalose did not change the antibacterial activity of GaPP against *S. aureus*; the MIC value of GaPP-LCNPs against *S. aureus* Xen 29 was similar to the original formulation (without trehalose) at 0.125 µg/mL, which was a significantly lower value compared to unformulated GaPP at 0.5 µg/mL. Moreover, rehydrated GaPP-LCNPs retained their antibacterial activity and inhibited bacterial growth at the same concentration (Table 2).

Table 2. Minimum inhibitory concentrations of GaPP in LCNPs before and after lyophilization process compared to unformulated GaPP dissolved in 1% DMSO. The data present better antibacterial activity of GaPP in LCNPs with no affect for the addition of trehalose (n = 6).

Formulation	Unformulated GaPP	GaPP-LCNP (Original)	GaPP-LCNP (2% w/v Trehalose) Before Freeze-Drying	GaPP-LCNP (2% w/v Trehalose) After Rehydration
MIC (μg/mL)	0.5	0.125	0.125	0.125

The better antibacterial activity of GaPP as an iron mimetic agent within LCNPs is attributed to the better solubility of GaPP molecules, which promotes their uptake via hemin receptors on *S. aureus* cell membranes [34], in addition to the curvature of the LCNP lipid bilayer that allows strong fusion abilities of LCNPs with bacterial barriers [35]. The success of rehydrated GaPP-LCNPs in retaining their antibacterial and photodynamic activities is a promising finding that will pave the way for future studies to investigate the shelf-life of LCNP formulations and test their antibacterial activity in more complex in vivo models, which will help scale up the manufacturing of GaPP-LCNPs and facilitate their utilization as a novel antimicrobial.

4. Conclusions

In this study, freeze-drying was used to produce a dry powder of GaPP-LCNPs. To the best of our knowledge, this is the first study to investigate the effect of lyophilization on the functionality of LCNPs loaded with a hydrophobic antimicrobial agent. This study demonstrated the ability of the loaded GaPP to retain its photodynamic and antimicrobial activities following freeze-drying and rehydration. Moreover, trehalose (2% w/v) was proven as an efficient cryoprotective agent for the formulation without altering the physicochemical characteristics. The rehydrated formulations were monodispersed with no significant change in LCNP concentration. Moreover, trehalose efficiently protected LCNPs without affecting the structure of the monooleate lipid bilayer. The efficient protective mechanism of trehalose preserved loaded GaPP with an entrapment efficiency of 99.2 ± 4.2% after rehydration. Most importantly, the functionality of GaPP-LCNPs as an antimicrobial agent and a photosensitizer was not changed after rehydration (Φ_Δ = 0.72, MIC = 125 μg/mL). This study paves the way for future investigations on the shelf-life and storage conditions of LCNP dispersions to promote their application as a delivery system.

Supplementary Materials: The following supporting information can be downloaded at https://www.mdpi.com/article/10.3390/antibiotics12091405/s1, Figure S1: Illustrative images showing the physical appearance of GaPP-LCNP steaky cakes cryoprotected with 0.5% and 1% w/v trehalose following freeze-drying (a & b) respectively and the dispersions (c & d) after rehydration showing some steaky aggregates on the glass vial walls.; Table S1: Summary of z-average diameter and polydispersity index of LCNP and GaPP-LCNP before and after the lyophilization process.

Author Contributions: Conceptualization, M.A., T.J.B. and C.A.P.; methodology, M.A.; formal analysis and investigation, M.A.; resources, C.A.P.; data curation, M.A.; writing—original draft preparation, M.A.; writing—review and editing, M.A., T.J.B. and C.A.P.; visualization, M.A.; supervision, C.A.P. and T.J.B.; project administration, C.A.P.; funding acquisition, C.A.P. All authors have read and agreed to the published version of the manuscript.

Funding: This research received no external funding.

Institutional Review Board Statement: Not applicable.

Informed Consent Statement: Not applicable.

Acknowledgments: The SAXS studies in this work were conducted on the SAXS/WAXS beamline at the Australian Synchrotron, part of the Australian Nuclear Science and Technology Organisation (ANSTO). We would like to acknowledge Achal B. Bhatt for his assistance during the SAXS studies. The authors acknowledge the instruments and scientific and technical assistance of Microscopy

Australia at Adelaide Microscopy, The University of Adelaide, a facility that is funded by the University, and State and Federal Governments.

Conflicts of Interest: The authors declare no conflict of interest.

References

1. Awad, M.; Thomas, N.; Barnes, T.J.; Prestidge, C.A. Nanomaterials enabling clinical translation of antimicrobial photodynamic therapy. *J. Control. Release* **2022**, *346*, 300–316. [CrossRef]
2. Thorn, C.R.; Thomas, N.; Boyd, B.J.; Prestidge, C.A. Nano-fats for bugs: The benefits of lipid nanoparticles for antimicrobial therapy. *Drug Deliv. Transl. Res.* **2021**, *11*, 1598–1624. [CrossRef]
3. Abourehab, M.A.S.; Ansari, M.J.; Singh, A.; Hassan, A.; Abdelgawad, M.A.; Shrivastav, P.; Abualsoud, B.M.; Amaral, L.S.; Pramanik, S. Cubosomes as an emerging platform for drug delivery: A review of the state of the art. *J. Mater. Chem. B* **2022**, *10*, 2781–2819. [CrossRef]
4. Boge, L.; Hallstensson, K.; Ringstad, L.; Johansson, J.; Andersson, T.; Davoudi, M.; Larsson, P.T.; Mahlapuu, M.; Håkansson, J.; Andersson, M. Cubosomes for topical delivery of the antimicrobial peptide LL-37. *Eur. J. Pharm. Biopharm.* **2019**, *134*, 60–67. [CrossRef]
5. Zhai, J.; Fong, C.; Tran, N.; Drummond, C.J. Non-Lamellar Lyotropic Liquid Crystalline Lipid Nanoparticles for the Next Generation of Nanomedicine. *ACS Nano* **2019**, *13*, 6178–6206. [CrossRef]
6. Awad, M.; Barnes, T.J.; Joyce, P.; Thomas, N.; Prestidge, C.A. Liquid crystalline lipid nanoparticle promotes the photodynamic activity of gallium protoporphyrin against S. aureus biofilms. *J. Photochem. Photobiol. B Biol.* **2022**, *232*, 112474. [CrossRef]
7. Awad, M.; Barnes, T.J.; Thomas, N.; Joyce, P.; Prestidge, C.A. Gallium Protoporphyrin Liquid Crystalline Lipid Nanoparticles: A Third-Generation Photosensitizer against Pseudomonas aeruginosa Biofilms. *Pharmaceutics* **2022**, *14*, 2124. [CrossRef]
8. Awad, M.; Kopecki, Z.; Barnes, T.J.; Wignall, A.; Joyce, P.; Thomas, N.; Prestidge, C.A. Lipid Liquid Crystal Nanoparticles: Promising Photosensitizer Carriers for the Treatment of Infected Cutaneous Wounds. *Pharmaceutics* **2023**, *15*, 305. [CrossRef]
9. Malheiros, B.; Dias de Castro, R.; Lotierzo, M.C.G.; Casadei, B.R.; Barbosa, L.R.S. Design and manufacturing of monodisperse and malleable phytantriol-based cubosomes for drug delivery applications. *J. Drug Deliv. Sci. Technol.* **2021**, *61*, 102149. [CrossRef]
10. Wessman, P.; Edwards, K.; Mahlin, D. Structural effects caused by spray-and freeze-drying of liposomes and bilayer disks. *J. Pharm. Sci.* **2010**, *99*, 2032–2048. [CrossRef] [PubMed]
11. Abdelwahed, W.; Degobert, G.; Stainmesse, S.; Fessi, H. Freeze-drying of nanoparticles: Formulation, process and storage considerations. *Adv. Drug Deliv. Rev.* **2006**, *58*, 1688–1713. [CrossRef] [PubMed]
12. Wang, J.-L.; Hanafy, M.S.; Xu, H.; Leal, J.; Zhai, Y.; Ghosh, D.; Williams, R.O., III; Smyth, H.D.C.; Cui, Z. Aerosolizable siRNA-encapsulated solid lipid nanoparticles prepared by thin-film freeze-drying for potential pulmonary delivery. *Int. J. Pharm.* **2021**, *596*, 120215. [CrossRef]
13. Salminen, H.; Ankenbrand, J.; Zeeb, B.; Badolato Bönisch, G.; Schäfer, C.; Kohlus, R.; Weiss, J. Influence of spray drying on the stability of food-grade solid lipid nanoparticles. *Food Res. Int.* **2019**, *119*, 741–750. [CrossRef] [PubMed]
14. Ali, M.E.; Lamprecht, A. Spray freeze drying as an alternative technique for lyophilization of polymeric and lipid-based nanoparticles. *Int. J. Pharm.* **2017**, *516*, 170–177. [CrossRef]
15. Glavas-Dodov, M.; Fredro-Kumbaradzi, E.; Goracinova, K.; Simonoska, M.; Calis, S.; Trajkovic-Jolevska, S.; Hincal, A.A. The effects of lyophilization on the stability of liposomes containing 5-FU. *Int. J. Pharm.* **2005**, *291*, 79–86. [CrossRef] [PubMed]
16. Christensen, D.; Foged, C.; Rosenkrands, I.; Nielsen, H.M.; Andersen, P.; Agger, E.M. Trehalose preserves DDA/TDB liposomes and their adjuvant effect during freeze-drying. *Biochim. Biophys. Acta (BBA)-Biomembr.* **2007**, *1768*, 2120–2129. [CrossRef]
17. Ingvarsson, P.T.; Yang, M.; Nielsen, H.M.; Rantanen, J.; Foged, C. Stabilization of liposomes during drying. *Expert Opin. Drug Deliv.* **2011**, *8*, 375–388. [CrossRef]
18. Dou, M.; Lu, C.; Sun, Z.; Rao, W. Natural cryoprotectants combinations of l-proline and trehalose for red blood cells cryopreservation. *Cryobiology* **2019**, *91*, 23–29. [CrossRef]
19. Stark, B.; Pabst, G.; Prassl, R. Long-term stability of sterically stabilized liposomes by freezing and freeze-drying: Effects of cryoprotectants on structure. *Eur. J. Pharm. Sci.* **2010**, *41*, 546–555. [CrossRef]
20. Pereira, C.S.; Hünenberger, P.H. Interaction of the sugars trehalose, maltose and glucose with a phospholipid bilayer: A comparative molecular dynamics study. *J. Phys. Chem. B* **2006**, *110*, 15572–15581. [CrossRef]
21. Abdelsalam, A.M.; Somaida, A.; Ambreen, G.; Ayoub, A.M.; Tariq, I.; Engelhardt, K.; Garidel, P.; Fawaz, I.; Amin, M.U.; Wojcik, M.; et al. Surface tailored zein as a novel delivery system for hypericin: Application in photodynamic therapy. *Mater. Sci. Eng. C* **2021**, *129*, 112420. [CrossRef]
22. Boge, L.; Västberg, A.; Umerska, A.; Bysell, H.; Eriksson, J.; Edwards, K.; Millqvist-Fureby, A.; Andersson, M. Freeze-dried and re-hydrated liquid crystalline nanoparticles stabilized with disaccharides for drug-delivery of the plectasin derivative AP114 antimicrobial peptide. *J. Colloid Interface Sci.* **2018**, *522*, 126–135. [CrossRef]
23. Avachat, A.M.; Parpani, S.S. Formulation and development of bicontinuous nanostructured liquid crystalline particles of efavirenz. *Colloids Surf. B Biointerfaces* **2015**, *126*, 87–97. [CrossRef]

24. Gerola, A.P.; Semensato, J.; Pellosi, D.S.; Batistela, V.R.; Rabello, B.R.; Hioka, N.; Caetano, W. Chemical determination of singlet oxygen from photosensitizers illuminated with LED: New calculation methodology considering the influence of photobleaching. *J. Photochem. Photobiol. A Chem.* **2012**, *232*, 14–21. [CrossRef]
25. Ludvíková, L.; Friš, P.; Heger, D.; Šebej, P.; Wirz, J.; Klán, P. Photochemistry of rose bengal in water and acetonitrile: A comprehensive kinetic analysis. *Phys. Chem. Chem. Phys.* **2016**, *18*, 16266–16273. [CrossRef]
26. Wiegand, I.; Hilpert, K.; Hancock, R.E.W. Agar and broth dilution methods to determine the minimal inhibitory concentration (MIC) of antimicrobial substances. *Nat. Protoc.* **2008**, *3*, 163–175. [CrossRef]
27. Elgindy, N.A.; Mehanna, M.M.; Mohyeldin, S.M. Self-assembled nano-architecture liquid crystalline particles as a promising carrier for progesterone transdermal delivery. *Int. J. Pharm.* **2016**, *501*, 167–179. [CrossRef]
28. Gustafsson, J.; Ljusberg-Wahren, H.; Almgren, M.; Larsson, K. Submicron particles of reversed lipid phases in water stabilized by a nonionic amphiphilic polymer. *Langmuir* **1997**, *13*, 6964–6971. [CrossRef]
29. Nakano, M.; Sugita, A.; Matsuoka, H.; Handa, T. Small-angle X-ray scattering and 13C NMR investigation on the internal structure of "cubosomes". *Langmuir* **2001**, *17*, 3917–3922. [CrossRef]
30. Nguyen, T.H.; Hanley, T.; Porter, C.J.H.; Larson, I.; Boyd, B.J. Phytantriol and glyceryl monooleate cubic liquid crystalline phases as sustained-release oral drug delivery systems for poorly water soluble drugs I. Phase behaviour in physiologically-relevant media. *J. Pharm. Pharmacol.* **2010**, *62*, 844–855. [CrossRef]
31. Muller, F.; Salonen, A.; Glatter, O. Phase behavior of Phytantriol/water bicontinuous cubic $Pn3m$ cubosomes stabilized by Laponite disc-like particles. *J. Colloid Interface Sci.* **2010**, *342*, 392–398. [CrossRef] [PubMed]
32. Mohanraj, V.J. Nanoparticle Coated Liposomes for Encapsulation and Delivery of Proteins. Doctoral Thesis, University of South Australia, Mawson Lakes, Australia, 2010.
33. Man, D.; Słota, R.; Broda, M.A.; Mele, G.; Li, J. Metalloporphyrin intercalation in liposome membranes: ESR study. *J. Biol. Inorg. Chem.* **2011**, *16*, 173–181. [CrossRef] [PubMed]
34. Morales-de-Echegaray, A.V.; Maltais, T.R.; Lin, L.; Younis, W.; Kadasala, N.R.; Seleem, M.N.; Wei, A. Rapid Uptake and Photodynamic Inactivation of Staphylococci by Ga (III)-Protoporphyrin IX. *ACS Infect. Dis.* **2018**, *4*, 1564–1573. [CrossRef] [PubMed]
35. Thorn, C.R.; de Souza Carvalho-Wodarz, C.; Horstmann, J.C.; Lehr, C.-M.; Prestidge, C.A.; Thomas, N. Tobramycin Liquid Crystal Nanoparticles Eradicate Cystic Fibrosis-Related Pseudomonas aeruginosa Biofilms. *Small* **2021**, *17*, 2100531. [CrossRef] [PubMed]

Disclaimer/Publisher's Note: The statements, opinions and data contained in all publications are solely those of the individual author(s) and contributor(s) and not of MDPI and/or the editor(s). MDPI and/or the editor(s) disclaim responsibility for any injury to people or property resulting from any ideas, methods, instructions or products referred to in the content.

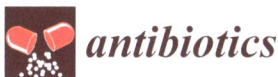

Article

Antibacterial Properties of the Antimicrobial Peptide Gallic Acid-Polyphemusin I (GAPI)

Olivia Lili Zhang [1], John Yun Niu [1], Iris Xiaoxue Yin [1], Ollie Yiru Yu [1], May Lei Mei [2] and Chun Hung Chu [1,*]

[1] Faculty of Dentistry, The University of Hong Kong, Hong Kong 999077, China; zhlili@connect.hku.hk (O.L.Z.); niuyun@hku.hk (J.Y.N.); irisxyin@hku.hk (I.X.Y.); ollieyu@hku.hk (O.Y.Y.)
[2] Faculty of Dentistry, The University of Otago, Dunedin 9054, New Zealand; may.mei@otago.ac.nz
* Correspondence: chchu@hku.hk

Abstract: A novel antimicrobial peptide, GAPI, has been developed recently by grafting gallic acid (GA) to polyphemusin I (PI). The objective of this study was to investigate the antibacterial effects of GAPI on common oral pathogens. This laboratory study used minimum inhibitory concentrations and minimum bactericidal concentrations to assess the antimicrobial properties of GAPI against common oral pathogens. Transmission electron microscopy was used to examine the bacterial morphology both before and after GAPI treatment. The results showed that the minimum inhibitory concentration ranged from 20 μM (*Lactobacillus rhamnosus*) to 320 μM (*Porphyromonas gingivalis*), whereas the minimum bactericidal concentration ranged from 80 μM (*Lactobacillus acidophilus*) to 640 μM (*Actinomyces naeslundii*, *Enterococcus faecalis*, and *Porphyromonas gingivalis*). Transmission electron microscopy showed abnormal curvature of cell membranes, irregular cell shapes, leakage of cytoplasmic content, and disruption of cytoplasmic membranes and cell walls. In conclusion, the GAPI antimicrobial peptide is antibacterial to common oral pathogens, with the potential to be used to manage oral infections.

Keywords: antimicrobial; caries; peptides; prevention

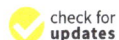

Citation: Zhang, O.L.; Niu, J.Y.; Yin, I.X.; Yu, O.Y.; Mei, M.L.; Chu, C.H. Antibacterial Properties of the Antimicrobial Peptide Gallic Acid-Polyphemusin I (GAPI). *Antibiotics* **2023**, *12*, 1350. https://doi.org/10.3390/antibiotics12091350

Academic Editor: Anisha D'Souza

Received: 27 March 2023
Revised: 16 August 2023
Accepted: 19 August 2023
Published: 22 August 2023

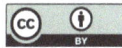

Copyright: © 2023 by the authors. Licensee MDPI, Basel, Switzerland. This article is an open access article distributed under the terms and conditions of the Creative Commons Attribution (CC BY) license (https://creativecommons.org/licenses/by/4.0/).

1. Introduction

Oral diseases are a global public health problem affecting over 3.5 billion people worldwide [1]. They can start in early childhood and progress throughout adolescence, adulthood, and old age [2]. Oral diseases have substantial negative effects on individuals, communities, and the wider society. The global economic burden of dental diseases amounts to more than USD 442 billion yearly [3]. The most prevalent oral diseases are dental caries and periodontal disease, which, when left untreated, can progress to tooth loss [4].

Dental caries and periodontal disease are infections resulting from the mixed biofilm (dental plaque) on teeth and periodontal tissues. Dental caries is the localised destruction of dental hard tissue, resulting from the acids that are produced from the sugar fermentation induced by bacteria [5]. *Streptococcus*, *Lactobacillus*, and *Actinomyces* are considered to be the primary cariogenic bacteria involved in the development of dental caries [6]. Pulp and periapical diseases are the secondary diseases of caries; pulpal inflammation and infection usually occur when the pulp is exposed to bacteria. *Enterococcus faecalis* is one of the most frequently found bacteria in teeth with pulp necrosis [7]. Periodontal disease is caused by bacteria, including *Porphyromonas gingivalis* and *Aggregatibacter actinomycetemcomitans* [8]. Thus, biofilm control is the key point for the treatment of oral diseases, such as caries and periodontal disease.

Highly effective antibacterial therapy for caries, endodontics, and periodontics should be applied to achieve optimal outcomes. It is well known that antibiotics are frequently prescribed for pathogens worldwide [9]. However, antibiotics are not clinically used to control cariogenic microorganisms [10]. Many systemic antibiotics, such as penicillin and tetracyclines, do not target oral bacteria specifically [11]. In addition, most antibiotics have side effects, especially for patients who are sensitive to chemical agents, including hypersensitivity and diarrhoea [12].

Furthermore, the spread of antibiotic resistance is the greatest problem in using antibiotics [11]. The World Health Organization (WHO) has reported that antibiotic resistance is one of the three greatest threats to public health [13]. Oral bacteria tend to be resistant to antibiotics, thus reducing antibiotics' efficacy [14]. In addition, alarms have been raised concerning the extensive use of adjunctive antibiotics to treat periodontal disease [15]. The European Federation of Periodontology called for a reasonably restrictive and judicious management of adjunctive systemic antibiotics [16].

Chlorhexidine is another active bactericidal agent that remains the gold standard of antibiofilm agents. However, it can cause genotoxicity and induce cellular apoptosis [17]. For long-term use, patients frequently report loss of taste, numbness, and extrinsic tooth staining. In endodontics, chlorhexidine is used as a root canal irrigant. However, it is ineffective at dissolving necrotic tissue [18]. In addition, low-level exposure to chlorhexidine may cause a cross-resistance to antibiotics [19]. Hence, the need for developing new antimicrobial agents as alternative therapies to fight oral infections is urgent.

Currently, antimicrobial peptides have captured attention. Researchers have adopted them as a novel and promising antimicrobial approach [20]. Abundant antimicrobial peptides are derived from multicellular organisms and are considered natural antibiotics [13]. Antimicrobial peptides have also been established as the first line of defence against various pathogens, including Gram-positive or -negative microbes, fungi, parasites, and viruses [20]. The mechanism of antimicrobial peptides against pathogens is that net positive-charge peptides can bind directly to the outer bacteria membrane of negatively charged headgroups [21]. Owing to the nonspecific mechanism, antimicrobial peptides have shown great promise, with little to no resistance [22]. Meanwhile, antimicrobial peptides can be effective for microbes that are resistant to conventional antibiotics, and they have low toxicity because their degradation products are natural amino acids [23]. Moreover, antimicrobial peptides can be functionally modified easily with chemical synthesis methods to obtain more small-molecule derivatives [24]. All these advantages make antimicrobial peptides excellent candidates for developing novel anti-infective agents [25], as well as serving as innovative products for immunomodulation and the promotion of wound healing [26]. Consequently, when considering that antimicrobial peptides have great prospects in terms of treating infections, it is relevant to also apply them for oral disease treatment [20].

Naturally, antimicrobial peptides can be found in various organisms, ranging from animals to bacteria, fungi, and plants [27]. Cathelicidin families, one of the most common antimicrobial peptides, are mainly found in mammals [28]. LL-37 is the only cathelicidin in human beings; it is active against various oral Gram-positive and -negative microorganisms due to its amphipathic structure [29]. In addition to its antimicrobial activity, LL-37 is also crucial in immunomodulatory and inflammatory responses [30]. Antimicrobial peptide LR-10, derived from the *Lactobacillus* species, can inhibit the growth of *S. mutans* by forming pores in bacterial membranes [31]. The fungi-derived antimicrobial peptide alamethicin is bacteriocidal against Gram-positive and -negative bacteria [32]. Fa-AMP1 and Fa-AMP2 are novel antimicrobial peptides that are purified from the seeds of buckwheat, and that have antibacterial and antifungal activity [33].

A bibliometric analysis shows a growing global interest in using antimicrobial peptides as functional biomaterials for caries management [34]. Dental caries management philosophy has shifted to minimally invasive dentistry [35,36]. Thus, different bioactive materials, such as biomimetic hydroxyapatite and peptide-based bioactive materials, are introduced to caries management [37,38]. Peptide-based bioactive materials play an important role in inhibiting biofilm growth and remineralising demineralised teeth [39]. For example, GA-KR12, a novel antimicrobial peptide, effectively inhibits *S. mutans* biofilm growth and promotes the remineralisation of artificial enamel and dentin caries [40,41]. Thus, researchers are interested in developing novel antimicrobial peptides for managing oral diseases [42].

Polyphemusin I (PI) is an antimicrobial peptide derived from horseshoe crabs. It can kill bacteria through binding to and by crossing cell membranes, thus rupturing the bacterial membrane [43]. Gallic acid is abundant in fruits and vegetables, and it can accelerate the regeneration of hydroxyapatites due to its pyrogallol group. In addition, gallic acid shows antimicrobial activities [44]. In our previous study, we synthesised a novel peptide (GAPI) by grafting antimicrobial peptide PI to gallic acid. GAPI peptide could be synthesised using the standard fluorenylmethoxycarbonyl solid-phase synthesis method. A multiple-species biofilm study demonstrated that GAPI impact the growth of cariogenic biofilm formation. However, its antimicrobial properties against other common oral pathogens are still unclear. Therefore, the objective of this study was to investigate the antibacterial effects of GAPI on several common oral pathogens.

2. Results

2.1. Minimum Inhibitory Concentration (MIC) and Minimum Bactericidal Concentration (MBC)

The MIC and MBC of GAPI against *Streptococcus mutans, Streptococcus sobrinus, Lactobacillus acidophilus, Lactobacillus rhamnosus, Actinomyces naeslundii, Enterococcus faecalis, Porphyromonas gingivalis,* and *Actinobacillus actinomycetemcomitans* are summarised in Table 1.

Table 1. The minimum inhibitory concentration (MIC) and minimum bactericidal concentration (MBC) of GAPI against common American Type Culture Collection (ATCC) oral pathogens.

Bacteria	ATCC	MIC (μM)	MBC (μM)
Actinobacillus actinomycetemcomitans	29523	160	320
Actinomyces naeslundii	12104	160	640
Enterococcus faecalis	29212	160	640
Lactobacillus acidophilus	9224	40	80
Lactobacillus rhamnosus	10863	20	160
Porphyromonas gingivalis	33277	320	640
Streptococcus mutans	35668	80	160
Streptococcus sobrinus	33478	80	320

The MICs of GAPI against *S. mutans* and *S. sobrinus* were 80 μM, whereas the MBCs for these two bacteria were 160 μM and 320 μM, respectively. For *L. acidophilus* and *L. rhamnosus*, the MICs were 40 μM and 20 μM, and the MBCs were 80 μM and 160 μM, respectively. The MICs and MBCs for *A. naeslundii* and *E. faecalis* were 160 μM and 640 μM, respectively. The MICs for *P. gingivalis* and *A. actinomycetemcomitans* were 320 μM and 160 μM, respectively. The MBCs for *P. gingivalis* and *A. actinomycetemcomitans* were 640 μM and 320 μM, respectively. The results indicated that GAPI showed strong antimicrobial activity against cariogenic bacteria.

2.2. Morphology of the Microorganisms

Figure 1 represents the morphology of various cariogenic bacteria that were treated with or without GAPI.

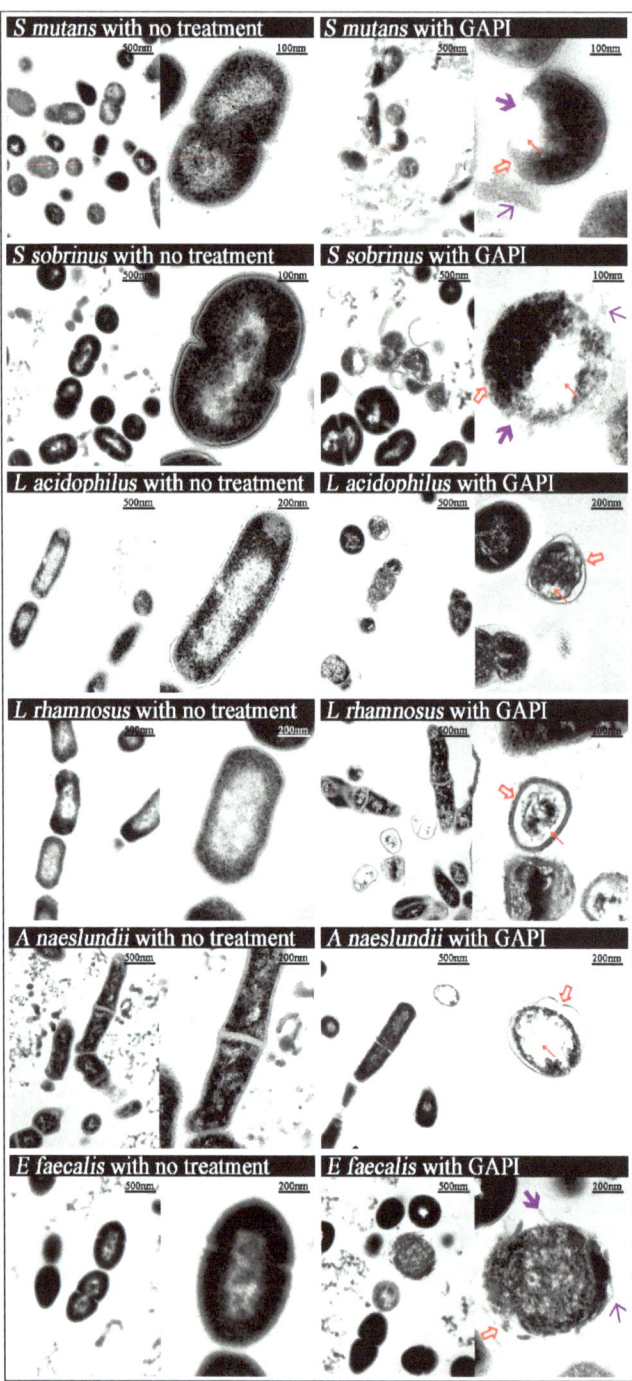

Figure 1. Micrographs of cariogenic pathogens both before and after GAPI treatment. ⇨ Abnormal cell membrane, ↖ Cytoplasmic clear zone, ⬆ Disrupted cell membrane, ↖ Cytoplasmic content leakage.

S. mutans was severely damaged after being treated with GAPI. The *S. mutans* cells lost their normal morphology, with effects including abnormal cell curvatures and irregular cell shapes. The cell wall separated from the cell membrane. In addition, the cells' cytoplasmic membranes were entirely disrupted, resulting in transparent cytoplasmic zones and the leakage of cytoplasmic contents.

For GAPI-treated *S. sobrinus*, the morphology changes were similar to GAPI-treated *S. mutans*: the abnormal curvature of cell membranes and irregular cell shapes, clear cytoplasmic zones, the disruption of the cytoplasmic membrane, and the leakage of cytoplasmic contents.

For *L. acidophilus*, *L. rhamnosus*, and *A. naeslundii*, the typical changes after treatment with GAPI included the abnormal curvature of cell membranes, irregular cell shapes, and cytoplasmic clear zones.

For *E. faecalis*, compared with untreated bacteria, higher magnification images showed that the bacteria in the GAPI group had abnormal morphological characteristics, including the disruption of the cytoplasmic membrane and the leakage of cytoplasmic contents.

Figure 2 represents the morphology of various periodontal-associated bacteria with or without GAPI treatment. For *P. gingivalis* and *A. actinomycetemcomitans*, after being treated with GAPI, the abnormal curvature of cell membranes, irregular cell shapes, and intra-bacterial vacuolisation can be identified. In addition, membrane disruption and the leakage of intracellular components were observed.

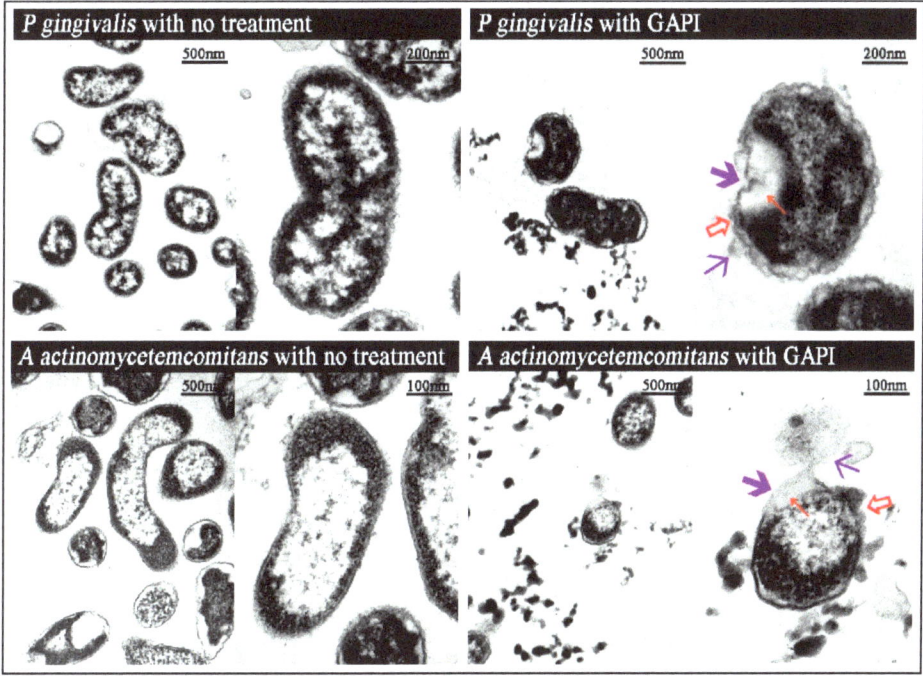

Figure 2. Micrographs of the periodontal pathogens both before and after GAPI treatment. ↘ Abnormal cell membrane, ↖ Cytoplasmic clear zone, ↖ Disrupted cell wall/membrane, ↖ Cytoplasmic content leakage.

3. Discussion

Antimicrobial peptides have been studied widely by researchers and are regarded as a new generation of antibiotics due to their broad-spectrum bactericidal activity [45]. In this study, we successfully synthesised GAPI, which consists of the peptide PI as an antimicrobial action domain. Furthermore, gallic acid has been demonstrated to have broad-spectrum antibacterial, antiviral, and antifungal activities [46]. It is a phenolic acid and is easily obtained in large amounts from plants. It has been widely used as an antioxidant additive in food. The addition of gallic acid has potentiated antimicrobials' effectiveness against various pathogenic bacteria [47]. Accordingly, gallic acid could be applied as a promising compound for new antimicrobial drug development. The antibacterial activity of the synthesised GAPI was investigated against several typical oral pathogenic microorganisms that are frequently found in oral environments.

Cariogenic microbes are essential for caries development. The definition of cariogenic microorganisms includes the following factors: (1) the bacteria have strong bond affinity to the tooth surface; (2) the bacteria can synthesise extracellular and intracellular polysaccharides; (3) the bacteria are acidogenic, transporting and metabolising various carbohydrates; and (4) the bacteria can tolerate acid environments [48]. *Streptococcus*, *Lactobacillus*, and *Actinomyces* species are three common cariogenic microorganisms' taxa.

It has been largely accepted that *S. mutans* plays a critical role in biofilm formation, depending on its core attributes [49]. *S. mutans* possesses multiple high-affinity surface adhesins, thereby enabling colonisation even in the absence of sucrose. It can synthesise large quantities of extracellular glucan polymers from sucrose, which is useful in the permanent colonisation of hard surfaces and in forming extracellular polymeric matrices in situ [50]. In addition, *S. mutans* can provide a favourable niche for other bacterial species to colonise in the oral cavity by altering the local environment [51]. Moreover, it has acidogenic characteristics. *S. sobrinus* is another common cariogenic bacterium in the *Streptococcus* taxa. Studies have shown that *S. sobrinus* is more associated with caries' development progress, especially in early childhood caries [52]. *S. sobrinus* is capable of producing acid and is acid tolerant [53]. Several studies have indicated a significant association between *S. sobrinus* and caries, thereby showing that *S. sobrinus* is more effective in promoting caries than *S. mutans* [54]. Regardless, *S. mutans* and *S. sobrinus* have been implicated as the primary cariogenic microorganisms in biofilm. Therefore, targeting *S. mutans* and *S. sobrinus* growth could be useful in preventing cariogenic biofilm formation.

Lactobacillus strains are frequently identified at active carious lesions in adults and children. Among the *Lactobacillus* species found from carious lesions, *L. acidophilus* and *L. rhamnosus* are two dominant microorganisms. *Lactobacillus* species can produce weak acids and tolerate low-pH environments [55]. They are strictly fermentative bacteria and are known for their high capacity for enzyme production. These enzymes enable the *Lactobacillus* species to rapidly break down various carbohydrates into acidic products, at least half of which is lactic acid. In addition, *Lactobacillus* species can grow and remain viable at a lower PH to cope with acid stresses [56]. Unlike *Streptococcus mutans*, which has been well characterised in terms of pathophysiology, the mechanisms of the *Lactobacillus* species still require further investigation.

A. naeslundii, a facultative anaerobic Gram-positive bacteria, is related to dental plaque ageing [57]. It can penetrate into dentinal tubules via exposed dentine, thus causing dentin or root caries, and promoting infections of root canal systems [58]. *E. faecalis* is the most commonly isolated bacteria from root canal systems in endodontic infection teeth. It is an anaerobic Gram-positive facultative microorganism that is highly resistant to antimicrobial agents and can survive in very harsh environments, such as low oxygen or poor nutrient supply [7].

P. gingivalis and *A. actinomycetemcomitans* are two of the most frequently associated bacteria with periodontitis [59]. *P. gingivalis*, as a keystone pathogen of periodontitis, can produce different kinds of virulence factors, such as lipopolysaccharide, vesicles, gingipains, and fimbriae [60]. These factors destroy not only periodontal tissue directly, but also cause secondary tissue damage by inducing an inflammatory reaction. In addition, *P. gingivalis* forms a dynamic balance and symbiotic relationship with the host, thereby allowing the bacteria to evade the host's immune reaction. Thus, *P. gingivalis* is regarded as a significant periodontal pathogen that is close to periodontitis' development, progression, severity, and recurrence [61]. *A. actinomycetemcomitans* is associated with chronic and aggressive periodontitis [62]. It can produce a variety of virulence factors, including endo- and exotoxins. These factors can directly damage host tissues, as well as protect the bacteria from host defences. In addition, *A. actinomycetemcomitans* can impersonate normal epithelial cell functions in order to induce its uptake and to also disseminate into neighbour epithelial cells.

Antimicrobial susceptibility is a key determinant in the process of antimicrobial drug selection, which can be tested via MIC. It is necessary in the application of MIC-guided antimicrobial therapy [63]. According to the results of the present study, GAPI exhibited significant antibacterial efficiency. The MICs and MBCs against eight bacteria were shown to range from 20 to 320 μM and 80 to 640 μM, respectively, which are better than the other peptides from existing studies (MICs and MBCs ranged from 160 to 320 μM and 640 to 1280 μM, respectively) [40].

Furthermore, TEM was used to show bacterial morphology changes after GAPI treatment in order to further understand GAPI's mechanism. The micrographs revealed that the GAPI disrupted the bacterial membrane, thus causing abnormal membrane curvature, irregular cell shapes, and intra-bacterial vacuolisation, and inducing cytoplasmic components to escape from the microorganism. The mechanism of action begins with GAPI binding to bacteria and then interacting with the cytoplasmic membrane, thereby crossing the cytoplasmic membrane and damaging the membrane integrity. The damage to the integrity of the cell membrane is an important mechanism, by which antibacterial methods deactivate microorganisms. Furthermore, the TEM images indicated that GAPI could damage the bacterial cell structure, causing cytoplasmic content leakage.

Indeed, this observation is consistent with previous studies showing that positively charged antimicrobial peptides can initially bind to negatively charged phospholipids on the outer leaflet of a bacterial membrane [40]. Most antimicrobial peptides contain hydrophilic and hydrophobic residues at either end. After the initial electrostatic interactions, the antimicrobial peptides accumulate at the surface until reaching a certain concentration. Then, the hydrophobic ends insert into the lipid bilayer, disrupting the bacterial cell membrane and resulting in the leakage of cytoplasmic contents, further resulting in the death of bacteria [21]. Different action models can describe this mechanism, including barrel-stave pore, carpet-like, and toroidal pore models. In addition, antimicrobial peptides can translocate to the inner cytoplasmic leaflet, potentially targeting intracellular components.

In the reaction stage, the specific cationic nature is critical. Studies have shown that there is a correlation between antibacterial activity and charge, as an increasing charge is related to strengthened antibacterial activity. However, too much charge may hinder the antimicrobial activity because the strong interaction of the peptide and lipid head group will inhibit the translocation of antimicrobial peptides into the membrane's inner leaflet. On the other hand, hydrophobic residues are another feature of antimicrobial peptides. Hydrophobicity determines the degree to which water-soluble antimicrobial peptides can move into the membrane lipid bilayer. Peptides lacking hydrophobic residues typically have poor membrane attachment. However, excessive hydrophobicity can cause cell toxicity and antimicrobial specificity loss [64].

It should be noted that negatively charged phospholipids are more commonly found in bacterial cell membranes when compared to neutral mammalian host cell membranes [65,66]. According to the significant difference in their respective bacterial cell envelopes, these bacteria are thus classified as Gram-positive and Gram-negative. Both have similar inner or cytoplasmic membranes. For Gram-negative bacteria, the outer membrane consists of two layers: the inner leaflet of this membrane contains phosphate lipids, while the outer leaflet is composed principally of lipopolysaccharide. Lipopolysaccharide molecules are highly decorated with negatively charged phosphate groups. In comparison, Gram-positive bacteria are surrounded by peptidoglycan layers that are many times thicker than Gram-negative bacteria. Teichoic acids embedded in peptidoglycan are long anionic polymers [67]. Thus, Welling et al. designed an in vivo study to test whether antimicrobial peptides can distinguish microbial cells and host tissues. They indicated that antimicrobial peptides could discriminate between microorganisms and host tissues and also can accumulate at infection sites. Overall, inherent structures or functions of microbial versus host cells contribute to the selective antimicrobial discretion of certain peptides [68].

As alternative antibacterial agents, antimicrobial peptides are also known as host defence peptides [69], as they can not only clear the infected bacteria, but also enhance the human immune response. Thus, antimicrobial peptides can selectively kill bacteria without damage to the host cell. In addition, studies have shown that antimicrobial peptides rarely produce microbial resistance because the antimicrobial peptide's hydrophobic tail can directly enter the bacterial liquid bilayer [66]. The membrane-active mechanism is particularly important when targeting antibiotic-resistant pathogens.

Antimicrobial peptides can be classified into four broad subclasses, including α-helical and β sheets, as well as αβ and non-αβ structures [24]. Moreover, β-hairpin antimicrobial peptides are abundant in animal species and can be isolated in invertebrates and vertebrates. Further, β-hairpin peptides are more active in crossing bacterial cell membranes and accessing intracellular targets [65]. It is noted that small-size β-hairpin antimicrobial peptides have a high resistance to proteolytic degradation [70]. In our study, peptide PI, from the American horseshoe crab *Limulus polyphemus*, is an antimicrobial cell-penetrating peptide with a β-hairpin structure. Additionally, the primary target of β-hairpin antimicrobial peptides is the cellular membrane. Under this premise, the cell-penetrating peptide PI can pass through a cell membrane without interaction with specific receptors. In the present study, the addition of gallic acid did not change the antimicrobial properties of the peptide. Therefore, the new antimicrobial peptide GAPI could be considered a promising alternative antibacterial agent to traditional antibiotics in treating dental diseases.

4. Materials and Methods

4.1. Peptide Synthesis

GAPI was synthesised using standard fluorenylmethoxycarbonyl synthesis by standard solid-phase peptide synthesis. The GAPI powder was dissolved in sterile deionised water to a specific concentration for study and was stored at $-20\,^\circ$C.

4.2. Microorganisms

Eight common oral pathogenic bacterial strains were selected for this study. They are *Streptococcus mutans* ATCC 35668, *Streptococcus sobrinus* ATCC 33478, *Lactobacillus acidophilus* ATCC 9224, *Lactobacillus rhamnosus* ATCC10863, *Actinomyces naeslundii* ATCC 12104, *Enterococcus faecalis* ATCC 29212, *Porphyromonas gingivalis* ATCC 33277, and *Actinobacillus actinomycetemcomitans* ATCC 29523. All the strains were cultured anaerobically.

4.3. MIC and MBC

Brain heart infusion (BHI) medium was used for culture of *S. mutans*, *S. sobrinus*, *L. acidophilus*, *L. rhamnosus*, *A. naeslundii*, *E. faecalis*, and *A. actinomycetemcomitans*, whereas p.g. broth was used for culture of *Porphyromonas gingivalis*. The standard dilution method in a 96-well microplate was conducted in order to evaluate the antimicrobial efficacy of GAPI. Each well was filled with 100 μL GAPI dilutions. In addition, serial twofold dilutions in concentrations ranging from 1280 μM to 1.25 μM were prepared. A 10 μL bacterial culture (10^6 CFU/mL) was added. Chlorhexidine was used as positive control, and medium was used as negative control. The plates were then anaerobically incubated at 37 $^\circ$C for 24 h. The absorbance was measured at a wavelength of 660 nm in order to analyse the growth of microorganisms. The MIC value was defined as the lowest concentration at which no visible growth was seen in the clear well. After the MIC determination, 10 μL fluid from each well, which showed no visible bacterial growth, was pipetted and seeded on blood agar, which were then put into an anaerobic incubator at 37 $^\circ$C for 48 h. The MBC endpoint was the lowest concentration at which 99.9% of the bacterial population was killed, which thus means the absence of bacteria.

4.4. Morphology of the Microorganisms

Bacteria morphology was observed using a transmission electron microscope (TEM, Philips CM100). GAPI was added to a bacterial culture of 10^8 CFU/mL, and the bacteria were harvested after incubating at 37 °C for 18 h. The semi-thin sections of cell were contained in grids and examined with the TEM.

5. Conclusions

This laboratory study showed that the novel antimicrobial peptide GAPI has promising antibacterial effects against common cariogenic and periodontal pathogens. It can also serve as an alternative to antibiotics in terms of managing dental infection.

Author Contributions: Conceptualisation, O.L.Z. and M.L.M.; methodology, O.L.Z. and O.Y.Y.; formal analysis, O.L.Z. and I.X.Y.; investigation, O.L.Z. and J.Y.N.; writing—original draft preparation, O.L.Z. and J.Y.N.; writing—review and editing, I.X.Y. and C.H.C.; supervision, O.Y.Y., M.L.M. and C.H.C.; project administration, C.H.C. All authors have read and agreed to the published version of the manuscript.

Funding: This research was funded by the National Natural Science Foundation of China (NSFC), General Program 81870812.

Institutional Review Board Statement: Not applicable.

Informed Consent Statement: Not applicable.

Data Availability Statement: The data are contained within the article.

Conflicts of Interest: The authors declare no conflict of interest.

References

1. Peres, M.A.; Macpherson, L.M.D.; Weyant, R.J.; Daly, B.; Venturelli, R.; Mathur, M.R.; Listl, S.; Celeste, R.K.; Guarnizo-Herreno, C.C.; Kearns, C.; et al. Oral diseases: A global public health challenge. *Lancet* **2019**, *394*, 249–260. [CrossRef] [PubMed]
2. Kassebaum, N.J.; Smith, A.G.C.; Bernabe, E.; Fleming, T.D.; Reynolds, A.E.; Vos, T.; Murray, C.J.L.; Marcenes, W.; GBD 2015 Oral Health Collaborators. Global, Regional, and National Prevalence, Incidence, and Disability-Adjusted Life Years for Oral Conditions for 195 Countries, 1990–2015: A Systematic Analysis for the Global Burden of Diseases, Injuries, and Risk Factors. *J. Dent. Res.* **2017**, *96*, 380–387. [CrossRef] [PubMed]
3. Listl, S.; Galloway, J.; Mossey, P.A.; Marcenes, W. Global Economic Impact of Dental Diseases. *J. Dent. Res.* **2015**, *94*, 1355–1361. [CrossRef]
4. Tonetti, M.S.; Bottenberg, P.; Conrads, G.; Eickholz, P.; Heasman, P.; Huysmans, M.C.; Lopez, R.; Madianos, P.; Muller, F.; Needleman, I.; et al. Dental caries and periodontal diseases in the ageing population: Call to action to protect and enhance oral health and well-being as an essential component of healthy ageing—Consensus report of group 4 of the joint EFP/ORCA workshop on the boundaries between caries and periodontal diseases. *J. Clin. Periodontol.* **2017**, *44* (Suppl. 18), S135–S144. [CrossRef] [PubMed]
5. Zhao, G.N.; Wong, H.M.; Wen, P.Y.F.; Wu, Y.; Zhong, Y.J.; Jiang, Y. Burden, Trends, and Inequality of Dental Caries in the U.S., 1990–2019. *Am. J. Prev. Med.* **2023**, *64*, 788–796. [CrossRef] [PubMed]
6. Mei, M.L.; Yan, Z.; Duangthip, D.; Niu, J.Y.; Yu, O.Y.; You, M.; Lo, E.C.M.; Chu, C.H. Effect of silver diamine fluoride on plaque microbiome in children. *J. Dent.* **2020**, *102*, 103479. [CrossRef]
7. Alghamdi, F.; Shakir, M. The Influence of Enterococcus faecalis as a Dental Root Canal Pathogen on Endodontic Treatment: A Systematic Review. *Cureus* **2020**, *12*, e7257. [CrossRef]
8. Cheng, W.C.; van Asten, S.D.; Burns, L.A.; Evans, H.G.; Walter, G.J.; Hashim, A.; Hughes, F.J.; Taams, L.S. Periodontitis-associated pathogens P. gingivalis and A. actinomycetemcomitans activate human CD14(+) monocytes leading to enhanced Th17/IL-17 responses. *Eur. J. Immunol.* **2016**, *46*, 2211–2221. [CrossRef]
9. Theuretzbacher, U.; Gottwalt, S.; Beyer, P.; Butler, M.; Czaplewski, L.; Lienhardt, C.; Moja, L.; Paul, M.; Paulin, S.; Rex, J.H.; et al. Analysis of the clinical antibacterial and antituberculosis pipeline. *Lancet Infect. Dis.* **2019**, *19*, e40–e50. [CrossRef]
10. Dai, L.L.; Mei, M.L.; Chu, C.H.; Lo, E.C.M. Antibacterial effect of a new bioactive glass on cariogenic bacteria. *Arch. Oral. Biol.* **2020**, *117*, 104833. [CrossRef]
11. Qiu, W.; Zhou, Y.; Li, Z.; Huang, T.; Xiao, Y.; Cheng, L.; Peng, X.; Zhang, L.; Ren, B. Application of Antibiotics/Antimicrobial Agents on Dental Caries. *Biomed. Res. Int.* **2020**, *2020*, 5658212. [CrossRef] [PubMed]
12. Mohsen, S.; Dickinson, J.A.; Somayaji, R. Update on the adverse effects of antimicrobial therapies in community practice. *Can. Fam. Physician* **2020**, *66*, 651–659.

13. Rai, A.; Ferrao, R.; Palma, P.; Patricio, T.; Parreira, P.; Anes, E.; Tonda-Turo, C.; Martins, M.C.L.; Alves, N.; Ferreira, L. Antimicrobial peptide-based materials: Opportunities and challenges. *J. Mater. Chem. B* **2022**, *10*, 2384–2429. [CrossRef] [PubMed]
14. Ardila, C.M.; Bedoya-Garcia, J.A. Antimicrobial resistance of *Aggregatibacter actinomycetemcomitans*, *Porphyromonas gingivalis* and *Tannerella forsythia* in periodontitis patients. *J. Glob. Antimicrob. Resist.* **2020**, *22*, 215–218. [CrossRef] [PubMed]
15. Ardila, C.M.; Bedoya-Garcia, J.A.; Arrubla-Escobar, D.E. Antibiotic resistance in periodontitis patients: A systematic scoping review of randomized clinical trials. *Oral. Dis.* 2022; ahead of print. [CrossRef] [PubMed]
16. Sanz, M.; Herrera, D.; Kebschull, M.; Chapple, I.; Jepsen, S.; Beglundh, T.; Sculean, A.; Tonetti, M.S.; Participants, E.F.P.W.; Methodological, C. Treatment of stage I-III periodontitis-The EFP S3 level clinical practice guideline. *J. Clin. Periodontol.* **2020**, *47* (Suppl. 22), 4–60. [CrossRef]
17. Karpinski, T.M.; Szkaradkiewicz, A.K. Chlorhexidine—pharmaco-biological activity and application. *Eur. Rev. Med. Pharmacol. Sci.* **2015**, *19*, 1321–1326.
18. Naenni, N.; Thoma, K.; Zehnder, M. Soft tissue dissolution capacity of currently used and potential endodontic irrigants. *J. Endod.* **2004**, *30*, 785–787. [CrossRef]
19. Cieplik, F.; Jakubovics, N.S.; Buchalla, W.; Maisch, T.; Hellwig, E.; Al-Ahmad, A. Resistance Toward Chlorhexidine in Oral Bacteria—Is There Cause for Concern? *Front. Microbiol.* **2019**, *10*, 587. [CrossRef]
20. Niu, J.Y.; Yin, I.X.; Mei, M.L.; Wu, W.K.K.; Li, Q.L.; Chu, C.H. The multifaceted roles of antimicrobial peptides in oral diseases. *Mol. Oral. Microbiol.* **2021**, *36*, 159–171. [CrossRef]
21. Kumar, P.; Kizhakkedathu, J.N.; Straus, S.K. Antimicrobial Peptides: Diversity, Mechanism of Action and Strategies to Improve the Activity and Biocompatibility In Vivo. *Biomolecules* **2018**, *8*, 4. [CrossRef] [PubMed]
22. Magana, M.; Pushpanathan, M.; Santos, A.L.; Leanse, L.; Fernandez, M.; Ioannidis, A.; Giulianotti, M.A.; Apidianakis, Y.; Bradfute, S.; Ferguson, A.L.; et al. The value of antimicrobial peptides in the age of resistance. *Lancet Infect. Dis.* **2020**, *20*, e216–e230. [CrossRef] [PubMed]
23. Rima, M.; Rima, M.; Fajloun, Z.; Sabatier, J.M.; Bechinger, B.; Naas, T. Antimicrobial Peptides: A Potent Alternative to Antibiotics. *Antibiotics* **2021**, *10*, 1095. [CrossRef] [PubMed]
24. Zhang, O.L.; Niu, J.Y.; Yu, O.Y.; Mei, M.L.; Jakubovics, N.S.; Chu, C.H. Peptide Designs for Use in Caries Management: A Systematic Review. *Int. J. Mol. Sci.* **2023**, *24*, 4247. [CrossRef]
25. Erdem Buyukkiraz, M.; Kesmen, Z. Antimicrobial peptides (AMPs): A promising class of antimicrobial compounds. *J. Appl. Microbiol.* **2022**, *132*, 1573–1596. [CrossRef]
26. Mahlapuu, M.; Bjorn, C.; Ekblom, J. Antimicrobial peptides as therapeutic agents: Opportunities and challenges. *Crit. Rev. Biotechnol.* **2020**, *40*, 978–992. [CrossRef]
27. Lei, J.; Sun, L.; Huang, S.; Zhu, C.; Li, P.; He, J.; Mackey, V.; Coy, D.H.; He, Q. The antimicrobial peptides and their potential clinical applications. *Am. J. Transl. Res.* **2019**, *11*, 3919–3931.
28. Kosciuczuk, E.M.; Lisowski, P.; Jarczak, J.; Strzalkowska, N.; Jozwik, A.; Horbanczuk, J.; Krzyzewski, J.; Zwierzchowski, L.; Bagnicka, E. Cathelicidins: Family of antimicrobial peptides. A review. *Mol. Biol. Rep.* **2012**, *39*, 10957–10970. [CrossRef]
29. Duplantier, A.J.; van Hoek, M.L. The Human Cathelicidin Antimicrobial Peptide LL-37 as a Potential Treatment for Polymicrobial Infected Wounds. *Front. Immunol.* **2013**, *4*, 143. [CrossRef]
30. Hancock, R.E.; Haney, E.F.; Gill, E.E. The immunology of host defence peptides: Beyond antimicrobial activity. *Nat. Rev. Immunol.* **2016**, *16*, 321–334. [CrossRef]
31. Liang, D.; Li, H.; Xu, X.; Liang, J.; Dai, X.; Zhao, W. Rational design of peptides with enhanced antimicrobial and anti-biofilm activities against cariogenic bacterium Streptococcus mutans. *Chem. Biol. Drug Des.* **2019**, *94*, 1768–1781. [CrossRef] [PubMed]
32. Leitgeb, B.; Szekeres, A.; Manczinger, L.; Vagvolgyi, C.; Kredics, L. The history of alamethicin: A review of the most extensively studied peptaibol. *Chem. Biodivers.* **2007**, *4*, 1027–1051. [CrossRef] [PubMed]
33. Fujimura, M.; Minami, Y.; Watanabe, K.; Tadera, K. Purification, characterization, and sequencing of a novel type of antimicrobial peptides, Fa-AMP1 and Fa-AMP2, from seeds of buckwheat (*Fagopyrum esculentum* Moench). *Biosci. Biotechnol. Biochem.* **2003**, *67*, 1636–1642. [CrossRef]
34. Zhang, O.L.; Niu, J.Y.; Yin, I.X.; Yu, O.Y.; Mei, M.L.; Chu, C.H. Growing Global Research Interest in Antimicrobial Peptides for Caries Management: A Bibliometric Analysis. *J. Funct. Biomater.* **2022**, *13*, 210. [CrossRef]
35. Yu, O.Y.; Lam, W.Y.; Wong, A.W.; Duangthip, D.; Chu, C.H. Nonrestorative Management of Dental Caries. *Dent. J.* **2021**, *9*, 121. [CrossRef] [PubMed]
36. Nizami, M.Z.I.; Yeung, C.; Yin, I.X.; Wong, A.W.Y.; Chu, C.H.; Yu, O.Y. Tunnel Restoration: A Minimally Invasive Dentistry Practice. *Clin. Cosmet. Investig. Dent.* **2022**, *14*, 207–216. [CrossRef]
37. Odorici, A.; Colombari, B.; Bellini, P.; Meto, A.; Venturelli, I.; Blasi, E. Novel Options to Counteract Oral Biofilm Formation: In Vitro Evidence. *Int. J. Environ. Res. Public Health* **2022**, *19*, 8056. [CrossRef]
38. Peppoloni, S.; Colombari, B.; Tagliazucchi, D.; Odorici, A.; Ventrucci, C.; Meto, A.; Blasi, E. Attenuation of Pseudomonas aeruginosa Virulence by Pomegranate Peel Extract. *Microorganisms* **2022**, *10*, 2500. [CrossRef]
39. Zhang, O.L.; Niu, J.Y.; Yin, I.X.; Yu, O.Y.; Mei, M.L.; Chu, C.H. Bioactive Materials for Caries Management: A Literature Review. *Dent. J.* **2023**, *11*, 59. [CrossRef]
40. Niu, J.Y.; Yin, I.X.; Wu, W.K.K.; Li, Q.L.; Mei, M.L.; Chu, C.H. A novel dual-action antimicrobial peptide for caries management. *J. Dent.* **2021**, *111*, 103729. [CrossRef]

41. Niu, J.Y.; Yin, I.X.; Wu, W.K.K.; Li, Q.L.; Mei, M.L.; Chu, C.H. Remineralising dentine caries using an artificial antimicrobial peptide: An in vitro study. *J. Dent.* **2021**, *111*, 103736. [CrossRef] [PubMed]
42. Niu, J.Y.; Yin, I.X.; Wu, W.K.K.; Li, Q.L.; Mei, M.L.; Chu, C.H. Antimicrobial peptides for the prevention and treatment of dental caries: A concise review. *Arch. Oral. Biol.* **2021**, *122*, 105022. [CrossRef] [PubMed]
43. Zhang, L.Y.; Fang, Z.H.; Li, Q.L.; Cao, C.Y. A tooth-binding antimicrobial peptide to prevent the formation of dental biofilm. *J. Mater. Sci. Mater. Med.* **2019**, *30*, 45. [CrossRef] [PubMed]
44. Niu, J.Y.; Yin, I.X.; Wu, W.K.K.; Li, Q.L.; Mei, M.L.; Chu, C.H. Efficacy of the dual-action GA-KR12 peptide for remineralising initial enamel caries: An in vitro study. *Clin. Oral. Investig.* **2022**, *26*, 2441–2451. [CrossRef]
45. Niu, J.Y.; Yin, I.X.; Wu, W.K.K.; Li, Q.L.; Mei, M.L.; Chu, C.H. *Data from: A Concise Review on Antimicrobial Peptides for Prevention and Treatment of Dental Caries*; Dryad: Moscow, Russia, 2021. [CrossRef]
46. Passos, M.R.; Almeida, R.S.; Lima, B.O.; Rodrigues, J.Z.S.; Macedo Neres, N.S.; Pita, L.S.; Marinho, P.D.F.; Santos, I.A.; da Silva, J.P.; Oliveira, M.C.; et al. Anticariogenic activities of *Libidibia ferrea*, gallic acid and ethyl gallate against Streptococcus mutans in biofilm model. *J. Ethnopharmacol.* **2021**, *274*, 114059. [CrossRef] [PubMed]
47. Cota, D.; Patil, D. Antibacterial potential of ellagic acid and gallic acid against IBD bacterial isolates and cytotoxicity against colorectal cancer. *Nat. Prod. Res.* **2022**, *37*, 1998–2002. [CrossRef]
48. Chen, X.; Daliri, E.B.; Kim, N.; Kim, J.R.; Yoo, D.; Oh, D.H. Microbial Etiology and Prevention of Dental Caries: Exploiting Natural Products to Inhibit Cariogenic Biofilms. *Pathogens* **2020**, *9*, 569. [CrossRef]
49. Cui, T.; Luo, W.; Xu, L.; Yang, B.; Zhao, W.; Cang, H. Progress of Antimicrobial Discovery Against the Major Cariogenic Pathogen Streptococcus mutans. *Curr. Issues Mol. Biol.* **2019**, *32*, 601–644. [CrossRef]
50. Lin, Y.; Chen, J.; Zhou, X.; Li, Y. Inhibition of Streptococcus mutans biofilm formation by strategies targeting the metabolism of exopolysaccharides. *Crit. Rev. Microbiol.* **2021**, *47*, 667–677. [CrossRef]
51. Lemos, J.A.; Palmer, S.R.; Zeng, L.; Wen, Z.T.; Kajfasz, J.K.; Freires, I.A.; Abranches, J.; Brady, L.J. The Biology of Streptococcus mutans. *Microbiol. Spectr.* **2019**, *7*, 7. [CrossRef]
52. Li, J.W.; Wyllie, R.M.; Jensen, P.A. A Novel Competence Pathway in the Oral Pathogen Streptococcus sobrinus. *J. Dent. Res.* **2021**, *100*, 542–548. [CrossRef]
53. Nascimento, M.M.; Lemos, J.A.; Abranches, J.; Goncalves, R.B.; Burne, R.A. Adaptive acid tolerance response of Streptococcus sobrinus. *J. Bacteriol.* **2004**, *186*, 6383–6390. [CrossRef]
54. Korona-Glowniak, I.; Skawinska-Bednarczyk, A.; Wrobel, R.; Pietrak, J.; Tkacz-Ciebiera, I.; Maslanko-Switala, M.; Krawczyk, D.; Bakiera, A.; Borek, A.; Malm, A.; et al. Streptococcus sobrinus as a Predominant Oral Bacteria Related to the Occurrence of Dental Caries in Polish Children at 12 Years Old. *Int. J. Environ. Res. Public Health* **2022**, *19*, 15005. [CrossRef]
55. Wen, Z.T.; Huang, X.; Ellepola, K.; Liao, S.; Li, Y. Lactobacilli and human dental caries: More than mechanical retention. *Microbiology* **2022**, *168*, 001196. [CrossRef] [PubMed]
56. Horiuchi, M.; Washio, J.; Mayanagi, H.; Takahashi, N. Transient acid-impairment of growth ability of oral Streptococcus, *Actinomyces*, and Lactobacillus: A possible ecological determinant in dental plaque. *Oral. Microbiol. Immunol.* **2009**, *24*, 319–324. [CrossRef] [PubMed]
57. Dame-Teixeira, N.; Parolo, C.C.; Maltz, M.; Tugnait, A.; Devine, D.; Do, T. *Actinomyces* spp. gene expression in root caries lesions. *J. Oral. Microbiol.* **2016**, *8*, 32383. [CrossRef] [PubMed]
58. Briseno-Marroquin, P.; Ismael, Y.; Callaway, A.; Tennert, C.; Wolf, T.G. Antibacterial effect of silver diamine fluoride and potassium iodide against *E. faecalis*, *A. naeslundii* and *P. micra*. *BMC Oral. Health* **2021**, *21*, 175. [CrossRef]
59. Taylor, J.J. Protein biomarkers of periodontitis in saliva. *ISRN Inflamm.* **2014**, *2014*, 593151. [CrossRef]
60. Jia, L.; Han, N.; Du, J.; Guo, L.; Luo, Z.; Liu, Y. Pathogenesis of Important Virulence Factors of *Porphyromonas gingivalis* via Toll-Like Receptors. *Front. Cell Infect. Microbiol.* **2019**, *9*, 262. [CrossRef]
61. Hajishengallis, G. Immunomicrobial pathogenesis of periodontitis: Keystones, pathobionts, and host response. *Trends Immunol.* **2014**, *35*, 3–11. [CrossRef]
62. Kononen, E.; Muller, H.P. Microbiology of aggressive periodontitis. *Periodontology* **2014**, *65*, 46–78. [CrossRef]
63. Lowman, W. Minimum inhibitory concentration-guided antimicrobial therapy—The Achilles heel in the antimicrobial stewardship agenda. *S. Afr. Med. J.* **2018**, *108*, 710–712. [CrossRef]
64. Yin, L.M.; Edwards, M.A.; Li, J.; Yip, C.M.; Deber, C.M. Roles of hydrophobicity and charge distribution of cationic antimicrobial peptides in peptide-membrane interactions. *J. Biol. Chem.* **2012**, *287*, 7738–7745. [CrossRef] [PubMed]
65. Amiss, A.S.; von Pein, J.B.; Webb, J.R.; Condon, N.D.; Harvey, P.J.; Phan, M.D.; Schembri, M.A.; Currie, B.J.; Sweet, M.J.; Craik, D.J.; et al. Modified horseshoe crab peptides target and kill bacteria inside host cells. *Cell Mol. Life Sci.* **2021**, *79*, 38. [CrossRef] [PubMed]
66. Li, J.; Koh, J.J.; Liu, S.; Lakshminarayanan, R.; Verma, C.S.; Beuerman, R.W. Membrane Active Antimicrobial Peptides: Translating Mechanistic Insights to Design. *Front. Neurosci.* **2017**, *11*, 73. [CrossRef]
67. Silhavy, T.J.; Kahne, D.; Walker, S. The bacterial cell envelope. *Cold Spring Harb. Perspect. Biol.* **2010**, *2*, a000414. [CrossRef]
68. Welling, M.M.; Lupetti, A.; Balter, H.S.; Lanzzeri, S.; Souto, B.; Rey, A.M.; Savio, E.O.; Paulusma-Annema, A.; Pauwels, E.K.; Nibbering, P.H. 99mTc-labeled antimicrobial peptides for detection of bacterial and Candida albicans infections. *J. Nucl. Med.* **2001**, *42*, 788–794. [PubMed]

69. Mookherjee, N.; Anderson, M.A.; Haagsman, H.P.; Davidson, D.J. Antimicrobial host defence peptides: Functions and clinical potential. *Nat. Rev. Drug Discov.* **2020**, *19*, 311–332. [CrossRef]
70. Panteleev, P.V.; Balandin, S.V.; Ivanov, V.T.; Ovchinnikova, T.V. A Therapeutic Potential of Animal beta-hairpin Antimicrobial Peptides. *Curr. Med. Chem.* **2017**, *24*, 1724–1746. [CrossRef]

Disclaimer/Publisher's Note: The statements, opinions and data contained in all publications are solely those of the individual author(s) and contributor(s) and not of MDPI and/or the editor(s). MDPI and/or the editor(s) disclaim responsibility for any injury to people or property resulting from any ideas, methods, instructions or products referred to in the content.

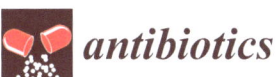

Review

Innovative Approaches for Maintaining and Enhancing Skin Health and Managing Skin Diseases through Microbiome-Targeted Strategies

Khadeejeh AL-Smadi [1], Vania Rodrigues Leite-Silva [1,2], Newton Andreo Filho [2,3], Patricia Santos Lopes [2] and Yousuf Mohammed [1,3,*]

1. Frazer Institute, Faculty of Medicine, The University of Queensland, Brisbane, QLD 4102, Australia; k.alsmadi@uqconnect.edu.au (K.A.-S.); vania.leite@unifesp.br (V.R.L.-S.)
2. Departamento de Ciências Farmacêuticas, Instituto de Ciências Ambientais, Químicas e Farmacêuticas, Universidade Federal de São Paulo, UNIFESP-Diadema, Diadema CEP 09913-030, SP, Brazil; n.andreofilho@uq.edu.au (N.A.F.); patricia.lopes@unifesp.br (P.S.L.)
3. School of Pharmacy, The University of Queensland, Brisbane, QLD 4102, Australia
* Correspondence: y.mohammed@uq.edu.au; Tel.: +61-433853534

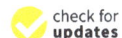

Citation: AL-Smadi, K.; Leite-Silva, V.R.; Filho, N.A.; Lopes, P.S.; Mohammed, Y. Innovative Approaches for Maintaining and Enhancing Skin Health and Managing Skin Diseases through Microbiome-Targeted Strategies. *Antibiotics* **2023**, *12*, 1698. https://doi.org/10.3390/antibiotics12121698

Academic Editor: Anisha D'Souza

Received: 31 October 2023
Revised: 29 November 2023
Accepted: 29 November 2023
Published: 4 December 2023

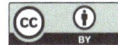

Copyright: © 2023 by the authors. Licensee MDPI, Basel, Switzerland. This article is an open access article distributed under the terms and conditions of the Creative Commons Attribution (CC BY) license (https://creativecommons.org/licenses/by/4.0/).

Abstract: The skin microbiome is crucial in maintaining skin health, and its disruption is associated with various skin diseases. Prebiotics are non-digestible fibers and compounds found in certain foods that promote the activity and growth of beneficial bacteria in the gut or skin. On the other hand, live microorganisms, known as probiotics, benefit in sustaining healthy conditions when consumed in reasonable quantities. They differ from postbiotics, which are by-product compounds from bacteria that release the same effects as their parent bacteria. The human skin microbiome is vital when it comes to maintaining skin health and preventing a variety of dermatological conditions. This review explores novel strategies that use microbiome-targeted treatments to maintain and enhance overall skin health while managing various skin disorders. It is important to understand the dynamic relationship between these beneficial microorganisms and the diverse microbial communities present on the skin to create effective strategies for using probiotics on the skin. This understanding can help optimize formulations and treatment regimens for improved outcomes in skincare, particularly in developing solutions for various skin problems.

Keywords: vitiligo; microbiome; prebiotics; probiotics; postbiotics

1. Introduction

The skin microbiome is a complex and dynamic ecology that resides in the skin, which is the largest organ of the human body. This varied group of microbes, which includes bacteria, fungi, and viruses, is essential to the homeostasis and health of the skin. A variety of skin diseases and disorders have been connected to disruptions of this critical microbial balance [1], such as psoriasis, vitiligo, and atopic dermatitis (AD) [2]. Promising new opportunities in the field of dermatology have recently arisen with the development of nanotechnology. Scientists and researchers have been investigating the development of innovative nanotechnology that provides efficacy in the restoration and control of the skin microbiome [3,4]. Nanoparticles can generally be utilized for delivering drugs in a way that improves their resistance to enzymatic degradation, targets specific locations, increases bioavailability, solubilizes them for intravascular transport, and maintains their effects [5]. These nanosystems or microbiome-targeted nanotherapeutics provide a novel approach that targets the related causes of skin disorders while reducing the adverse effects associated with traditional therapies.

The field of microbiome-targeted nanotherapeutics has been growing rapidly, and many nanosystems are being investigated for the regeneration and maintenance of the microbiota [6,7]. The nanostructures can be engineered to interact with the microbiome, either by modulating the microbial composition or delivering therapeutic agents that influence the microbiome, which affects the progression of certain skin conditions [8]. However, careful consideration of unexpected effects, biocompatibility, regulatory challenges, and long-term impacts is essential to ensuring the safety and efficacy of these innovative treatments [9]. Nanoparticles and nanoemulsions are the most popular nanosystems for targeting microbiomes because of their small size, modified properties, and efficient delivery capabilities. Their unique characteristics enable precise interactions with microbial communities and facilitate effective, customized interventions for improved dermatological treatments [3,10]. Nanoparticles typically range in size from 1 to 100 nanometers and are solid, colloidal particles. They can be made from a variety of materials, such as metals, polymers, and lipids. They include lipid nanoparticles (liposomes and solid lipid nanoparticles), polymeric micelles, metal nanoparticles, and polymeric nanoparticles (Figure 1). They are utilized in drug delivery since they may protect and deliver drugs to particular target locations within the body, enhancing medication effectiveness and minimizing adverse effects.

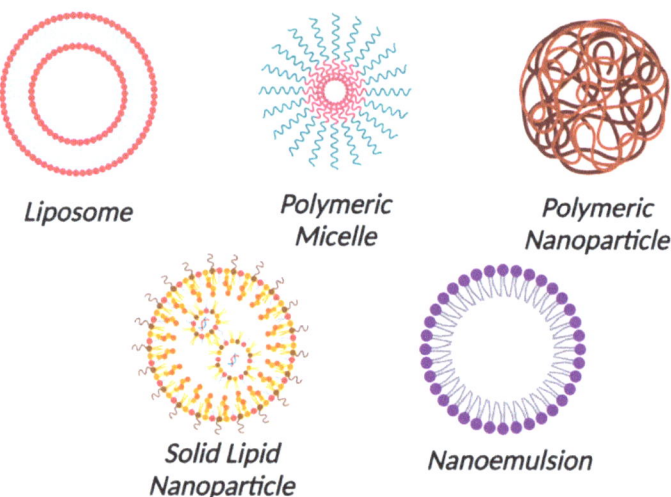

Figure 1. Nanoparticles and Nanoemulsions. Created with Biorender.com.

Furthermore, nanoparticles are employed to improve the performance of sunscreens, lotions, and other skincare products [11–13]. On the other hand, nanoemulsions are small oil droplets, typically ranging in size from 20 to 200 nanometers, distributed in an aqueous phase and frequently stabilized by surfactants in a process known as nanoemulsions formulations. They are either oil-in-water (O/W) or water-in-oil (W/O) nanoemulsions. The solubility and bioavailability of poorly water-soluble drugs can be enhanced by using nanoemulsions. In addition, they are used to improve the stability of some products as well as to encapsulate flavors, vitamins, and other bioactive components. In cosmetics, nanoemulsions are utilized in order to enhance the texture and stability of lotions and skincare items [14,15]. When creating medications in nanoform to increase absorption and effectiveness, three main variables need to be considered. These include FDA quality-related standards, drug transport, degradation mechanisms, and the stability of the manufactured drug. The pharmaceutical industry has limitations while utilizing nanoformulations because of this. The primary cause of the low therapeutic efficacy of nano-formulations is their propensity to self-aggregate at low drug concentrations, which compromises the formulation's stability and increases the variability of drug entrapment because of polydispersity. Unformulated liposomes are more stable, but when a medicine is built into them, the stability decreases as the ionic strength grows. Starting with smaller nanoparticles (<20 nm) for the formulation could solve this issue such that even after loading the drug, it remains below 100 nm [16,17]. Although around 100 nm-sized nanoparticles have increased surface reactivity, they can have adverse biological effects like protein unfolding, membrane impairment, DNA damage, and inflammatory reactions. Additionally, several size-dependent processes, such as clathrin-mediated entry and caveolae-mediated pathways, allow particles in the 10–500 nm range, including those about 100 nm, to be absorbed into cells. Particle size preferences vary throughout cells; endothelial cells prefer particles that are around 100 nm in size, while professional phagocytes prefer larger particles [18,19].

Oxidative stress affects mitochondrial function and promotes the production of reactive oxygen species (ROS) and pro-inflammatory cytokines [20]. Increased ROS in the skin destroys melanocytes by damaging their DNA and associated cellular structures [21]. In addition, ROS causes a variety of oxidation products, including oxidized protein products and glycation products, that alter the structure of melanocytes [22]. It has been suggested that the main cause of melanocyte loss is mitochondrial malfunction driven by oxidative stress. Increased carbonylation in vitiligo melanocytes causes mitochondrial dysregulation, which could lead to severe mitochondrial dysfunction and melanocyte apoptosis [23]. The microbiome may influence the skin's general durability and response to oxidative stress or contribute to the modulation of oxidative stress and inflammation [24].

In the exploration of skin health, emerging research underscores the role of the skin microbiome in various dermatological conditions. Among these conditions, vitiligo is an autoimmune condition characterized by depigmented macules and patches of various forms, which is caused by the death of melanocytes or the loss of their activity to produce natural skin pigments [25]. Consequently, discolored white spots appear on the skin, hair, and mucous membranes in various parts of the body. The prevalence of vitiligo in the general population of the world ranges from 0.06% to 2.28% [26]. Vitiligo can be classified into different types based on the characteristics of the lesions. Acrofacial vitiligo is characterized by lesions occasionally appearing on the extremities and face. Mixed vitiligo involves a combination of non-segmental and segmental patterns. Focal vitiligo is distinguished by small and isolated lesions. Mucosal vitiligo occurs in or around mucosal membranes. Universal vitiligo is a type where lesions develop and spread over the entire body [27,28]. Numerous mechanisms have been connected to the degeneration of melanocytes and the emergence of white patches in vitiligo. These mechanisms include neuronal, genetic, autoimmune, oxidative stress, environmental triggers, and the creation of inflammatory mediators [29]. The most prevalent and well-established explanation proposes that a defect in the immune response results in the destruction of melanocytes by autoimmune effector mechanisms, either memory cytotoxic T cells or autoantibodies directed against melanocyte surface antigens. Numerous studies have demonstrated a link between vitiligo and other autoimmune diseases such as Addison's disease, pernicious anemia, diabetes, systemic lupus erythematosus, rheumatoid arthritis, psoriasis, and alopecia areata [30,31]. Topical corticosteroids (TCSs) and Topical calcineurin inhibitors (TCIs) are often used and recognized as a common treatment for many types of vitiligo [32]. When concerns regarding the reported adverse effects of prolonged usage of potent TCSs and TCIs arise, both have demonstrated a high degree of repigmentation but are not safe treatment options. TCIs often result in erythema, pruritus, and burning sensations as side effects, while TCSs increase the possibility of skin atrophy, striae, and telangiectasia [33,34]. Alternative treatments and outcomes have improved as a result of the introduction of numerous therapeutic approaches, such as phototherapy, excimer laser, vitamin D, and epidermal grafts [35,36]. However, there is occasionally hesitancy to suggest treatment because, historically, vitiligo was thought to respond to treatment quite poorly and infrequently [37]. Another common pathogenic trigger for melanocyte destruction in vitiligo patients is oxidative stress, which is also a key element in the onset and progression of the disease [38].

Psoriasis is a chronic inflammatory skin disease developed by the influence of a genetic predisposition and external variables. It has several different kinds; however, they are all identified by erythematous plaques that are frequently itchy [39]. The cutaneous immune system's improper activation against a presumed infection is the main theory regarding the development of psoriasis. The innate and adaptive immune systems are both implicated in the pathogenesis of the disease, which also involves abnormal keratinocyte development and immune cell infiltration in the dermis and epidermis, with dendritic cells and T cells performing significant roles [40].

AD is the most prevalent inflammatory skin disorder worldwide. It affects a substantial portion of the global population, impacting around 15% to 20% of children and 1% to 3% of adults [41]. This chronic inflammatory skin condition is characterized by itchy and dry inflamed lesions. It stems from a range of hereditary mutations in skin barrier proteins and immunological defects specific to allergens. Individuals with AD often exhibit symptoms such as skin dryness, redness, and the development of erythematous lesions. Moreover, AD frequently presents with related issues like eczema, skin scaling, and persistent itching. Additionally, it can be associated with comorbidities such as allergic rhinoconjunctivitis and asthma [42].

Recently, evidence showed that altered skin microbiomes (dysbiosis) contribute to the pathogenesis of vitiligo by influencing immunological homeostasis, oxidative stress, and skin barrier [43,44]. Further, research on the skin lesions of psoriasis patients has revealed an imbalance in the skin microbiome. The authors report that inflammation results from a dysbiosis disruption of the skin's immunological responses. *Streptococcus* bacteria are frequently overabundant, while *Cutibacterium* is less present in these lesions [39]. Studies are increasingly focusing on combining probiotics and nanotechnology to treat skin infections. Improved drug delivery, moisture retention, controlling the release of active compounds, and anti-infective properties have been demonstrated by nanotechnology, especially nanoparticle-based methods [45]. Some research suggests that topical probiotics emollient and bacteria-derived formulations may be an effective alternative for the treatment of AD [46]. Due to their capacity to have a favorable effect on the skin microbiome, these formulations can decrease inflammation and enhance the general health of the skin barrier by creating a balance in the microbial communities on the skin. [47]. Additionally, the controlled probiotic release offered by nanoparticles and nanotechnology delivers enormous potential for treating human infections. Although beneficial results have been observed, further human research is required to investigate their effectiveness in dermatological applications and to address the problem of bacterial resistance [48,49]. Therefore, in this review, we aim to provide a comprehensive evaluation of the use of topical probiotics, prebiotics, and postbiotics in treating skin disorders due to the increasing popularity of these topical treatments and the lack of clinical trials or efficacy studies to support their therapeutic value. Also, examine innovative approaches involving the use of microbiome-targeted techniques to maintain and improve overall skin health while addressing the management of different skin diseases.

2. Prebiotics, Probiotics and Postbiotics

Prebiotics are specific fermented substances or dietary supplements that are not digested, enhancing intestinal health by encouraging the growth of commensal bacteria [50]. On the other hand, probiotics are non-pathogenic live microorganisms, frequently yeast or bacteria, that, when administered in sufficient amounts, confer a health benefit to the host [51,52]. Probiotics from the first generation are commonly available products to treat microecological disorders. The next level of development is the production of "metabiotics", which are small molecules or chemicals obtained from probiotic microorganisms. The bioactive compounds produced by symbiotic microorganisms (a combination of probiotics and prebiotics) from naturally occurring probiotic strains, or natural sources can be used to synthesize or semi-synthesize these metabiotics. They are known as "metabolic probiotics", "postbiotics", "biological drugs", or "pharmacobiotics". These compounds have the potential to impact the microbiota, human metabolic processes, signaling pathways, and physiological activities related to the host. Postbiotics have recognized chemical structures that may improve the composition and functionality of the host's native microbiota as well as components involved in immunology, neurohormone biology, and metabolic and behavioral responses [53]. For instance, many commensal bacteria produce butyrate, a postbiotic that is a major source of energy for the colon and is essential for intestinal growth, differentiation, and inflammation control [54,55]. Moreover, postbiotics are probiotic-derived effector chemicals secreted by bacteria or released after lysis and capable of exerting qualities identical to those of the original probiotics [56,57] (Figure 2). They attempt to imitate the benefits of probiotics without taking the risk of administering live bacteria. While these probiotics, prebiotics, and postbiotics are commonly associated with dietary supplements targeting the gut microbiome, their application extends beyond the digestive system to various body parts, including the skin. In dermatology, particularly in addressing skin conditions, these concepts find relevance as researchers explore their potential in topical formulations and skincare products.

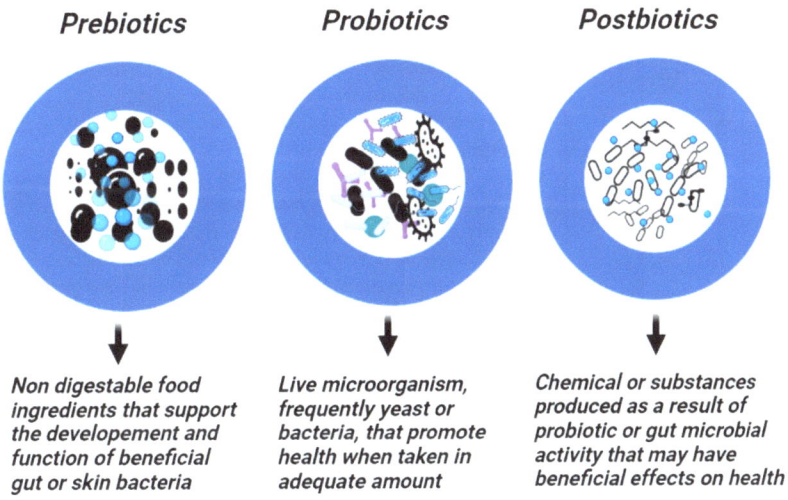

Figure 2. Prebiotics, Probiotics, and Postbiotics. Created with Biorender.com.

3. Skin Microbiome

The connection between microbial communities and the host tissue is symbiotic in the skin. The importance of resident microbial communities in maintaining the skin's and immune system's normal, healthy function has been demonstrated recently [58,59]. A diverse group of microorganisms known as the skin microbiome work together to maintain a complicated connection on the skin [1]. A large and diverse community of bacteria, viruses, and eukaryotes, including fungi and arthropods, comprise the human skin microbiota [60,61]. The heterogeneity of the skin microbiota, both in terms of its composition and prevalence, can be demonstrated in the significant variances between individuals and between different skin regions. These differences can be attributable to a complex interaction of elements, including genetic predisposition, dietary habits, choice of lifestyle, gender, age, ethnic background, and environmental circumstances [62,63]. The skin provides essential nutrients to establish its microbiota, including amino acids, fatty acids, and lactic acids from various sources like proteins, the stratum corneum, sweat, lipid hydrolysis, and sebum [64]. This relationship between the host and commensal microorganisms is vital for various physiological processes. To maintain this symbiotic relationship, commensal-specific T cells play a role in distinguishing between resident microorganisms and potential pathogens, thereby promoting tolerance towards the commensal microbiota [65]. The skin microbiome is made up of several different bacterial species. Microorganism imbalances can lead to skin diseases such as acne, AD, psoriasis, and rosacea [66]. Probiotic bacteria have been used to make a variety of treatments, nutritional items, and additives that support human health [67]. They provide several functions, one of which is serving as the first line of defense against invasive diseases and are also used to prevent both acute and chronic disorders or prophylaxis [68]. This shows that probiotics are used as an avoidance strategy for some disorders. In addition, specific health conditions, such as acute or chronic diarrhea and intestinal inflammation that can cause allergies, atherosclerosis, and cancer, are also treated with probiotic medications [69]. Coagulation-negative Staphylococci are also prevalent on human skin, and they act via a number of mechanisms including the epidermal barrier environment and the innate and adaptive immune systems found in the epidermis and dermis [70]. Further, the bacteriocins produced by this species have anti-inflammatory, and antibacterial characteristics that reduce the survival of harmful bacteria on the skin surface [41]. Endogenous urocanic acid found in the stratum corneum of the skin acts similarly to sunscreens in preventing damaging Ultraviolet (UV) radiation from penetrating the epidermis [67,71].

The microorganisms that make up the skin microbiome cooperate to keep the skin safe. However, due to many factors, such as external ones, commensal microorganisms may transform into pathogenic microbes, causing inflammation, itching, scaling, and other medical symptoms that point to an imbalance between our skin and its microbiome [72]. The word "dysbiosis" is used to describe how the microbiome of the skin has changed. Functional dysbiosis disturbs the interactions between bacteria and hosts and causes skin issues. Age, sex, hygiene, the use of particular pharmaceuticals, skin pH, sweating propensity, hair development on the skin, sebum production, usage of skin cosmetics, and lifestyle are only a few of the host factors that have an impact on the microbiome host interaction [73]. The potential of oral probiotics as a treatment for skin conditions has increased as research has revealed a connection between disrupted gut microbiota and inflammatory skin conditions [74]. Researchers are actively investigating the relationships among changes in the gut microbiota, immune system dysregulation, and the development or aggravation of autoimmune skin disorders, aiming to identify biomarkers and molecular pathways for potential therapeutic targeting [75–77]. Studies on probiotics have been performed using a concept known as the gut–brain–skin axis idea. These studies have demonstrated the efficacy of probiotics in the management of some dermatological conditions, including psoriasis, acne, vitiligo, and AD [2,78]. For example, AD is characterized by cutaneous dysbiosis and a greater presence of *Staphylococci* like *S. aureus* and *Malassezia* spp. These microorganisms release toxic chemicals and nanovesicles that trigger cytokines, which contribute to the persistence and aggravation of AD symptoms.

Transplanting specific strains of *S. epidermidis* and *S. hominis* that produce antimicrobial peptides resulted in significant decreases in the levels of *S. aureus* in individuals with AD. This implies a promising therapeutic strategy for addressing AD by influencing the skin's microbiome to regulate and reduce the overgrowth of *S. aureus* [79]. The local skin microbiome plays a role in psoriasis pathogens. Psoriasis patients have a similar major species of bacteria in their skin flora compared to non-psoriasis individuals but with reduced diversity and changes in the relative abundance of certain bacteria. Specifically, lower concentrations of *Cutibacterium acnes* (formerly *Propionibacterium*) and *Actinobacteria* species are found in psoriasis patients, while higher concentrations of *Firmicutes*, *Proteobacteria*, *Acidobacteria*, *Schlegelella*, *Streptococcaceae*, *Rhodobacteraceae*, *Campylobacteraceae*, and *Moraxellaceae* species are observed when compared to controls. This suggests that alterations in the skin microbiome may contribute to psoriasis alongside immune system dysfunction [80,81]. As a result, these skin disorders present greater opportunities for probiotic research regarding topical benefits. In general, the gut microbiota is responsible for the body's appropriate immunity and defense against harmful microbes. Therefore, alterations that are considered harmful at the intestinal microbiota level may result in infections and autoimmune diseases in a variety of organs outside of the colon, including the skin [82]. A recent study [83] shows that patients with vitiligo have a different microbial composition from healthy people, with a considerably lower Bacteroidetes to Firmicutes ratio. They also differ significantly from healthy people in 23 blood metabolites, and these metabolites are linked to particular microbial indicators. Commensal bacteria are vital components of the skin microbiome and play a crucial role in skin health. Another study [84] highlights that vitiligo-affected skin exhibits a dysbiosis in microbial community diversity, with lesional areas showing reduced taxonomic richness and evenness. Notably, Actinobacterial species are dominant in normal skin, while Firmicutes species dominate in vitiligo lesions, suggesting that these microbial changes could influence the development and severity of vitiligo.

4. Mechanisms of Action for Topical Prebiotics, Postbiotics and Probiotics

Many low-molecular-weight (LMW) bioactive substances, such as bacteriocins and other antimicrobial compounds, short-chain fatty acids, various fatty and organic acids, biosurfactants, polysaccharides, peptidoglycans, teichoic acids, lipo- and glycoproteins, vitamins, antioxidants, nucleic acids, amino acids, and different proteins, including enzymes and lectins, can be derived from different probiotic strains [85,86]. The applicable agents of these groups of LMW compounds isolated from symbiotic microorganisms or their cultural liquids may be used to produce functional foods, drugs for the prophylaxis and treatment of chronic human diseases, as well as sports and anti-aging foods [87,88]. The application of the probiotics concept in biotechnology has made it possible to include several thousand additional strains from the human-dominant intestinal phyla (Bacteroides, Firmicutes, Proteobacteria, Actinobacteria, and Archae) for nutritional and therapeutic purposes in addition to *Bifidobacteria*, *Lactobacilli*, *Escherichia*, and *Enterococci* sp. [89,90].

Microbiome development and changes are influenced by various factors such as childbirth, diet, drugs, and diseases [91]. The skin microbiota varies significantly across different body regions due to the presence of unique glands and hair follicles, creating distinct conditions for microbial growth. Specific bacterial and fungal species dominate various areas, such as lipophilic bacteria in sebaceous regions and fungal communities on the feet. Additionally, the facial skin microbiota is mainly composed of Proteobacteria, Firmicutes, Actinobacteria, and Bacteroidetes, with variations linked to age, and diversity differs by facial location, with cheek sites having the highest richness scores. Postbiotics like acetate, propionate, and butyrate play a crucial role in intestinal health by providing energy, enhancing the epithelial barrier, regulating immunity, and preventing pathogen invasion [92]. Immune diseases, inflammation, and gut dysbiosis can result from a dysregulation of this balance [93]. The gut–skin axis is proposed as a connection between emotional states, gut health, and skin conditions. Increased intestinal permeability can activate T cells, disrupt immunosuppressive factors, and lead to systemic inflammation, potentially affecting skin homeostasis [94]. Gut microbes can also communicate with other organs through neurotransmitter production. Therefore, changes in the gut microbiome may directly impact systemic inflammation [92]. In the last century, the ability to identify microorganisms based on their appearance or biochemical traits and improvements in cell culture techniques have allowed for the expansion of study into the microbial variety of human skin. Researchers have identified numerous genera of bacteria that are typically found on healthy skin using culture-dependent methods. These genera include *Staphylococci*, *Micrococci*, *Corynebacteria*, *Brevibacteria*, *Propionibacteria*, and *Acinetobacter* [95]. *Staphylococcus aureus*, *Streptococcus pyogenes*, and *Pseudomonas aeruginosa* were identified at the species level using culture techniques, such as colonizers in unusual conditions [96]. The skin microbiome is primarily made up of two main types of bacteria: the resident and transient microbiota types. The resident microbiota is the most significant and persistent group and may regenerate after any disturbances [97]. In contrast, the transitory microbiome is environment-dependent and only stays on the skin for a few hours or days [98]. Both of these microbiota types are harmless in healthy skin. Actinobacteria, Firmicutes, Proteobacteria, and Bacteroides are some of the most prevalent phyla on the skin, while the most common genera are *Corynebacterium*, *Propionibacterium*, and *Staphylococci* [66,99].

5. Clinical Verification and Effectiveness

The effectiveness of probiotic products used topically has received very little investigation. However, in the past ten years, the number of commercially available topical probiotics has dramatically increased [100], and probiotics have been applied topically and orally to treat various skin disorders [53] Table 1. The gut microbiota significantly affects the immune system, and many studies [2,101,102] have shown the importance of dysregulations in the skin and gut microbiome in immune-related diseases. Immune dysregulation driven by imbalances in the gut microbiota may involve an excessive immune response that targets melanocytes and contributes to their destruction in vitiligo [103]. It is thought that both genetic and environmental factors play a role in the vitiligo development process. Recent research indicates that vitiligo patients have altered immune responses and increased stress-induced production of Interferon-gamma (IFN-γ), which leads to melanocyte apoptosis [104]. Dysbiosis in the gut microbiome is observed in vitiligo patients, with reduced Bacteroides populations and changes in microbiota diversity, which are associated with mitochondrial damage and peripheral changes in innate immunity [105]. Skin microbiota composition also differs between vitiligo patients and healthy controls, particularly in vitiligo lesions, where there is a reduction in *Staphylococcus* and *Cutibacterium* and an increase in *Proteobacteria* associated with inflammation [103].

Table 1. Examples of Probiotic-Containing Commercial Products.

Probiotics	Oral	Topical	Benefits Claimed
Lactobacillus			
		Lactobacillus Ferment Essence	A skincare brand containing *Lactobacillus ferment* for skin nourishment
	Probiotic Complex with *Lactobacillus Acidophilus*		a health brand promoting overall well-being, including potential benefits for the skin
Bifidobacterium			
		BifidoBalance Cream	A skincare company formulated with *Bifidobacterium* to support skin microbiome balance
	Gut Health Probiotic Blend with *Bifidobacterium*		A nutritional supplement brand aimed at promoting gut health with potential skin benefits
Streptococcus thermophilus			
		Thermal Probiotic Cream	Skincare line featuring *Streptococcus thermophilus* for enhancing the diversity of the skin microbiome
Saccharomyces boulardii			
	Saccharomyces boulardii Probiotic Capsules		A wellness brand specifically designed to support gut health and potentially improve skin conditions
Probiotic Blends			
		Probiotic Power Serum	A skincare brand incorporating a blend of *Lactobacillus*, *Bifidobacterium*, and *Streptococcus thermophilus* for a comprehensive skin health approach
	Daily Probiotic Blend Capsules		A health and wellness company offering a mix of various probiotic strains for overall health, including potential benefits for the skin

The topical application of probiotic bacteria may help enhance the skin's natural barrier by directly affecting the site of application. This may be performed by the resident bacteria and the probiotic bacteria that produce certain antimicrobial amino peptides that benefit the immune responses in the skin and help eliminate pathogens [106]. The administration of probiotic species that are not native to a particular ecosystem can potentially cause adverse effects [107]. They are commonly included in over-the-counter cosmeceutical products, but their effectiveness may be compromised by their high bacterial load and the preservatives used, which can impact the skin's microbiota [108]. Probiotics have been utilized in a variety of cosmetic items, including lotions, intimate hygiene products, shampoos, and toothpaste. These strains include *Bacillus subtilis*, *Lactobacillus acidophilus*, *Lactobacillus casei*, and *Lactobacillus plantarum*. These probiotics provide several benefits for skin health, including moisturizing effects, reducing toxic metabolites, enhancing antibody production, restoring immune system balance, and regulating cytokine synthesis [109,110]. In addition, topically applied probiotics can serve as a protective barrier on the skin by competing with and inhibiting the binding of potential pathogens to skin sites. This competitive inhibition helps prevent the colonization of harmful microorganisms on the skin, further contributing to skin health and protection [100].

Postbiotics, formed from microbial growth by-products or inactive dead strains, positively benefit skin health because they contain bioactive substances such as bacteriocins, lipoteichoic acids, and organic acids [111]. Species of *Lactobacillus*, including those found in cosmetics, create lactic acid, which aids in moisturization and anti-aging [112]. *Streptococcus* and *Bifidobacterium* strains have also been demonstrated to increase skin hydration and elasticity, with *Bifidobacterium* contributing to the production of hyaluronic acid for improved skin appearance [113,114].

Novel strategies in the field of dermatology employ nanocarriers to improve the topical applications of probiotics and prebiotics [4,6]. These nanocarriers, often in the form of nanoparticles or nanoemulsions, serve as efficient vehicles for loading and delivering probiotic strains to the skin. This advanced delivery system not only protects the viability of probiotics during formulation but also enhances their penetration into the skin, maximizing their potential to establish a protective barrier.

6. Formulations and Delivery Methods

Skin microbiota can be preserved and restored by probiotics, prebiotics, or combination supplements (symbiotic) [106] Table 2. In other words, probiotics, prebiotics, and symbiotics are the three treatment modalities currently employed to maintain and restore the gut microbial ecology [90,115]. In cosmetic formulations, prebiotics can selectively increase the activity and growth of beneficial skin probiotics [116]. Some cosmetic formulations may help foster the normal skin microbiome by being selective in their activity [106]. It has recently been demonstrated that incorporating antioxidants and probiotics in combination with other therapies can accelerate repigmentation. One study on AD skin showed that topical formulations with particular probiotic strains helped reduce skin lesions [117]. Another study conducted by Chaudhry et al. [118] combined TCI with an antioxidant and probiotic diet as an adjuvant. They demonstrated that full repigmentation could be achieved in just six weeks and that no relapses were noted for 52 weeks following the treatment. Certain lactic acid bacteria, specifically *Streptococcus thermophiles*, have been found to enhance ceramide production in the skin when topically applied as a cream. Ceramides are lipids that play a crucial role in maintaining the skin's barrier function and hydration levels, and this is particularly beneficial for individuals with acne-prone skin because acne treatments can sometimes lead to dryness and irritation. Additionally, it shows antimicrobial activity against *Cutibacterium acnes*, a bacterium associated with the development of acne [119].

Table 2. Overview of Formulations and Delivery Methods in Skin Microbiota Preservation.

Treatment Modality	Delivery Method	Key Components	Results and Applications
Probiotics	Topical application	Live bacteria (Probiotics)	Reduction of skin lesions in AD; potential for repigmentation
Prebiotics	Oral administration	Substances promoting beneficial bacteria growth (e.g., fructooligosaccharides)	Improved psoriasis scores when combined with topical hydrocortisone; positive effects on gut microbiota linked to AD
Symbiotics	Oral administration	Combination of probiotics and prebiotics (e.g., Lactocare®)	Improved psoriasis scores when used alongside topical hydrocortisone
Postbiotics	Topical application	Cell-free supernatants, lysates, bioactive peptides	Acceleration of epithelization, reduction of skin inflammation, antioxidant capabilities against UVB-induced damage; multiple positive effects on skin health

Incorporating live bacteria, such as probiotics, into cosmetic products is a complex process that requires significant adjustments in production, storage, and distribution procedures [120]. These adjustments are necessary because formulation processes can potentially deactivate probiotics and alter their intended functions. Different dehydration techniques are frequently employed in probiotic manufacture to overcome this [121]. In contrast to oral probiotic formulations, topical probiotic products often need reconstitution in a vehicle, such as creams, gels, and emulsions, before use, allowing them to be applied to the skin and integrated into specific pharmaceutical bases [122,123] Figure 3. Additionally, many factors can influence the probiotic quality during storage or delivery because of their susceptibility to temperature, humidity, and cooling conditions [124]. Prebiotics and postbiotics have recently been proposed as alternative options to address these concerns.

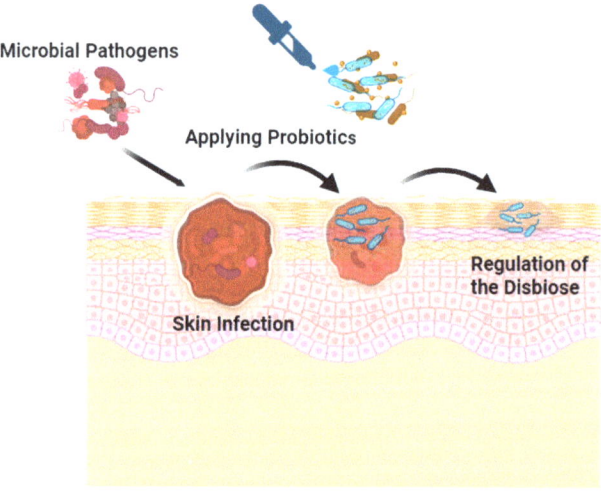

Figure 3. Probiotics Application During Skin Infection. Created with Biorender.com.

Prebiotics or symbiotics have been demonstrated to improve skin health significantly. For instance, Lactocare®, a symbiotic composition, combined with topical hydrocortisone improved psoriasis scores when administered orally [125]. A different study showed that giving mice with AD olive-derived antioxidant dietary fiber caused enhancements in the gut microbiota's composition, cytokine profiles, and butyrate synthesis, which improved the immune system response linked to AD [126]. Prebiotic polysaccharides such as fructo-oligosaccharides, galacto-oligosaccharides, and milk-derived oligosaccharides are fermented by bacteria (probiotics) in the human colon, resulting in the production of short-chain fatty acids (SCFAs), such as acetate, propionate, and butyrate [127–129]. These SCFAs increase blood flow in the colon, improve fluid and electrolyte absorption in the gut, promote the growth of intestinal cells, decrease bowel inflammation, influence enzyme activity, and reduce the risk of cancer and pathogen colonization [130,131]. Intestinal cells use butyrate as an energy source, which stimulates proliferation, increases the production of protective mucin, strengthens the intestinal barrier, and enhances immune system performance [129,131]. The human gut contains a variety of strains from the *Lactobacillus* and *Bifidobacterium* genera, which have a range of advantageous benefits. Additionally, these bacteria are used to generate probiotics [127].

Postbiotics produced from several probiotic strains have demonstrated potential therapeutic advantages for various skin issues and disorders. Cell-free supernatants, lysates, and bioactive peptides are some examples of postbiotics that have been examined for their effects on skin health and have shown a variety of beneficial results [132]. Postbiotics from *Lactobacillus fermentum*, *Lactobacillus reuteri*, and *Lactobacillus subtilis* natto are being investigated as a novel method to promote earlier full epithelization and decrease skin inflammation when applied topically with a cold cream [133]. A cell-free supernatant of fermented milk from the *L. helveticus* strain demonstrated substantial antioxidant capabilities against UVB-induced skin damage, including decreasing lipid peroxidation and inhibiting melanin formation [132]. A customized blend of probiotic strains (*Lactobacillus plantarum*, *Lactobacillus casei*, and *S. thermophilus*) has shown promise in reducing pore size and wrinkle depth, as well as maintaining hydration and skin smoothness [134]. *S. thermophiles* lysate with sphingomyelinase has been demonstrated to strengthen the lipid barrier of the skin, elevate stratum corneum ceramide levels, and lower water loss [135]. In order to stimulate the expression of moisturizing factors in the skin, *L. plantarum* ferment lysate and *L. plantarum* K8 strain lysate have been proposed as functional ingredients for moisturizing cosmetics [136]. Improvements in acne lesions have been seen, along with decreases in transepidermal water loss and sebum production, when using *L. plantarum* ferment lysate [137]. Multiple positive effects of *Vitreoscilla filiformis* lysate on skin health have been observed, including modulation of skin immunity, inflammation reduction, and skin barrier enhancement [138]. LactoSporin® formulation, containing cell-free supernatants of *Bacillus coagulans* and inactivated cells of *Bacillus longum*, has been effective in managing mild-to-moderate acne lesions and seborrheic conditions, surpassing benzoyl peroxide in some cases [139]. A skincare cream containing fermented lysate derived from Lactobacillus plantarum can effectively and safely cure mild-to-moderate acne vulgaris after four weeks of topical treatment [140]. By potentially enhancing the skin barrier and regulating the skin's immune system, a postbiotic derived from *Bifidobacterium lactis* has shown effectiveness in reducing dandruff [141]. A topical formulation containing plantaricin A bioactive peptides, postbiotics, and *Lactobacillus kunkeei* isolated from bee bread, along with *Tropaeolum majus* flower/leaf/stem extract, has shown significant improvement in patients with alopecia areata [142] Figure 4.

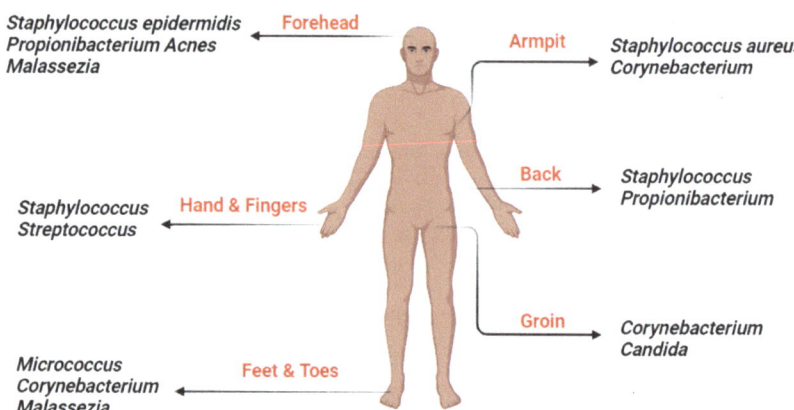

Figure 4. Skin Microbiome Diversity at Different Body Regions that can be Targeted. Created with Biorender.com.

7. Challenges in Maintaining Probiotic and Prebiotic Viability and Stability

Microbiomes can directly protect the host against pathogens, manage inflammation, and modify the functions of the adaptive immune system [143]. Microbial populations within the human body differ across various body sites. These variations can be influenced by the immune system, environment, and interactions between various microbial species [144]. The potential health benefits of probiotics have sparked interest in developing dermo-cosmetics derived from them. However, there are significant technological and legal challenges in using live microbes on the skin [145].

Furthermore, given that many people use cosmetics daily, these products can influence the skin microbiota. While cosmetics do not need to be completely sterile, they must adhere to current regulatory standards to ensure they do not carry harmful bacteria. Nevertheless, the inclusion of antimicrobial preservatives in formulations may affect the skin microbiome, potentially leading to long-term consequences such as the emergence of antibiotic-resistant bacteria [146]. In recent research, biomolecules such as polysaccharides (chitosan, xanthan, dextrin, and carrageenan) and milk proteins have been used to microencapsulate probiotics and other bioactive components. Sodium alginate is used more because of its cheapness and easy availability [147]. Therefore, it is important to keep in mind that it can be challenging to create and maintain the stability of probiotics in skincare products. Probiotics' viability and efficacy can be affected by variables such as pH, temperature, and exposure to air and light. Thus, while developing a formulation for topical treatment, it is crucial to ensure that the selected probiotic strains can maintain their viability and activity within the formulation.

8. Conclusions

The significance of microbiome restoration as a potential therapeutic strategy is highlighted by the skin microbiome's role in preserving skin homeostasis and its connections to numerous skin disorders. The possible use of probiotics, prebiotics, and postbiotics in topical preparations for many skin disorders is now the subject of investigation and study. Prebiotics contribute to improved gastrointestinal well-being by exhibiting anti-inflammatory and immunomodulating effects. They prevent the colonization of harmful microorganisms, support the integrity of the intestinal barrier, and enhance overall immune function, which can be considered a novel alternative therapy for many immune-related skin diseases. Postbiotics derived from probiotic strains and bacterial lysates have shown promise in various aspects of skin health, including moisturization and inflammation reduction. New techniques may employ nanocarriers to improve probiotic and prebiotic topical administration by protecting their viability, enabling effective loading, and enhancing skin penetration. These findings suggest the potential for postbiotic-based skincare products and treatments in addressing a wide range of dermatological concerns. However, it is essential to acknowledge the challenges ahead. Regulatory considerations and safety concerns surrounding the use of microbiome in skincare require careful attention. While oral probiotics have a clear legal definition tied to bacteria and yeast, the lack of such a definition for skin probiotics underscores a regulatory gap, signaling a pressing need for guidelines in this rapidly advancing field. Further research is also needed to understand their long-term effects and optimal formulations.

Author Contributions: K.A.-S.; writing-preparation of the original draft and drawing figures and tables. N.A.F., V.R.L.-S. and Y.M.; review and editing. P.S.L. and Y.M.; supervision. All authors have read and agreed to the published version of the manuscript.

Funding: This research received no external funding.

Institutional Review Board Statement: Not applicable.

Informed Consent Statement: Not applicable.

Data Availability Statement: Not applicable.

Acknowledgments: We thank CNPq (National Council for Scientific and Technological Development) for allowing Leite-Silva to work with us at the University of Queensland and FAPESP (The São Paulo Research Foundation, Brazil) process number # 2022/07541-6 for allowing Andreo-Filho to work with us at the University of Queensland.

Conflicts of Interest: The authors declare no conflict of interest.

References

1. Dréno, B.; Araviiskaia, E.; Berardesca, E.; Gontijo, G.; Sanchez Viera, M.; Xiang, L.F.; Martin, R.; Bieber, T. Microbiome in healthy skin, update for dermatologists. *J. Eur. Acad. Dermatol. Venereol.* **2016**, *30*, 2038–2047. [CrossRef]
2. Ni, Q.; Zhang, P.; Li, Q.; Han, Z. Oxidative Stress and Gut Microbiome in Inflammatory Skin Diseases. *Front. Cell Dev. Biol.* **2022**, *10*, 849985. [CrossRef]
3. Lin, Y.-K.; Yang, S.-C.; Hsu, C.-Y.; Sung, J.-T.; Fang, J.-Y. The antibiofilm nanosystems for improved infection inhibition of microbes in skin. *Molecules* **2021**, *26*, 6392. [CrossRef]
4. Lúcio, M.; Giannino, N.; Barreira, S.; Catita, J.; Gonçalves, H.; Ribeiro, A.; Fernandes, E.; Carvalho, I.; Pinho, H.; Cerqueira, F. Nanostructured lipid carriers enriched hydrogels for skin topical administration of quercetin and omega-3 fatty acid. *Pharmaceutics* **2023**, *15*, 2078. [CrossRef]
5. Basu, B.; Garala, K.; Bhalodia, R.; Joshi, B.; Mehta, K. Solid lipid nanoparticles: A promising tool for drug delivery system. *J. Pharm. Res.* **2010**, *3*, 84–92.
6. Zupančič, Š.; Rijavec, T.; Lapanje, A.; Petelin, M.; Kristl, J.; Kocbek, P. Nanofibers with incorporated autochthonous bacteria as potential probiotics for local treatment of periodontal disease. *Biomacromolecules* **2018**, *19*, 4299–4306. [CrossRef]
7. Chen, H.-J.; Lin, D.-a.; Liu, F.; Zhou, L.; Liu, D.; Lin, Z.; Yang, C.; Jin, Q.; Hang, T.; He, G. Transdermal delivery of living and biofunctional probiotics through dissolvable microneedle patches. *ACS Appl. Bio Mater.* **2018**, *1*, 374–381. [CrossRef]
8. Li, Z.; Wang, Y.; Liu, J.; Rawding, P.; Bu, J.; Hong, S.; Hu, Q. Chemically and biologically engineered bacteria-based delivery systems for emerging diagnosis and advanced therapy. *Adv. Mater.* **2021**, *33*, 2102580. [CrossRef]
9. Duncan, R.; Gaspar, R. Nanomedicine (s) under the microscope. *Mol. Pharm.* **2011**, *8*, 2101–2141. [CrossRef]
10. Nastiti, C.M.R.R.; Ponto, T.; Abd, E.; Grice, J.E.; Benson, H.A.E.; Roberts, M.S. Topical nano and microemulsions for skin delivery. *Pharmaceutics* **2017**, *9*, 37. [CrossRef]
11. Marcato, P.D.; Durán, N. New aspects of nanopharmaceutical delivery systems. *J. Nanosci. Nanotechnol.* **2008**, *8*, 2216–2229. [CrossRef] [PubMed]
12. Naahidi, S.; Jafari, M.; Edalat, F.; Raymond, K.; Khademhosseini, A.; Chen, P. Biocompatibility of engineered nanoparticles for drug delivery. *J. Control. Release* **2013**, *166*, 182–194. [CrossRef]
13. Mishra, D.; Hubenak, J.R.; Mathur, A.B. Nanoparticle systems as tools to improve drug delivery and therapeutic efficacy. *J. Biomed. Mater. Res. Part A Off. J. Soc. Biomater. Jpn. Soc. Biomater. Aust. Soc. Biomater. Korean Soc. Biomater.* **2013**, *101*, 3646–3660. [CrossRef] [PubMed]
14. Solans, C.; Izquierdo, P.; Nolla, J.; Azemar, N.; Garcia-Celma, M.J. Nano-emulsions. *Curr. Opin. Colloid Interface Sci.* **2005**, *10*, 102–110. [CrossRef]
15. Solans, C.; Solé, I. Nano-emulsions: Formation by low-energy methods. *Curr. Opin. Colloid Interface Sci.* **2012**, *17*, 246–254. [CrossRef]

16. Choi, S.H.; Lee, J.-H.; Choi, S.-M.; Park, T.G. Thermally reversible pluronic/heparin nanocapsules exhibiting 1000-fold volume transition. *Langmuir* **2006**, *22*, 1758–1762. [CrossRef] [PubMed]
17. Barenholz, Y.C. Doxil®—The first FDA-approved nano-drug: Lessons learned. *J. Control. Release* **2012**, *160*, 117–134. [CrossRef] [PubMed]
18. Akinc, A.; Battaglia, G. Exploiting endocytosis for nanomedicines. *Cold Spring Harb. Perspect. Biol.* **2013**, *5*, a016980. [CrossRef]
19. Nel, A.; Xia, T.; Madler, L.; Li, N. Toxic potential of materials at the nanolevel. *Science* **2006**, *311*, 622–627. [CrossRef]
20. Tannahill, G.M.; Curtis, A.M.; Adamik, J.; Palsson-McDermott, E.M.; McGettrick, A.F.; Goel, G.; Frezza, C.; Bernard, N.J.; Kelly, B.; Foley, N.H. Succinate is an inflammatory signal that induces IL-1β through HIF-1α. *Nature* **2013**, *496*, 238–242. [CrossRef]
21. Lampropoulou, V.; Sergushichev, A.; Bambouskova, M.; Nair, S.; Vincent, E.E.; Loginicheva, E.; Cervantes-Barragan, L.; Ma, X.; Huang, S.C.-C.; Griss, T. Itaconate links inhibition of succinate dehydrogenase with macrophage metabolic remodeling and regulation of inflammation. *Cell Metab.* **2016**, *24*, 158–166. [CrossRef] [PubMed]
22. Mitra, S.; De Sarkar, S.; Pradhan, A.; Pati, A.K.; Pradhan, R.; Mondal, D.; Sen, S.; Ghosh, A.; Chatterjee, S.; Chatterjee, M. Levels of oxidative damage and proinflammatory cytokines are enhanced in patients with active vitiligo. *Free Radic. Res.* **2017**, *51*, 986–994. [CrossRef] [PubMed]
23. Yi, X.; Guo, W.; Shi, Q.; Yang, Y.; Zhang, W.; Chen, X.; Kang, P.; Chen, J.; Cui, T.; Ma, J. SIRT3-dependent mitochondrial dynamics remodeling contributes to oxidative stress-induced melanocyte degeneration in vitiligo. *Theranostics* **2019**, *9*, 1614–1633. [CrossRef] [PubMed]
24. Iddir, M.; Brito, A.; Dingeo, G.; Fernandez Del Campo, S.S.; Samouda, H.; La Frano, M.R.; Bohn, T. Strengthening the immune system and reducing inflammation and oxidative stress through diet and nutrition: Considerations during the COVID-19 crisis. *Nutrients* **2020**, *12*, 1562. [CrossRef] [PubMed]
25. Czajkowski, R.; Męcińska-Jundziłł, K. Current aspects of vitiligo genetics. *Adv. Dermatol. Allergol./Postępy Dermatol. I Alergol.* **2014**, *31*, 247–255. [CrossRef] [PubMed]
26. Krüger, C.; Schallreuter, K.U. A review of the worldwide prevalence of vitiligo in children/adolescents and adults. *Int. J. Dermatol.* **2012**, *51*, 1206–1212. [CrossRef] [PubMed]
27. Ezzedine, K.; Lim, H.W.; Suzuki, T.; Katayama, I.; Hamzavi, I.; Lan, C.C.E.; Goh, B.K.; Anbar, T.; Silva de Castro, C.; Lee, A.Y. Revised classification/nomenclature of vitiligo and related issues: The Vitiligo Global Issues Consensus Conference. *Pigment Cell Melanoma Res.* **2012**, *25*, E1–E13. [CrossRef]
28. Bergqvist, C.; Ezzedine, K. Vitiligo: A review. *Dermatology* **2020**, *236*, 571–592. [CrossRef]
29. Al-smadi, K.; Imran, M.; Leite-Silva, V.R.; Mohammed, Y. Vitiligo: A Review of Aetiology, Pathogenesis, Treatment, and Psychosocial Impact. *Cosmetics* **2023**, *10*, 84. [CrossRef]
30. Alkhateeb, A.; Fain, P.R.; Thody, A.; Bennett, D.C.; Spritz, R.A. Epidemiology of vitiligo and associated autoimmune diseases in Caucasian probands and their families. *Pigment Cell Res.* **2003**, *16*, 208–214. [CrossRef]
31. Laberge, G.; Mailloux, C.M.; Gowan, K.; Holland, P.; Bennett, D.C.; Fain, P.R.; Spritz, R.A. Early disease onset and increased risk of other autoimmune diseases in familial generalized vitiligo. *Pigment Cell Res.* **2005**, *18*, 300–305. [CrossRef] [PubMed]
32. Taieb, A.; Alomar, A.; Böhm, M.; Dell'Anna, M.L.; De Pase, A.; Eleftheriadou, V.; Ezzedine, K.; Gauthier, Y.; Gawkrodger, D.J.; Jouary, T. Guidelines for the management of vitiligo: The European Dermatology Forum consensus. *Br. J. Dermatol.* **2013**, *168*, 5–19. [CrossRef] [PubMed]
33. Lee, J.H.; Kwon, H.S.; Jung, H.M.; Lee, H.; Kim, G.M.; Yim, H.W.; Bae, J.M. Treatment outcomes of topical calcineurin inhibitor therapy for patients with vitiligo: A systematic review and meta-analysis. *JAMA Dermatol.* **2019**, *155*, 929–938. [CrossRef] [PubMed]
34. Horn, E.J.; Domm, S.; Katz, H.I.; Lebwohl, M.; Mrowietz, U.; Kragballe, K.; International Psoriasis, Council. Topical corticosteroids in psoriasis: Strategies for improving safety. *J. Eur. Acad. Dermatol. Venereol.* **2010**, *24*, 119–124. [CrossRef] [PubMed]
35. Forschner, T.; Buchholtz, S.; Stockfleth, E. Current state of vitiligo therapy–evidence-based analysis of the literature. *JDDG J. Dtsch. Dermatol. Ges.* **2007**, *5*, 467–475. [CrossRef] [PubMed]
36. Al-Smadi, K.; Ali, M.; Alavi, S.E.; Jin, X.; Imran, M.; Leite-Silva, V.R.; Mohammed, Y. Using a Topical Formulation of Vitamin D for the Treatment of Vitiligo: A Systematic Review. *Cells* **2023**, *12*, 2387. [CrossRef] [PubMed]
37. Klaassen, C.D. Heavy metals and heavy-metal antagonists. In *Goodman and Gilman's the Pharmacological Basis of Therapeutics*, 11th ed.; McGraw-Hill: New York, NY, USA, 2006; pp. 1753–1775.
38. Wang, Y.; Li, S.; Li, C. Perspectives of new advances in the pathogenesis of vitiligo: From oxidative stress to autoimmunity. *Med. Sci. Monit. Int. Med. J. Exp. Clin. Res.* **2019**, *25*, 1017–1023. [CrossRef] [PubMed]
39. Thio, H.B. The microbiome in psoriasis and psoriatic arthritis: The skin perspective. *J. Rheumatol. Suppl.* **2018**, *94*, 30–31. [CrossRef]
40. Greb, J.E.; Goldminz, A.M.; Elder, J.T.; Lebwohl, M.G.; Gladman, D.D.; Wu, J.J.; Mehta, N.N.; Finlay, A.Y.; Gottlieb, A.B. Psoriasis (Primer). *Nat. Rev. Dis. Primers* **2016**, *2*, 1. [CrossRef]
41. Nakatsuji, T.; Gallo, R.L. The role of the skin microbiome in atopic dermatitis. *Ann. Allergy Asthma Immunol.* **2019**, *122*, 263–269. [CrossRef]
42. Pothmann, A.; Illing, T.; Wiegand, C.; Hartmann, A.A.; Elsner, P. The microbiome and atopic dermatitis: A review. *Am. J. Clin. Dermatol.* **2019**, *20*, 749–761. [CrossRef] [PubMed]

43. Chen, Y.; Zhang, J.Y.; Gao, S.; Li, Y.R.; Wu, Y.F. Research progress of microbiome and pathogenesis of vitiligo. *Life Res.* **2021**, *4*, 13. [CrossRef]
44. Pellicciotta, M.; Rigoni, R.; Falcone, E.L.; Holland, S.M.; Villa, A.; Cassani, B. The microbiome and immunodeficiencies: Lessons from rare diseases. *J. Autoimmun.* **2019**, *98*, 132–148. [CrossRef] [PubMed]
45. Mihranyan, A.; Ferraz, N.; Strømme, M. Current status and future prospects of nanotechnology in cosmetics. *Prog. Mater. Sci.* **2012**, *57*, 875–910. [CrossRef]
46. Park, S.B.; Im, M.; Lee, Y.; Lee, J.H.; Lim, J.; Park, Y.-H.; Seo, Y.J. Effect of emollients containing vegetable-derived lactobacillus in the treatment of atopic dermatitis symptoms: Split-body clinical trial. *Ann. Dermatol.* **2014**, *26*, 150–155. [CrossRef] [PubMed]
47. Ambrożej, D.; Kunkiel, K.; Dumycz, K.; Feleszko, W. The use of probiotics and bacteria-derived preparations in topical treatment of atopic dermatitis—A systematic review. *J. Allergy Clin. Immunol. Pract.* **2021**, *9*, 570–575. [CrossRef] [PubMed]
48. Salvioni, L.; Morelli, L.; Ochoa, E.; Labra, M.; Fiandra, L.; Palugan, L.; Prosperi, D.; Colombo, M. The emerging role of nanotechnology in skincare. *Adv. Colloid Interface Sci.* **2021**, *293*, 102437. [CrossRef]
49. Bekiaridou, E.; Karlafti, E.; Oikonomou, I.M.; Ioannidis, A.; Papavramidis, T.S. Probiotics and their effect on surgical wound healing: A systematic review and new insights into the role of nanotechnology. *Nutrients* **2021**, *13*, 4265. [CrossRef]
50. Patel, S.; Goyal, A. The current trends and future perspectives of prebiotics research: A review. *3 Biotech* **2012**, *2*, 115–125. [CrossRef]
51. Morelli, L.; Capurso, L. FAO/WHO guidelines on probiotics: 10 years later. *J. Clin. Gastroenterol.* **2012**, *46*, S1–S2. [CrossRef]
52. Sanders, M.E.; Gibson, G.R.; Gill, H.S.; Guarner, F. Probiotics: Their potential to impact human health. *Counc. Agric. Sci. Technol. Issue Pap.* **2007**, *36*, 1–20.
53. França, K. Topical probiotics in dermatological therapy and skincare: A concise review. *Dermatol. Ther.* **2021**, *11*, 71–77. [CrossRef] [PubMed]
54. Swaby, A.M.; Agellon, L.B. The Potential Role of Commensal Microbes in Optimizing Nutrition Care Delivery and Nutrient Metabolism. *Recent Prog. Nutr.* **2022**, *2*, 1–16. [CrossRef]
55. Novik, G.; Savich, V. Beneficial microbiota. Probiotics and pharmaceutical products in functional nutrition and medicine. *Microbes Infect.* **2020**, *22*, 8–18. [CrossRef] [PubMed]
56. Gao, J.; Li, Y.; Wan, Y.; Hu, T.; Liu, L.; Yang, S.; Gong, Z.; Zeng, Q.; Wei, Y.; Yang, W. A novel postbiotic from Lactobacillus rhamnosus GG with a beneficial effect on intestinal barrier function. *Front. Microbiol.* **2019**, *10*, 477. [CrossRef] [PubMed]
57. Abbasi, A.; Rad, A.H.; Ghasempour, Z.; Sabahi, S.; Kafil, H.S.; Hasannezhad, P.; Rahbar Saadat, Y.; Shahbazi, N. The biological activities of postbiotics in gastrointestinal disorders. *Crit. Rev. Food Sci. Nutr.* **2022**, *62*, 5983–6004. [CrossRef] [PubMed]
58. Hill, D.A.; Artis, D. Intestinal bacteria and the regulation of immune cell homeostasis. *Annu. Rev. Immunol.* **2009**, *28*, 623–667. [CrossRef]
59. Belkaid, Y.; Tamoutounour, S. The influence of skin microorganisms on cutaneous immunity. *Nat. Rev. Immunol.* **2016**, *16*, 353–366. [CrossRef]
60. Boxberger, M.; Cenizo, V.; Cassir, N.; La Scola, B. Challenges in exploring and manipulating the human skin microbiome. *Microbiome* **2021**, *9*, 125. [CrossRef]
61. Bay, L.; Barnes, C.J.; Fritz, B.G.; Thorsen, J.; Restrup, M.E.M.; Rasmussen, L.; Sørensen, J.K.; Hesselvig, A.B.; Odgaard, A.; Hansen, A.J. Universal dermal microbiome in human skin. *MBio* **2020**, *11*, 10–1128. [CrossRef]
62. Ogai, K.; Nana, B.C.; Lloyd, Y.M.; Arios, J.P.; Jiyarom, B.; Awanakam, H.; Esemu, L.F.; Hori, A.; Matsuoka, A.; Nainu, F. Skin microbiome profile of healthy Cameroonians and Japanese. *Sci. Rep.* **2022**, *12*, 1364. [CrossRef] [PubMed]
63. Lee, H.-J.; Kim, M. Skin barrier function and the microbiome. *Int. J. Mol. Sci.* **2022**, *23*, 13071. [CrossRef] [PubMed]
64. Wilson, M. *The Human Microbiota in Health and Disease: An Ecological and Community-Based Approach*; Garland Science: New York, NY, USA, 2018.
65. Harrison, O.J.; Linehan, J.L.; Shih, H.-Y.; Bouladoux, N.; Han, S.-J.; Smelkinson, M.; Sen, S.K.; Byrd, A.L.; Enamorado, M.; Yao, C. Commensal-specific T cell plasticity promotes rapid tissue adaptation to injury. *Science* **2019**, *363*, eaat6280. [CrossRef] [PubMed]
66. Navarro-López, V.; Núñez-Delegido, E.; Ruzafa-Costas, B.; Sánchez-Pellicer, P.; Agüera-Santos, J.; Navarro-Moratalla, L. Probiotics in the therapeutic arsenal of dermatologists. *Microorganisms* **2021**, *9*, 1513. [CrossRef]
67. Scharschmidt, T.C.; Fischbach, M.A. What lives on our skin: Ecology, genomics and therapeutic opportunities of the skin microbiome. *Drug Discov. Today Dis. Mech.* **2013**, *10*, e83–e89. [CrossRef]
68. Günther, J.; Seyfert, H.-M. The first line of defence: Insights into mechanisms and relevance of phagocytosis in epithelial cells. In *Seminars in Immunopathology*; Springer: Berlin/Heidelberg, Germany, 2018; pp. 555–565.
69. Nazir, Y.; Hussain, S.A.; Abdul Hamid, A.; Song, Y. Probiotics and their potential preventive and therapeutic role for cancer, high serum cholesterol, and allergic and HIV diseases. *BioMed Res. Int.* **2018**, *2018*, 3428437. [CrossRef]
70. Cogen, A.L.; Yamasaki, K.; Sanchez, K.M.; Dorschner, R.A.; Lai, Y.; MacLeod, D.T.; Torpey, J.W.; Otto, M.; Nizet, V.; Kim, J.E. Selective antimicrobial action is provided by phenol-soluble modulins derived from *Staphylococcus epidermidis*, a normal resident of the skin. *J. Investig. Dermatol.* **2010**, *130*, 192–200. [CrossRef]
71. Gibbs, N.K.; Norval, M. Urocanic acid in the skin: A mixed blessing? *J. Investig. Dermatol.* **2011**, *131*, 14–17. [CrossRef]
72. Sfriso, R.; Egert, M.; Gempeler, M.; Voegeli, R.; Campiche, R. Revealing the secret life of skin-with the microbiome you never walk alone. *Int. J. Cosmet. Sci.* **2020**, *42*, 116–126. [CrossRef]
73. Schommer, N.N.; Gallo, R.L. Structure and function of the human skin microbiome. *Trends Microbiol.* **2013**, *21*, 660–668. [CrossRef]

74. Szántó, M.; Dózsa, A.; Antal, D.; Szabó, K.; Kemény, L.; Bai, P. Targeting the gut-skin axis—Probiotics as new tools for skin disorder management? *Exp. Dermatol.* **2019**, *28*, 1210–1218. [CrossRef] [PubMed]
75. Yamada, M.; Mohammed, Y.; Prow, T.W. Advances and controversies in studying sunscreen delivery and toxicity. *Adv. Drug Deliv. Rev.* **2020**, *153*, 72–86. [CrossRef] [PubMed]
76. Yousef, S.; Mohammed, Y.; Namjoshi, S.; Grice, J.; Sakran, W.; Roberts, M. Mechanistic evaluation of hydration effects on the human epidermal permeation of salicylate esters. *AAPS J.* **2017**, *19*, 180–190. [CrossRef] [PubMed]
77. Tapfumaneyi, P.; Imran, M.; Mohammed, Y.; Roberts, M.S. Recent advances and future prospective of topical and transdermal delivery systems. *Front. Drug Deliv.* **2022**, *2*, 957732. [CrossRef]
78. Sarao, L.K.; Arora, M. Probiotics, prebiotics, and microencapsulation: A review. *Crit. Rev. Food Sci. Nutr.* **2017**, *57*, 344–371. [CrossRef] [PubMed]
79. Nakatsuji, T.; Chen, T.H.; Narala, S.; Chun, K.A.; Two, A.M.; Yun, T.; Shafiq, F.; Kotol, P.F.; Bouslimani, A.; Melnik, A.V. Antimicrobials from human skin commensal bacteria protect against Staphylococcus aureus and are deficient in atopic dermatitis. *Sci. Transl. Med.* **2017**, *9*, eaah4680. [CrossRef]
80. Alekseyenko, A.V.; Perez-Perez, G.I.; De Souza, A.; Strober, B.; Gao, Z.; Bihan, M.; Li, K.; Methé, B.A.; Blaser, M.J. Community differentiation of the cutaneous microbiota in psoriasis. *Microbiome* **2013**, *1*, 31. [CrossRef]
81. Gallo, R.L.; Nakatsuji, T. Microbial symbiosis with the innate immune defense system of the skin. *J. Investig. Dermatol.* **2011**, *131*, 1974–1980. [CrossRef]
82. Chilicka, K.; Dzieńdziora-Urbińska, I.; Szyguła, R.; Asanova, B.; Nowicka, D. Microbiome and probiotics in acne vulgaris—A narrative review. *Life* **2022**, *12*, 422. [CrossRef]
83. Ni, Q.; Ye, Z.; Wang, Y.; Chen, J.; Zhang, W.; Ma, C.; Li, K.; Liu, Y.; Liu, L.; Han, Z. Gut microbial dysbiosis and plasma metabolic profile in individuals with vitiligo. *Front. Microbiol.* **2020**, *11*, 592248. [CrossRef]
84. Ganju, P.; Nagpal, S.; Mohammed, M.H.; Nishal Kumar, P.; Pandey, R.; Natarajan, V.T.; Mande, S.S.; Gokhale, R.S. Microbial community profiling shows dysbiosis in the lesional skin of Vitiligo subjects. *Sci. Rep.* **2016**, *6*, 18761. [CrossRef] [PubMed]
85. Holmes, E.; Li, J.V.; Athanasiou, T.; Ashrafian, H.; Nicholson, J.K. Understanding the role of gut microbiome–host metabolic signal disruption in health and disease. *Trends Microbiol.* **2011**, *19*, 349–359. [CrossRef] [PubMed]
86. Reid, G.; Younes, J.A.; Van der Mei, H.C.; Gloor, G.B.; Knight, R.; Busscher, H.J. Microbiota restoration: Natural and supplemented recovery of human microbial communities. *Nat. Rev. Microbiol.* **2011**, *9*, 27–38. [CrossRef] [PubMed]
87. Sonnenburg, J.L.; Fischbach, M.A. Community health care: Therapeutic opportunities in the human microbiome. *Sci. Transl. Med.* **2011**, *3*, ps12–ps78. [CrossRef] [PubMed]
88. Caselli, M.; Vaira, G.; Calo, G.; Papini, F.; Holton, J.; Vaira, D. Structural bacterial molecules as potential candidates for an evolution of the classical concept of probiotics. *Adv. Nutr.* **2011**, *2*, 372–376. [CrossRef] [PubMed]
89. Shenderov, B.A. Modern condition and prospective host microecology investigations. *Microb. Ecol. Health Dis.* **2007**, *19*, 145–149.
90. Shenderov, B.A. Metabiotics: Novel idea or natural development of probiotic conception. *Microb. Ecol. Health Dis.* **2013**, *24*, 20399. [CrossRef] [PubMed]
91. Zimmermann, M.; Zimmermann-Kogadeeva, M.; Wegmann, R.; Goodman, A.L. Mapping human microbiome drug metabolism by gut bacteria and their genes. *Nature* **2019**, *570*, 462–467. [CrossRef]
92. Dodd, D.; Spitzer, M.H.; Van Treuren, W.; Merrill, B.D.; Hryckowian, A.J.; Higginbottom, S.K.; Le, A.; Cowan, T.M.; Nolan, G.P.; Fischbach, M.A. A gut bacterial pathway metabolizes aromatic amino acids into nine circulating metabolites. *Nature* **2017**, *551*, 648–652. [CrossRef]
93. Fan, Y.; Pedersen, O. Gut microbiota in human metabolic health and disease. *Nat. Rev. Microbiol.* **2021**, *19*, 55–71. [CrossRef]
94. Wang, Y.; Kasper, L.H. The role of microbiome in central nervous system disorders. *Brain Behav. Immun.* **2014**, *38*, 1–12. [CrossRef] [PubMed]
95. Fredricks, D.N. Microbial ecology of human skin in health and disease. *J. Investig. Dermatol. Symp. Proc.* **2001**, *6*, 167–169. [CrossRef] [PubMed]
96. Byrd, A.L.; Belkaid, Y.; Segre, J.A. The human skin microbiome. *Nat. Rev. Microbiol.* **2018**, *16*, 143–155. [CrossRef] [PubMed]
97. Foulongne, V.; Sauvage, V.; Hebert, C.; Dereure, O.; Cheval, J.; Gouilh, M.A.; Pariente, K.; Segondy, M.; Burguière, A.; Manuguerra, J.-C. Human skin microbiota: High diversity of DNA viruses identified on the human skin by high throughput sequencing. *PLoS ONE* **2012**, *7*, e38499. [CrossRef] [PubMed]
98. Christensen, G.J.M.; Brüggemann, H. Bacterial skin commensals and their role as host guardians. *Benef. Microbes.* **2014**, *5*, 201–215. [CrossRef] [PubMed]
99. Gomes, J.A.P.; Frizon, L.; Demeda, V.F. Ocular surface microbiome in health and disease. *Asia-Pac. J. Ophthalmol.* **2020**, *9*, 505–511. [CrossRef] [PubMed]
100. Lee, G.R.; Maarouf, M.; Hendricks, A.J.; Lee, D.E.; Shi, V.Y. Topical probiotics: The unknowns behind their rising popularity. *Dermatol. Online J.* **2019**, *25*, 13030. [CrossRef]
101. Boyajian, J.L.; Ghebretatios, M.; Schaly, S.; Islam, P.; Prakash, S. Microbiome and human aging: Probiotic and prebiotic potentials in longevity, skin health and cellular senescence. *Nutrients* **2021**, *13*, 4550. [CrossRef]
102. Petra, A.I.; Panagiotidou, S.; Hatziagelaki, E.; Stewart, J.M.; Conti, P.; Theoharides, T.C. Gut-microbiota-brain axis and its effect on neuropsychiatric disorders with suspected immune dysregulation. *Clin. Ther.* **2015**, *37*, 984–995. [CrossRef]

103. Bzioueche, H.; Sjödin, K.S.; West, C.E.; Khemis, A.; Rocchi, S.; Passeron, T.; Tulic, M.K. Analysis of matched skin and gut microbiome of patients with vitiligo reveals deep skin dysbiosis: Link with mitochondrial and immune changes. *J. Investig. Dermatol.* **2021**, *141*, 2280–2290. [CrossRef]
104. Tulic, M.K.; Cavazza, E.; Cheli, Y.; Jacquel, A.; Luci, C.; Cardot-Leccia, N.; Hadhiri-Bzioueche, H.; Abbe, P.; Gesson, M.; Sormani, L. Innate lymphocyte-induced CXCR3B-mediated melanocyte apoptosis is a potential initiator of T-cell autoreactivity in vitiligo. *Nat. Commun.* **2019**, *10*, 2178. [CrossRef] [PubMed]
105. Dellacecca, E.R.; Cosgrove, C.; Mukhatayev, Z.; Akhtar, S.; Engelhard, V.H.; Rademaker, A.W.; Knight, K.L.; Le Poole, I.C. Antibiotics drive microbial imbalance and vitiligo development in mice. *J. Investig. Dermatol.* **2020**, *140*, 676–687. [CrossRef] [PubMed]
106. Al-Ghazzewi, F.H.; Tester, R.F. Impact of prebiotics and probiotics on skin health. *Benef. Microbes.* **2014**, *5*, 99–107. [CrossRef] [PubMed]
107. Wallen-Russell, C.; Wallen-Russell, S. Topical Probiotics Do Not Satisfy New Criteria for Effective Use Due to Insufficient Skin Microbiome Knowledge. *Cosmetics* **2021**, *8*, 90. [CrossRef]
108. Renuka, S.R.; Kumar, N.A.; Manoharan, D.; Naidu, D.K. Probiotics: A Review on Microbiome That Helps for Better Health–A Dermatologist's Perspective. *J. Pharmacol. Pharmacother.* **2023**, 0976500X231175225. [CrossRef]
109. Fuchs-Tarlovsky, V.; Marquez-Barba, M.F.; Sriram, K. Probiotics in dermatologic practice. *Nutrition* **2016**, *32*, 289–295. [CrossRef] [PubMed]
110. Reisch, M.S. Cosmetics: The next microbiome frontier. *Mitsui Chem. Catal. Sci. Award* **2017**, *95*, 30–34.
111. Vinderola, G.; Sanders, M.E.; Salminen, S. The concept of postbiotics. *Foods* **2022**, *11*, 1077. [CrossRef]
112. Zommiti, M.; Feuilloley, M.G.J.; Connil, N. Update of probiotics in human world: A nonstop source of benefactions till the end of time. *Microorganisms* **2020**, *8*, 1907. [CrossRef]
113. Miyazaki, K.; Hanamizu, T.; Iizuka, R.; Chiba, K. *Bifidobacterium*-fermented soy milk extract stimulates hyaluronic acid production in human skin cells and hairless mouse skin. *Ski. Pharmacol. Physiol.* **2003**, *16*, 108–116. [CrossRef]
114. Miyazaki, K.; Hanamizu, T.; Sone, T.; Chiba, K.; Kinoshita, T.; Yoshikawa, S. Topical application of *Bifidobacterium*-fermented soy milk extract containing genistein and daidzein improves rheological and physiological properties of skin. *J. Cosmet. Sci.* **2004**, *55*, 473–480. [CrossRef] [PubMed]
115. Roberfroid, M.; Gibson, G.R.; Hoyles, L.; McCartney, A.L.; Rastall, R.; Rowland, I.; Wolvers, D.; Watzl, B.; Szajewska, H.; Stahl, B. Prebiotic effects: Metabolic and health benefits. *Br. J. Nutr.* **2010**, *104*, S1–S63. [CrossRef] [PubMed]
116. Frei, R.; Akdis, M.; O'Mahony, L. Prebiotics, probiotics, synbiotics, and the immune system: Experimental data and clinical evidence. *Curr. Opin. Gastroenterol.* **2015**, *31*, 153–158. [CrossRef]
117. Myles, I.A.; Castillo, C.R.; Barbian, K.D.; Kanakabandi, K.; Virtaneva, K.; Fitzmeyer, E.; Paneru, M.; Otaizo-Carrasquero, F.; Myers, T.G.; Markowitz, T.E. Therapeutic responses to Roseomonas mucosa in atopic dermatitis may involve lipid-mediated TNF-related epithelial repair. *Sci. Transl. Med.* **2020**, *12*, eaaz8631. [CrossRef] [PubMed]
118. Chaudhry, A.; Rabiee, B.; Festok, M.; Gaspari, M.; Chaudhry, A. *Combination of Topical Tacrolimus, Antioxidants, and Probiotics in the Treatment of Periorbital Vitiligo*; Trinity Health Mid-Atlantic, Nazareth Hospital, Department of Ophthalmology: Darby, PA, USA, 2022; Available online: https://scholarcommons.towerhealth.org/cgi/viewcontent.cgi?article=1008&context=schc_researchday (accessed on 30 October 2023).
119. Podrini, C.; Schramm, L.; Marianantoni, G.; Apolinarska, J.; McGuckin, C.; Forraz, N.; Milet, C.; Desroches, A.-L.; Payen, P.; D'Aguanno, M. Topical Administration of Lactiplantibacillus plantarum (SkinDuoTM) Serum Improves Anti-Acne Properties. *Microorganisms* **2023**, *11*, 417. [CrossRef] [PubMed]
120. Simmering, R.; Breves, R. Prebiotic cosmetics. In *Nutrition for Healthy Skin: Strategies for Clinical and Cosmetic Practice*; Springer: Berlin/Heidelberg, Germany, 2010; pp. 137–147.
121. Baral, K.C.; Bajracharya, R.; Lee, S.H.; Han, H.-K. Advancements in the pharmaceutical applications of probiotics: Dosage forms and formulation technology. *Int. J. Nanomed.* **2021**, *16*, 7535–7556. [CrossRef] [PubMed]
122. Vargason, A.M.; Anselmo, A.C. Live biotherapeutic products and probiotics for the skin. *Adv. NanoBiomed Res.* **2021**, *1*, 2100118. [CrossRef]
123. Jung, N.; Namjoshi, S.; Mohammed, Y.; Grice, J.E.; Benson, H.A.; Raney, S.G.; Roberts, M.S.; Windbergs, M. Application of confocal Raman microscopy for the characterization of topical semisolid formulations and their penetration into human skin ex vivo. *Pharm. Res.* **2022**, *39*, 935–948. [CrossRef]
124. Ayichew, T.; Belete, A.; Alebachew, T.; Tsehaye, H.; Berhanu, H.; Minwuyelet, A. Bacterial probiotics their importances and limitations: A review. *J. Nutr. Health Sci.* **2017**, *4*, 202.
125. Akbarzadeh, A.; Alirezaei, P.; Doosti-Irani, A.; Mehrpooya, M.; Nouri, F. The Efficacy of Lactocare® Synbiotic on the Clinical Symptoms in Patients with Psoriasis: A Randomized, Double-Blind, Placebo-Controlled Clinical Trial. *Dermatol. Res. Pract.* **2022**, *2022*, 4549134. [CrossRef]
126. Lee, Y.H.; Kalailingam, P.; Delcour, J.A.; Fogliano, V.; Thanabalu, T. Olive-Derived Antioxidant Dietary Fiber Modulates Gut Microbiota Composition and Attenuates Atopic Dermatitis Like Inflammation in Mice. *Mol. Nutr. Food Res.* **2023**, *67*, 2200127. [CrossRef] [PubMed]

127. Barrangou, R.; Altermann, E.; Hutkins, R.; Cano, R.; Klaenhammer, T.R. Functional and comparative genomic analyses of an operon involved in fructooligosaccharide utilization by Lactobacillus acidophilus. *Proc. Natl. Acad. Sci. USA* **2003**, *100*, 8957–8962. [CrossRef] [PubMed]
128. Goh, Y.J.; Klaenhammer, T.R. Genetic mechanisms of prebiotic oligosaccharide metabolism in probiotic microbes. *Annu. Rev. Food Sci. Technol.* **2015**, *6*, 137–156. [CrossRef] [PubMed]
129. Topping, D.L.; Clifton, P.M. Short-chain fatty acids and human colonic function: Roles of resistant starch and nonstarch polysaccharides. *Physiol. Rev.* **2001**, *81*, 1031–1064. [CrossRef] [PubMed]
130. Florowska, A.; Krygier, K.; Florowski, T.; Dłużewska, E. Prebiotics as functional food ingredients preventing diet-related diseases. *Food Funct.* **2016**, *7*, 2147–2155. [CrossRef] [PubMed]
131. Bouhnik, Y.; Vahedi, K.; Achour, L.; Attar, A.; Salfati, J.; Pochart, P.; Marteau, P.; Flourie, B.; Bornet, F.; Rambaud, J.-C. Short-chain fructo-oligosaccharide administration dose-dependently increases fecal *Bifidobacteria* in healthy humans. *J. Nutr.* **1999**, *129*, 113–116. [CrossRef] [PubMed]
132. Rong, J.; Shan, C.; Liu, S.; Zheng, H.; Liu, C.; Liu, M.; Jin, F.; Wang, L. Skin resistance to UVB-induced oxidative stress and hyperpigmentation by the topical use of Lactobacillus helveticus NS8-fermented milk supernatant. *J. Appl. Microbiol.* **2017**, *123*, 511–523. [CrossRef] [PubMed]
133. Golkar, N.; Ashoori, Y.; Heidari, R.; Omidifar, N.; Abootalebi, S.N.; Mohkam, M.; Gholami, A. A novel effective formulation of bioactive compounds for wound healing: Preparation, in vivo characterization, and comparison of various postbiotics cold creams in a rat model. *Evid.-Based Complement. Altern. Med.* **2021**, *2021*, 8577116. [CrossRef]
134. Catic, T.; Pehlivanovic, B.; Pljakic, N.; Balicevac, A. The moisturizing efficacy of a proprietary dermo-cosmetic product (cls02021) versus placebo in a 4-week application period. *Med. Arch.* **2022**, *76*, 108. [CrossRef]
135. Dimarzio, L.; Cinque, B.; Cupelli, F.; De Simone, C.; Cifone, M.G.; Giuliani, M. Increase of skin-ceramide levels in aged subjects following a short-term topical application of bacterial sphingomyelinase from *Streptococcus thermophilus*. *Int. J. Immunopathol. Pharmacol.* **2008**, *21*, 137–143. [CrossRef]
136. Kim, H.; Jeon, B.; Kim, W.J.; Chung, D.-K. Effect of paraprobiotic prepared from Kimchi-derived Lactobacillus plantarum K8 on skin moisturizing activity in human keratinocyte. *J. Funct. Foods* **2020**, *75*, 104244. [CrossRef]
137. Cui, H.; Guo, C.; Wang, Q.; Feng, C.; Duan, Z. A pilot study on the efficacy of topical lotion containing anti-acne postbiotic in subjects with mild-to-moderate acne. *Front. Med.* **2022**, *9*, 1064460. [CrossRef] [PubMed]
138. Gueniche, A.; Liboutet, M.; Cheilian, S.; Fagot, D.; Juchaux, F.; Breton, L. *Vitreoscilla filiformis* extract for topical skin care: A review. *Front. Cell. Infect. Microbiol.* **2021**, *11*, 1253. [CrossRef] [PubMed]
139. Majeed, M.; Majeed, S.; Nagabhushanam, K.; Mundkur, L.; Rajalakshmi, H.R.; Shah, K.; Beede, K. Novel topical application of a postbiotic, LactoSporin®, in mild to moderate acne: A randomized, comparative clinical study to evaluate its efficacy, tolerability and safety. *Cosmetics* **2020**, *7*, 70. [CrossRef]
140. Cui, H.; Feng, C.; Guo, C.; Duan, Z. Development of novel topical anti-acne cream containing postbiotics for mild-to-moderate acne: An observational study to evaluate its efficacy. *Indian J. Dermatol.* **2022**, *67*, 667–673. [PubMed]
141. de Jesus, G.F.A.; Rossetto, M.P.; Voytena, A.; Feder, B.; Borges, H.; da Costa Borges, G.; Feuser, Z.P.; Dal-Bó, S.; Michels, M. Clinical evaluation of paraprobiotic-associated *Bifidobacterium* lactis CCT 7858 anti-dandruff shampoo efficacy: A randomized placebo-controlled clinical trial. *Int. J. Cosmet. Sci.* **2023**, *45*, 572–580. [CrossRef]
142. Rinaldi, F.; Trink, A.; Pinto, D. Efficacy of postbiotics in a PRP-like cosmetic product for the treatment of alopecia area Celsi: A randomized double-blinded parallel-group study. *Dermatol. Ther.* **2020**, *10*, 483–493. [CrossRef]
143. Cogen, A.L.; Nizet, V.; Gallo, R.L. Skin microbiota: A source of disease or defence? *Br. J. Dermatol.* **2008**, *158*, 442–455. [CrossRef]
144. Mousa, W.K.; Chehadeh, F.; Husband, S. Recent advances in understanding the structure and function of the human microbiome. *Front. Microbiol.* **2022**, *13*, 825338. [CrossRef]
145. Gueniche, A.; Perin, O.; Bouslimani, A.; Landemaine, L.; Misra, N.; Cupferman, S.; Aguilar, L.; Clavaud, C.; Chopra, T.; Khodr, A. Advances in microbiome-derived solutions and methodologies are founding a new era in skin health and care. *Pathogens* **2022**, *11*, 121. [CrossRef]
146. Holland, K.T.; Bojar, R.A. Cosmetics: What is their influence on the skin microflora? *Am. J. Clin. Dermatol.* **2002**, *3*, 445–449. [CrossRef] [PubMed]
147. Amiri, S.; Kohneshahri, S.R.A.; Nabizadeh, F. The effect of unit operation and adjunct probiotic culture on physicochemical, biochemical, and textural properties of Dutch Edam cheese. *Lebensm.-Wiss. Technol.* **2022**, *155*, 112859. [CrossRef]

Disclaimer/Publisher's Note: The statements, opinions and data contained in all publications are solely those of the individual author(s) and contributor(s) and not of MDPI and/or the editor(s). MDPI and/or the editor(s) disclaim responsibility for any injury to people or property resulting from any ideas, methods, instructions or products referred to in the content.

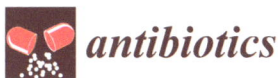

Article

Development, Optimization, and In Vitro/In Vivo Evaluation of Azelaic Acid Transethosomal Gel for Antidermatophyte Activity

Ali M. Nasr [1,2], Noha M. Badawi [3,4,*], Yasmine H. Tartor [5,*], Nader M. Sobhy [6] and Shady A. Swidan [3,4]

1. Department of Pharmaceutics, Faculty of Pharmacy, Port Said University, Port Said 42526, Egypt
2. Department of Pharmaceutics and Industrial Pharmacy, Faculty of Pharmacy, Galala University, New Galala 43713, Egypt
3. Department of Pharmaceutics and Pharmaceutical Technology, Faculty of Pharmacy, The British University in Egypt, El-Sherouk City, Cairo 11837, Egypt
4. The Centre for Drug Research and Development (CDRD), Faculty of Pharmacy, The British University in Egypt, El-Sherouk City, Cairo 11837, Egypt
5. Department of Microbiology, Faculty of Veterinary Medicine, Zagazig University, Zagazig 44511, Egypt
6. Department of Animal Medicine, Faculty of Veterinary Medicine, Zagazig University, Zagazig 44511, Egypt
* Correspondence: noha.alaa@bue.edu.eg (N.M.B.); yasminehtartor@zu.edu.eg (Y.H.T.)

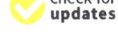

Abstract: Treatment of dermatophytosis is quite challenging. This work aims to investigate the antidermatophyte action of Azelaic acid (AzA) and evaluate its efficacy upon entrapment into transethosomes (TEs) and incorporation into a gel to enhance its application. Optimization of formulation variables of TEs was carried out after preparation using the thin film hydration technique. The antidermatophyte activity of AzA-TEs was first evaluated in vitro. In addition, two guinea pig infection models with *Trichophyton* (*T.*) *mentagrophytes* and *Microsporum* (*M.*) *canis* were established for the in vivo assessment. The optimized formula showed a mean particle size of 219.8 ± 4.7 nm and a zeta potential of −36.5 ± 0.73 mV, while the entrapment efficiency value was 81.9 ± 1.4%. Moreover, the ex vivo permeation study showed enhanced skin penetration for the AzA-TEs (3056 µg/cm^2) compared to the free AzA (590 µg/cm^2) after 48 h. AzA-TEs induced a greater inhibition in vitro on the tested dermatophyte species than free AzA (MIC$_{90}$ was 0.01% vs. 0.32% for *T. rubrum* and 0.032% for *T. mentagrophytes* and *M. canis* vs. 0.56%). The mycological cure rate was improved in all treated groups, specially for our optimized AzA-TEs formula in the *T. mentagrophytes* model, in which it reached 83% in this treated group, while it was 66.76% in the itraconazole and free AzA treated groups. Significant ($p < 0.05$) lower scores of erythema, scales, and alopecia were observed in the treated groups in comparison with the untreated control and plain groups. In essence, the TEs could be a promising carrier for AzA delivery into deeper skin layers with enhanced antidermatophyte activity.

Keywords: transethosomes; azelaic acid; antidermatophyte; thin film hydration; guinea pig model; *Trichophyton mentagrophytes*; *Microsporum canis*

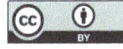

1. Introduction

Studies have shown that the greatest number of dermatological disorders occur as superficial fungal infections at a high rate in developing countries, and can in some cases lead to death [1]. Dermatophytic infection affects millions of people worldwide every year [2]. Recent years have seen a rise in the incidence of fungal topical infections which have proven to face significant obstacles in their treatment. Dermatophytosis is among the most prevalent forms of infectious diseases globally, accounting for almost 25% of all skin mycoses worldwide [3,4]. Dermatophytosis is a superficial fungal infection of the keratinized structures including skin, hair, nails, or animal hoof and claws caused by a dermatophyte mold which is most commonly of the Trichophyton and Microsporum genus. The infection can be transmitted to humans by anthropophilic species, geophilic species from the soil, or zoophilic species through contact with animals [5].

Treatment of dermatophytosis might be quite challenging and needs a cautious approach in certain population groups including pregnant women, children, and the elderly. Recently, there is a tendency to limit treatment to topical therapies owing to their negligible systemic absorption. Future research on newer medications or topical drug formulations with a "depot" impact may contribute to a reduction in the treatment duration as well as recurrences [4]. The main difficulties with the treatment of dermatological fungal infections are how to bypass the stratum corneum (SC) barrier, the long time required for treatment, and recurring infection. Due to the presence of tight junctions and the highly organized structure of the SC, dermatophytosis treatment is complicated. Efficient treatment requires the presence of antifungal drugs with a high concentration on the epidermis and dermis [6]. There is a preference for the use of topical antifungal drugs over systemic ones since the drug is delivered directly to the affected site leading to fewer adverse effects [7].

Further approaches were carried out to develop a drug delivery system that enables various antifungal drugs to bypass the SC's barrier function. Among these novel drug delivery systems, lipid-based nanoformulations such as liposomes have proven to be promising drug carriers for dermatological delivery and attracted the attention of many researchers in this field [8]. It should be noted, however, that the liposomal rigid structure and their large size have limited drug diffusion into deeper skin layers [9]. As a consequence, an improvement over liposomal strategy was developed recently and novel approaches of lipid-based vesicles such as the ultra-deformable liposomes (transfersomes), ethosomes, and transethosomes (TEs) have been designed as enhanced versions of liposomes [10]. Transfersomes are liposomal formulations that contain edge activators. An advantage of this approach is that these edge activators destabilize the liposomal lipid bilayer and improve the flexibility of liposomes [11]. Ethosomes, on the other hand, are novel flexible malleable vesicles that consist of phospholipids, water, and a high concentration of ethanol [12]. Ethosomes enhance the penetration rate of drugs across the SC and can bypass this critical barrier where ethanol increases the vesicles' flexibility by fluidizing the lipid bilayers, allowing them to squeeze through the skin pores which are much smaller than their original diameters [13]. Thus, if we can formulate a system that combines the benefits of transfersomes and ethosomes, it will be an invaluable carrier in delivering the drugs to deeper skin layers. This was achieved recently with the development of nanovesicles TEs. TEs are vesicular systems containing phospholipid (e.g., soy lecithin), water, and high concentration of ethanol along with an edge activator (EA) or permeation enhancer [14]. The EA plays an important role as it preserves the integrity of the vesicles when going across small channels, thus increasing stability and the deformity is consequently procured [15]. The particle size of TEs is the most important factor for their skin penetration. Recent studies stated that a size below 500 nm is necessary for the efficient diffusion of nanocolloids through the SC [16]. Additionally, hydrogels have been widely utilized as potential strategies for drug delivery. This could be attributed to their outstanding biocompatibility, biodegradability, wide mechanical properties that match various soft tissues in the human body, and controllable drug release capabilities [17–19].

Azelaic acid (AzA) is straight-chained dicarboxylic acid approved for acne vulgaris and inflammatory (papulopustular) rosacea treatment. Owing to its poor water solubility, about 0.24 g/100 mL at 25 °C, as well as limited skin penetration across the SC, various formulations have been developed, including liposome, microemulsion, ethosomes, and liquid crystal [20]. Since relatively little is known about the antidermatophyte activity of AzA, we investigated for the first time its in vitro and in vivo effects on dermatophyte species in comparison with its nano transethosomal formulation (AzA-TEs) and itraconazole as a positive control.

To date, no attempt has been made to investigate the potential of TEs as carriers for AzA, and no trials have been carried out to examine the antidermatophyte effect of the AzA-TEs nanocarriers. The current investigation aimed to develop a nanotransethosomal gel of AzA for efficient cutaneous delivery, in order to improve its biopharmaceutical profile and enhance therapeutic efficacy as an antifungal for dermatophytosis treatment. The overall study was carried out in two steps. AzA-TEs were developed and formulated in the first step using the quality by design methodology. Additionally, the morphology, vesicle size, zeta potential, polydispersity index, and physical state of the optimized formulation were characterized. The second stage included the incorporation of the optimized TEs vesicles into a Carbopol-based gel for enhanced skin adherence. Two guinea pig models are performed in the in vivo study of AzA-TEs. Various dermatophyte species including *T. mentagrophytes* and *M. canis* have been utilized successfully in the current study animal models as they cause acute inflammatory infections which are easy to be clinically evaluated.

2. Materials and Methods

2.1. Materials

Azelaic acid was a kind gift from Medical Union Pharmaceuticals (MUP, Ismailia, Egypt), Labrafil M 1944 SC, and was kindly gifted by Gattefossé, (Saint-Priest, France). Soy leci-thin, Sodium deoxycholate (SDC) and Dialysis tubing cellulose membrane (molecular weight cut off 12,000–14,000 Dalton) were purchased from Sigma Aldrich Chemical Co. (St. Louis, MO, USA). Oleic acid and Carbopol 934 were purchased from El-Nasr Pharmaceutical Company (Cairo, Egypt). Dichloromethane and ethanol were purchased from Fisher Scientific (Loughborough, UK). All other materials were of analytical grade.

2.2. Methods

2.2.1. Experimental Design

A 2^3 full factorial design was generated for the optimization of AzA-TEs using the Design-Expert 11 program (Stat-Ease, Inc., Minneapolis, MN, USA). Eight runs were created in this model by the design. Three independent variables were selected to be studied including SAA type (X1), SAA:Lecithin ratio (X2), in addition to ethanol concentration% (X3). The outcome responses for this design were particle size (PS) (Y1), zeta potential (ZP) (Y2), and entrapment efficiency (EE%) (Y3). Table 1 presents the independent and dependent variables utilized in the current study as well as their levels and desirability constraints.

Table 1. Full factorial design (2^3) used for preparation and optimization of AzA-TEs.

Independent Variables	Low	High
X1: SAA type	Labrafil	SDC
X2: SAA:Lecithin ratio	15:85	5:95
X3: Ethanol concentration%	20	40
Dependent Variables	Desirability Constraints	
Y1: PS	Minimize	
Y2: ZP	Maximize	
Y3: EE%	Maximize	

Abbreviations: AzA: Azelaic acid, TEs: Transethosomes; SAA: Surfactant; SDC: Sodium deoxycholate; PS, particle size; ZP, zeta potential, and EE%, entrapment efficiency percentage.

2.2.2. Preparation of AzA-Loaded TEs

AzA-TEs vesicles were prepared via the thin-film hydration method [21]. Precisely weighed amounts of Soy Lecithin, SAA, oleic acid, and AzA were added to 10 mL dichloromethane in a long-necked round-bottom flask as shown in Table 2. The solvent mixture was then evaporated under vacuum at 60 °C and 90 rpm speed via Heidolph rotary evaporator (P/N Hei-AP Precision ML/G3, Schwabach, Germany). The vacuum was applied until the solvent was evaporated totally and a thin film was formed on the round flask wall. The dried film was then hydrated by adding 10 mL distilled water containing ethanol, at 60 °C which is above the lipid phase transition temperature (Tc), and stirred for 45 min. Finally, the prepared dispersion was sonicated for 10 min using a probe sonicator (Vibra Cell-Sonics Material, 130 W, 20 kHz, Newtown, CT, USA) at 70% amplitude to obtain the AzA-loaded TEs. The dispersed vesicles were then stored for further investigations at 4 °C.

Table 2. Composition of the prepared TEs loaded with AzA.

Formulae Code	AzA Amount (mg)	Oleic Acid Amount (mg)	SAA Type	SAA: Lecithin Ratio	Ethanol Concentration (%)
F1	50	10	Labrafil	5:95	20
F2	50	10	SDC	15:85	40
F3	50	10	Labrafil	5:95	40
F4	50	10	SDC	15:85	20
F5	50	10	Labrafil	15:85	20
F6	50	10	SDC	5:95	40
F7	50	10	SDC	5:95	20
F8	50	10	Labrafil	15:85	40

Abbreviations: AzA: Azelaic acid; TEs: Transethosomes; SAA: Surfactant; SDC: Sodium deoxycholate.

2.2.3. Characterization and Optimization of the Prepared AzA-Loaded TEs Formulations

Particle Size (PS), Polydispersity Index (PDI), and Zeta Potential (ZP) Measurement

The average PS, PDI, and ZP of the fabricated AzA-TEs formulations were attained via dynamic light scattering technique using a Zeta-sizer 3000 PCS (Malvern Instruments Ltd., Worcestershire, UK). Before analysis, the samples were diluted with de-ionized water. The obtained values were the means of triplicate measurements at 25 ± 1 °C [22].

Entrapment Efficiency (EE%) Measurement

EE% of AzA-TEs were calculated using the centrifugation method. Firstly, the vesicular dispersions of the prepared formulae were centrifuged at 20,000 rpm at a temperature of 4 °C for 2 h utilizing a cooling centrifuge (Sigma 3K 30, Osterede am Harz, Germany). After that, the supernatant was separated and collected to be analyzed λ_{max} 204 nm using a UV-Vis spectrophotometer (Shimadzu UV1650 Spectrophotometer, Kyoto, Japan) [23]. Determination of EE% was carried out using the following equation [24]:

$$EE\% = \left(\frac{\text{Total AzA concentration} - \text{Free AzA concentartion}}{\text{Total Aza concentration}} \right) \times 100\%$$

2.2.4. Optimization of Formulation Variables

For selecting the optimized formula to be subjected to further studies, the desirability function that expects the optimum levels of the response variables was calculated. The principle for choosing the optimum formula was attaining the least PS and the highest ZP and EE%.

Transmission Electron Microscopy

The morphology of the optimized AzA-TEs was inspected via a transmission electron microscope (Joel JEM 1230, Tokyo, Japan). Firstly, the application of the vesicular dispersion was carried out on a carbon-coated copper grid and left to be dried in order to produce a thin film. A drop of 2% aqueous solution of uranyl acetate was placed for 1 min. The remaining solution was swept and the sample was air-dried at room temperature and then viewed and photographed [25].

Fourier Transform Infrared (FTIR) Spectroscopy

Infrared spectra of the free drug AzA, medicated optimized formula and the plain formula (without drug) were attained using FTIR spectrophotometer VERTEX 70 (Bruker Corporation, Karlsruhe, Germany) [26]. The spectra were analyzed in the range of 500 to 4000 cm^{-1}. The spectrum of air was used as a background before the analysis of each sample. Sample spectra in addition to the background were taken in a room with a temperature of 22–24 °C, at a spectral resolution of 4 cm^{-1}. For each measurement, 32 scans were carried out.

In Vitro Release of AzA from the Optimized Formula

The in vitro release behavior of the AzA-TEs optimized formula was performed via the dialysis bag technique and compared with free AzA [27]. Before using the cellulose dialysis bag, it was soaked in phosphate-buffered saline pH 7.4 for 24 h. AzA-Tes equivalent to 10 mg of AzA was accurately weighed and the same amount of free AzA was dispersed in phosphate-buffered saline pH 7.4 and then subjected to 5 min vortexing. Afterward, samples were placed in the dialysis bags, and the bag's ends were tightly closed. The bags which acted as the donor cell were kept in a phosphate-buffered saline pH 7.4 (50 mL) that represented the receptor cell and then placed in a shaker water bath (WSB-18, Dahan Scientific Co., Ltd., Seoul, Korea), with a rotation speed of 50 rpm and temperature of 37 ± 0.5 °C. Ethanol (30% v/v) was added to the phosphate-buffered saline pH 7.4 to maintain the sink condition [28]. Aliquots were withdrawn at different time intervals from 1 to 48 h, substituted with fresh buffer to maintain the sink condition, and then analyzed spectrophotometrically at 204 nm. Triplicate samples were analyzed and the average concentration was utilized.

Ex Vivo Permeation of AzA from the Optimized Formula

Mouse skin was utilized as a model to simulate human skin [29]. The ex vivo permeation experiment was performed via Franz diffusion cells with a diffusional area of 1.76 cm^2 using the same conditions of the in vitro drug release study, except that the cellulose membrane was substituted by dorsal hairless mouse skin [27,29]. The sacrifice of male mice (weighing between 25–30 g) was first carried out, followed by hair removal, and excision of the ventral and dorsal abdominal skins. Afterward, tweezers were utilized to get rid of the subcutaneous fat, and the skin membrane fragments were washed with buffer. Subsequently, the skin fragments were kept at -20 °C until they were used [29]. The skin was placed between the two compartments (receptor and donor) of the Franz cell after being defrosted and soaked in phosphate-buffered saline pH 7.4. Following, 25 mL of phosphate-buffered saline pH 7.4 was transferred to the receptor compartment and then magnetically stirred in the water bath (37 ± 1 °C). The optimized formula was placed in the donor compartment. Then, samples (1 mL) were withdrawn from the receptor medium at different time intervals (from 1 to 48 h), and the drug concentrations were spectrophotometrically measured at λmax 204 nm. After withdrawing each sample, an equivalent volume of the fresh buffer solution was substituted. All samples were compared to a blank (without drug) to avoid any interference. This experiment was performed in triplicate and the average concentrations were used. The permeation flux (Jmax) at 48 h and the enhancement ratio (ER) were calculated according to the following equations [30]:

$$\text{Jmax} = \left(\frac{\text{Amount of drug permeated}}{\text{Time} \times \text{Area of the membrane}} \right)$$

$$\text{ER} = \left(\frac{\text{Jmax of the nanovesicles}}{\text{Jmax of drug suspension}} \right)$$

2.2.5. Formulation of AzA and AzA-TEs Gels

AzA suspension and AzA-TEs optimal formula were converted into gels to enhance the skin application. The optimized formula and the free drug suspension were added to Carbopol gel and then mixed with the assistance of a magnetic stirrer (Thennolyne Corporation, Dubuque, IA, USA) to form gels with good consistency and final AzA concentration of 0.5% [31].

2.2.6. Evaluation of Antidermatophyte Activity

The antidermatophyte activity of the optimized AzA-TEs formulation was evaluated both in vitro and in vivo.

Dermatophyte Clinical Isolates

T. mentagrophytes and *T. rubrum* (n = 10 of each) that were isolated from cases of tinea corporis and *M. canis* (n = 10) recovered from tinea capitis and ringworm lesions in cats were included. Isolates were identified based on their macro- and micro-morphological, and physiological characteristics, as previously described [32]. A suspension was prepared in sterile saline from colonies of each isolate grown on mycobiotic agar medium (CONDA, Madrid, Spain) at 25 °C for a week, and adjusted to 10^6 CFU/mL using a hemocytometer.

In Vitro Evaluation of Antidermatophyte Activity of AzA-TEs

The antidermatophyte activity of AzA-TEs was evaluated using an agar well diffusion test against isolates of *T. mentagrophytes*, *T. rubrum*, and *M. canis* [33]. The fungal suspensions (10^6 CFU/mL) were evenly distributed on the surface of mycobiotic agar medium plates. With a sterile cork borer, 6 mm diameter wells were cut in the agar plate. Then, 100 µL of AzA-TEs formula (5 mg/mL), and free AzA were dissolved in 10% tween 20 (Sigma Aldrich, St. Louis, MO, USA) and adjusted to 5 mg/mL, gel (1.25 mg/mL) was placed in wells. The test was performed in triplicate and a negative control (tween 20) and a positive control (10 µg itraconazole disc; Hi-Media Laboratories, Mumbai, India) were included. The diameter of the zones of inhibition was measured and recorded after 96 h of incubation at 25 °C, and the mean values were interpreted as sensitive (inhibition zone $\geq$ 10 mm) [34].

Minimum inhibitory concentration (MIC) values were determined using different concentrations (0.1, 0.32, 1, 3.2, and 5 mg/mL) of both AzA-TEs and free AzA as previously described [35,36]. The MICs of itraconazole (Janssen Research Foundation Beerse, Belgium) were determined according to Clinical Laboratory Standards Institute M38 guidelines [37]. The MIC_{50} and MIC_{90} values, which, respectively, prevented the growth of 50% and 90% of the tested isolates [38].

In Vivo Evaluation of Antidermatophyte Activity of AzA-TEs

The effectiveness of the optimized AzA-TEs formula in comparison with the free AzA and itraconazole for the treatment of dermatophytosis was investigated in two infected guinea pig models. For establishing infection, in the two models, with *M. canis* and *T. mentagrophytes*, hair from the mid-dorsal region (diameter of 1.50 cm) of 60 guinea pigs (weight 250–300 g) was shaved using a manual razor. Then, 50 µL of *M. canis* or *T. mentagrophytes* suspension (10^7 cells/mL) was applied to the shaved skin. On the third day following inoculation, antifungal therapy was started on shaved regions and continued for 12 days [39].

In each model, guinea pigs were divided into five groups (6 animals/group): group 1 (G1); infected untreated control group, G2; infected and treated with 10 mg/kg itraconazole once daily by oral gavage [39]. AzA-TEs gel (5 mg/kg) (G3), AzA gel (G4), and plain gel (G5) were applied topically twice a day.

The infected and treated animals were evaluated clinically on days 3, 7, 10, and 14 post-treatment (PT) by scoring lesions (redness, scales, and hair loss) and mycologically by microscopy and culture on days 3, 7, and 14 PT. Animals were kept under observation up to day 28 PT to evaluate the final clinical cure rate.

The inoculated areas were disinfected with 70% ethyl alcohol and skin scrapings and hair samples were collected using a sterile toothbrush for subsequent microscopical examination using 20% potassium hydroxide (KOH) and culture on mycobiotic agar medium slants and dermatophyte test medium (DTM) plus dermato supplement (Himedia, India). Cultures were incubated at 25 °C for four weeks and observed twice a week. Based on macro- and micro-morphological features, isolates were identified to the species level. If cultures of the collected samples from the infected regions were negative, the animals were considered mycologically cured [40].

2.2.7. Data Analysis

Data were edited in Microsoft Excel (Microsoft Corporation, Redmond, WA, USA). Exact Wilcoxon test was used to compare untreated versus treated animals per day (3, 7, 10, and 14 PT) regarding the clinical score. The effect of the treatments was evaluated for each day (3, 7, and 14) by the frequency of positive microscopy and cultures in treated animals versus untreated control group according to the fisher exact test. Figures were fitted by the Graph-Pad Prism software 5.0 (Graph Pad, San Diego, CA, USA). Statistical significance was set at p-value less than 0.05.

3. Results and Discussion

3.1. Effect of Formulation Variables on the Observed Responses

3.1.1. Particle Size and Size Distribution

As seen from Table 3, the mean particle size ranged from 219.8 to 403.5 nm for formulae F3 and F4, respectively. Formulations F4 and F1 showed the widest and narrowest particle size distributions with PDI values of 0.249 and 0.414, respectively. Only one formula exceeded the PDI value of 0.4 and none exceeded the value of 0.5. The obtained values are acceptable and indicate relatively homogenous vesicular size distribution). According to Soleimanian et al., a PDI higher than 0.5 is not considered acceptable and reflects heterogeneous, wide size distribution values [41]. Regarding the particle size, a smaller size was achieved using a higher ethanol concentration. The model that best fits the particle size data is a quadratic model and the equations that best describe the model for different surfactants are:

$$PS = SAA\ type\ Labrafil + 364.38750 + 4.53750\ SAA:Lecithin - 3.96625\ Ethanol\ Conc$$

$$PS = SAA\ type\ SDC + 396.96250 + 4.53750\ SAA:Lecithin + 3.96625\ Ethanol\ Conc$$

Table 3. Observed responses for the prepared TEs formulations.

	PS (nm)	PDI	ZP (mV)	EE (%)
F1	309.0 ± 7.8	0.414 ± 0.067	−37.5 ± 0.35	69.5 ± 2.0
F2	281.2 ± 3.7	0.390 ± 0.002	−31.9 ± 0.23	71.6 ± 1.3
F3	219.8 ± 4.7	0.372 ± 0.015	−36.5 ± 0.73	81.9 ± 1.4
F4	403.5 ± 8.5	0.249 ± 0.022	−33.9 ± 0.77	57.6 ± 0.8
F5	335.9 ± 3.9	0.292 ± 0.029	−37.3 ± 0.61	59.7 ± 0.9
F6	270.2 ± 8.0	0.375 ± 0.013	−34.5 ± 1.03	77.2 ± 3.1
F7	338.5 ± 1.0	0.346 ± 0.014	−33.0 ± 0.66	62.8 ± 1.1
F8	298.4 ± 1.6	0.269 ± 0.013	−34.6 ± 0.78	77.1 ± 2.4

Abbreviations: TEs: Transethosomes; PS, particle size; ZP, zeta potential; and EE%, entrapment efficiency percentage.

The model was found significant (p-value 0.0170) (Figure 1A,B). Regarding the variables studied, it was found that increasing the ethanol concentration led to a decrease in the particle size. This effect might be due to the interaction between the ethanol and lipid bilayer [42]. Another explanation was presented by Vasanth and colleagues who suggested that high ethanol concentration causes interpenetration of the Lecithin hydrocarbon chain, which leads to a further reduction in the thickness of the membrane of the TEs vesicles and causes a decrease in mean particle size [43]. This was in agreement with Salem et al., who found a generalized reduction in the mean vesicle size by increasing ethanol content from 10 to 30%. Ahmed et al. found the same antagonistic effect of ethanol concentration; they offered an additional explanation that upon increasing the ethanol content, it causes a reduction in the main transition temperature of the phospholipids, which leads to partial fluidization of the TEs vesicles and the formation of small nanovesicles [44]. The same observation was found during the preparation of ethosomes by Limsuwan et al., who found that the highest ethanol concentration led to a smaller size of the prepared ethosomes [45]. High concentrations of ethanol—higher than 40%—were not attempted as it was mentioned previously that higher concentrations as 45% lead to the failure of vesicle formation or rapture of formed vesicles [46]. The other factor that was significant on the PS of the vesicles was the SAA to Lecithin ratio. It was found that decreasing the ratio led to a decrease in the PS. The same finding was observed by Qushawy et al., who found that the SAA:Lecithin ratio of 10:90 resulted in a smaller size of transfersomes compared to the 20:80 ratio [47]. Vasanth et al., who studied the same variable on transfersomes stated that the higher concentration of soy lecithin led to smaller vesicle size [43]. It is worth mentioning that some other studies found that this effect was insignificant on the vesicular size of TEs [27] and transfersomes [48]. No significant effect was found when either SDC or Labrafil M 1944 Cs were used on the vesicular size.

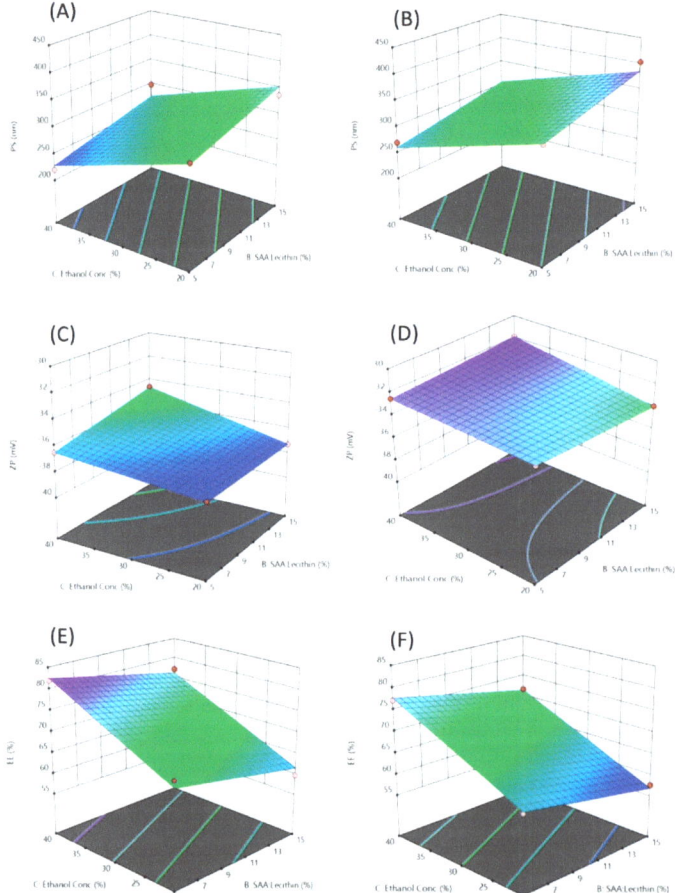

Figure 1. 3D-response surface plots showing the effect of the independent variables on PS (**A**,**B**), ZP (**C**,**D**), and EE% (**E**,**F**). (**A**,**C**,**E**) where the used SAA is Labrafil, (**B**,**D**,**F**) where the used SAA is SDC.

3.1.2. Zeta Potential

As expected from the composition, the TEs have negative charges due to the presence of oleic acid and the phosphate group in soy lecithin. As seen from Table 3, all prepared formulations show a ZP value over -30, which indicates high stability and a low tendency to agglomerate using all tried ingredients in all levels of the variables used. This leads to higher stability of TEs dispersion.

ZP = SAA type Labrafil − 37.9 − 0.135 SAA:Lecithin + 0.0125 Ethanol Conc + 0.008 SAA:Lecithin × Ethanol Conc

ZP = SAA type SDC − 32.15 − 0.255 SAA:Lecithin − 0.0175 Ethanol Conc + 0.008 SAA:Lecithin × Ethanol Conc

The model used was significant (p-value 0.027) (Figure 1C,D). It was mentioned by Ogiso et al. that the negative charge of the zeta potential of ethosomal systems is attributed mostly to the high ethanolic content in these nanovesicles. Ethanol provides negative charges to the polar head groups of the phospholipids that would create an electrostatic repulsion [49]. Formulations containing Labrafil M 1944 CS with the chemical formula mono-, di- and triglycerides, and PEG-6 (MW 300) mono- and diesters of oleic (C18:1) acid showed higher ZP than those containing SDC as surfactant. No significant effect of the SAA:Lecithin ratio on the ZP.

3.1.3. Entrapment Efficiency

High entrapment efficiencies of AzA up to 81.9% for formulation F3 were obtained. The least EE% value was in F4 with only 57.6% AzA entrapped. The model to optimize the AzA-TEs was highly significant (p-value = 0.0004) (Figure 1E,F). In addition, all variables showed a significant effect on the EE% of the prepared TEs. This could be explained by the co-solvent effect of the ethanol which has a high effect in increasing the solubility of lipophilic drugs—such as AzA—in the polar phase of the TEs. This also allows an additional amount of AzA in the aqueous core of the nano transethosomal dispersion to be accommodated [50]. Another explanation that was presented by Salem et al. is that the solubilization effect of ethanol increases the fluidity of the membrane of the TEs vesicles leading to a more entrapped AzA [51]. An interesting finding was obtained as decreasing SAA:Lecithin ratio resulted in higher EE%. In a lower ratio, higher lecithin concentration in the vesicular membrane might increase the entrapment of the hydrophobic AzA. The obtained results were in good agreement with Balata et al., who found that increasing surfactant concentration was accompanied by a decrease in EE%. They suggested that this might be due to the increased efficiency of surfactant incorporation within the lipids forming a more permeable vesicles membrane, hence lowering the EE% [48,52]. Formation of mixed micelles upon the addition of higher SAA concentrations is another explanation for lower EE% as they are more rigid and smaller in size [53]. Labrafil M 1944 SC with an HLB of 9 was found to achieve higher EE% compared to SDC. SDC is an anionic surfactant with a high HLB of 16. An explanation of the lower EE% in formulations containing SDC can be offered by discussing the findings of Amnuaikit et al., who found that high EE% of transfersomes contains the cationic drug phenylethyl resorcinol using SDC as SAA. They concluded that the high EE% was due to electrostatic attraction between the negatively charged drug and the positively charged SDC [54]. Using the same concept, the anionic AzA showed electrostatic repulsion with the anionic SDC resulting in the expulsion of the drug from the transethosomal vesicles, which lead to decreased EE%. The model equations for each surfactant type were

EE = SAA type Labrafil + 56.575 − 0.635 SAA:Lecithin + 0.7275 Ethanol Conc

EE = SAA type SDC + 51.825 − 0.635 SAA:Lecithin + 0.7275 Ethanol Conc

3.2. Optimization of Formulation Variables

Based on the analysis of the studied variables, the optimization was carried out using the desirability function approach. When several responses were evaluated in an experimental design, the optimum responses reached individually for each factor did not coincide in a single run in all cases. To solve multiple response problems, different statistical methods can be used; one of the most commonly used methods is the desirability function [55]. To find the most desirable formulation fulfilling all constraints of all studied variables, a weight factor of 1 was chosen for all individual desirabilities in this work. The best selected solution with the highest desirability (0.920) was found to be the same as the composition of F3. The selected solution and the predicted and practically performed formulations are listed in Table 4. Labrafil M 1944 SC was used as SAA with a ratio to lecithin of 5:95, respectively, and 40% ethanol concentration. As seen from Table 4 a small acceptable residual error was obtained indicating the validity of the model for the preparation of AzA-TEs. The selected formula was further characterized and investigated both in vitro, ex vivo, and in vivo for antidermatophyte effect.

Table 4. Validation of the optimization model using the desirability function.

	Independent Variables			Responses			Desirability
	SAA Type	SAA Ratio	Ethanol Conc.	PS	ZP	EE%	
Predicted formula	Labrafil	5.0	40.0	228.425	−36.475	82.5	
Practically prepared formula	Labrafil	5.0	40.0	219.8	−36.5	81.9	0.920
Residual error (%)				3.78%	0.07%	−0.73%	

Abbreviations: SAA, Surfactant; PS, particle size; ZP, zeta potential; and EE%, entrapment efficiency percentage.

3.2.1. Transmission Electron Microscopy

As seen in Figure 2A, the AzA-TEs vesicles are spherical in shape and homogenous in size. They are present as separate entities without agglomeration.

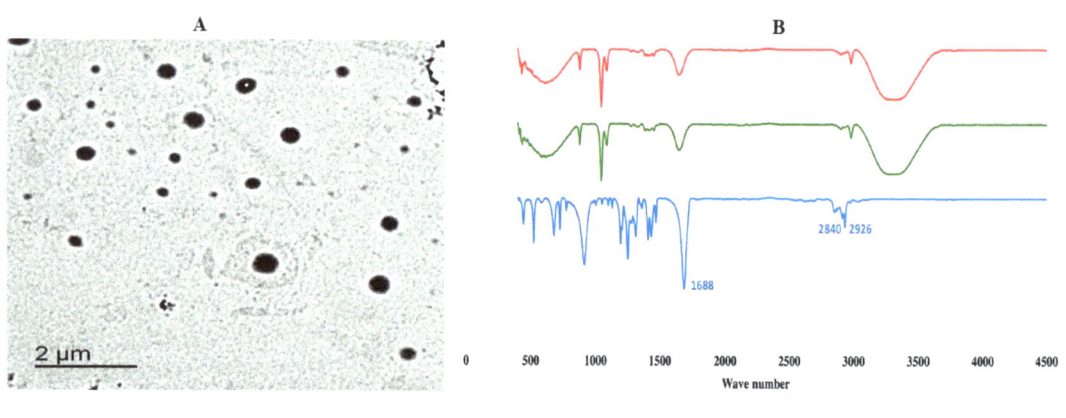

Figure 2. Characterization of the optimized formula; (**A**) Transmission electron microscopy of the optimized AzA-TEs; (**B**) FTIR spectra of the free AzA, plain formula, and optimized AzA-TEs.

3.2.2. Fourier Transform Infrared (FTIR) Spectroscopy

Figure 2B showed the FTIR spectrum of the free AzA, plain formula, and the optimized AzA-TEs. The FTIR spectrum of the AzA reveals typical bands coming from the aliphatic chain at 2926 cm^{-1} and 2840 cm^{-1}. There is also a band of high intensity coming from two free carboxyl groups at about 1700 cm^{-1} situated at the end of the molecule [56]. FTIR spectrum of AzA-TEs showed that the characteristic absorption peaks of AzA disappeared indicating the drug encapsulation within the nanovesicles. In addition, the peaks of the

AzA-TEs optimized formula and the plain drug free formula were identical, which confirms that AzA was successfully encapsulated in the nanovesicles [57].

3.2.3. In Vitro Release of AzA from the Optimized Formula

The in vitro release study of AzA-TEs optimized formula and free AzA was performed in a release media of phosphate-buffered saline pH 7.4 and ethanol (30%) and the data are plotted in Figure 3A. The attained data demonstrated that the optimized formulation reached 89% cumulative release after 48 h, in comparison to 45% only of the free AzA. The release behavior of AzA from AzA-TEs optimized formula showed a controlled release manner during the 48 h of the study in comparison to the free AzA that exhibited an uncontrolled release behavior. The dissolution rate of AzA-TEs was found to be faster than those of free AzA. The increase in the amount released could be due to the small PS of the TEs nanovesicles that led to the higher surface area, and hence improved dissolution rate. Additionally, the free drug solubility could be improved by reducing the PS according to the Oswald–Freundlich equation [58]. The abovementioned findings are in accordance with a study that used telmisartan ethosomal gel [27].

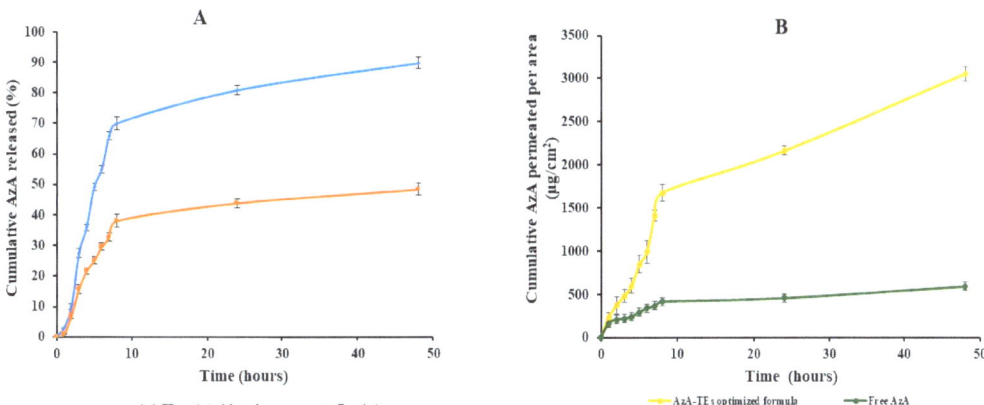

Figure 3. In vitro and ex vivo characterizations of the optimized formula; (**A**) In vitro drug release of the free AzA and the optimized AzA-TEs; (**B**) Ex vivo fluxes of the free AzA and the optimized AzA-TEs.

3.2.4. Ex Vivo Permeation of AzA from the Optimized Formula

The cumulative amount of AzA permeated from AzA-TEs optimized formula compared to the free AzA after 48 h is depicted in Figure 3B. It was detected that the amount of AzA permeated from the optimized formula (3056 µg/cm^2) was higher than the amount permeated from free AzA suspension (590 µg/cm^2) after 48 h, which may be due to that AzA can overcome the SC barrier and reach the deeper layers of the skin more efficiently than AzA in its free form. This behavior may be attributed to the presence of ethanol in the TEs nanovesicles which act as penetration enhancer and thus imparts flexibility to TEs and therefore is responsible for the high penetration [59]. It was reported that TEs employ pull and push effects on the intercellular interface of the SC cells and thus could enhance the drug penetration [59]. The push effect is a thermodynamic effect of ethanol evaporation, and the pull effect is a result of ethanol fluidizing SC lipids, which results in the formation of additional penetration pathways [30,59]. It is also worth noting that AzA-TEs obtained higher permeability parameters with a Jmax of 35.95 µg/cm^2/h compared to 6.94 µg/cm^2/h of free AzA with an ER of 5.18.

3.3. Evaluation of Antidermatophyte Activity

3.3.1. In Vitro Evaluation of Antidermatophyte Activity of AzA-TEs

This study records the antidermatophyte activity of an optimized AzA-TEs formula against three dermatophyte species. It exhibited the maximum inhibition of all strains tested, while the free AzA showed the minimum growth suppression. It was found that AzA-TEs liquid dispersion induces a significantly greater inhibition of the tested dermatophyte species than free AzA, whereas the mean inhibition zone diameters were 27.9 ± 0.15, 25.17 ± 0.05, and 26.15 ± 0.35 mm versus 16.8 ± 0.7, 15.83 ± 0.73, and 19 ± 0.21 for *T. rubrum*, *T. mentagrophytes*, and *M. canis*, respectively.

The MIC values obtained with the AzA-TEs formula were lower than those of free AzA for all test dermatophyte species (MIC_{90} was 0.01% vs. 0.32% for *T. rubrum* and 0.032% for *T. mentagrophytes* and *M. canis* vs. 0.56%). MIC range for itraconazole was 0.25–2, 0.03–1, and 0.125–1 µg/mL for *T. rubrum*, *T. mentagrophytes*, and *M. canis*, respectively.

This supports the findings of an earlier study that reported the antifungal activity of AzA (0.56%) against dermatophytes and *Scopulariopsis brevicaulis*. Moreover, 0.032% concentration of AzA did inhibit the strains tested, and testing the in vivo antifungal activity of this agent was encouraged [35]. Since *T. mentagrophytes* and *M. canis* produce acute inflammatory infections which are easy to clinically evaluate [60,61], we have established two dermatophytosis infection models using both species to be evaluated in vivo.

AzA-TEs showed an effective antifungal effect, which may be due to their unique subcellular size which can effectively increase the distribution of antifungal agents in fungal cells; therefore, greater antifungal activity was achieved [62].

3.3.2. In Vivo Evaluation of Antidermatophyte Activity of AzA-TEs

As presented in Figure 4, the infection progressed in the untreated control group (G1) and plain-gel-treated group (G5) with increasing lesion scores, while decreasing scores of erythema, scales, and alopecia were observed in the treated groups (G2, G3, and G4). Maximum response of erythema in G1 and G5 was on day 10 in the *M. canis* model and day 7 in the *T. mentagrophytes* model. While maximum responses of scales and alopecia were on days 10–14 in G1 and G5 in the *T. mentagrophytes* model and on day 14 maximum alopecia was observed in the *M. canis* model. There is a significant ($p < 0.05$) lower erythema and lesion scores in the AzA-TEs gel-, AzA gel-, itraconazole-, and plain-gel-treated groups versus the untreated control group (Figure 4).

Animals in the treated groups were positive in direct microscopy during the 14 days observation period, whereas most of the culture from AzA-TEs gel (G3) and AzA gel (G4)-treated groups in the *M. canis* model were negative during the 14-day observation period (Table 5). Although five cultures from treated groups in the *T. mentagrophytes* model were negative on day 3 and day 7 PT, two cultures from itraconazole and AzA gel treated animals were positive on day 14 PT (mycological cure rate was 66.76%). Nonetheless, the mycological cure rate was 83% in AzA-TEs gel-treated group after 14 days from the onset of treatment. Cultures of untreated control and plain-gel-treated animals were persistently positive in both *T. mentagrophytes* and *M. canis* models. Therefore, there is a significant difference between treated groups versus untreated control and plain-gel-treated ones.

Guinea pigs are used in animal models for dermatophytosis because they are predisposed to cutaneous fungal infections with clinical characteristics similar to those found in humans [63,64]. In *M. canis-* and *T. mentagrophytes*-infected animals, significantly lower clinical scores were observed in treated as compared to untreated animals (Figure 4). The ability of AzA-TEs gel (G3) and AzA (G4) to reduce the erythema, scales, and hair loss in the treated animals could be directly related to its anti-inflammatory and antikeratinizing activity (decrease in the size and quantity of keratohyalin granules and tonofilament bundles due to alteration of epidermal keratinization, which is especially detrimental to the terminal phases of epidermal differentiation) [65].

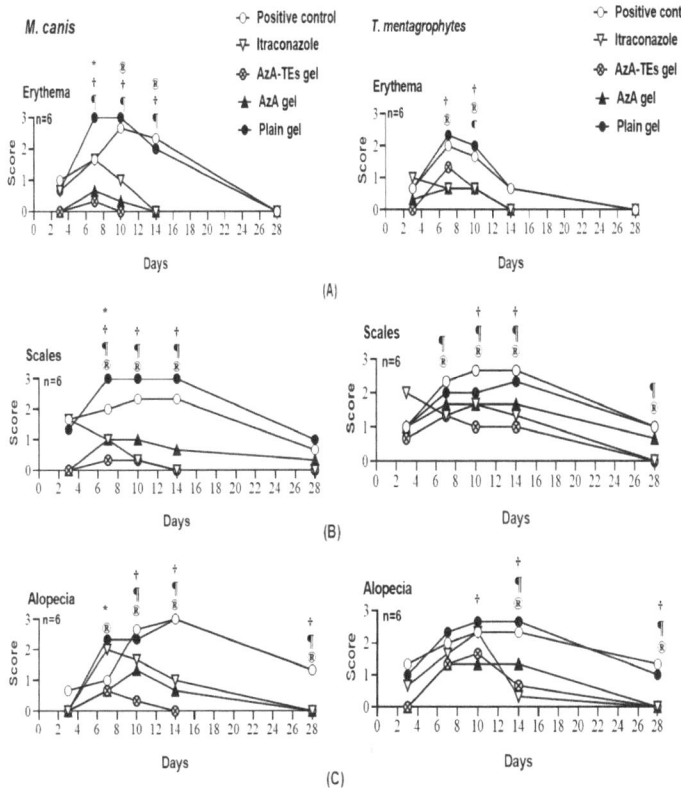

Figure 4. Means of erythema (**A**), scales (**B**), and alopecia (**C**) scores in *Microsporum canis* and *Trichophyton mentagrophytes* infected guinea pigs in different groups. * $p < 0.05$ (plain gel); † $p < 0.05$ (AZA gel); ® $p < 0.05$ (itraconazole); ¶ $p < 0.05$ (AzA-TEs gel) versus untreated positive controls. *p*-value was estimated using exact Wilcoxon test.

Table 5. Mycological evaluation of dermatophytosis treatments in a guinea pig model.

		Day 3					Day 7					Day 14				
		G1	G2	G3	G4	G5	G1	G2	G3	G4	G5	G1	G2	G3	G4	G5
T. menta-grophytes	M	6	6	6	6	5	5	4	1†	4	5	6	2†	1†	2†	6
	C	5	1†	1†	1†	4	6	1†	1†	1†	6	6	2†	1†	2†	6
	M&C	5	1†	1†	1†	4	6	1†	1†	1†	6	6	2†	1†	2†	6
M. canis	M	6	6	6	6	6	6	6	3	3	6	6	1†	3	3	6
	C	3	2	0	0	3	6	4	1†	1†	6	6	1†	1†	1†	6
	M&C	3	2	0	0	3	6	4	1†	1†	6	6	1†	1†	1†	6

Treated groups versus positive controls were compared using Fisher's exact test per day. † differs significantly with positive control $p < 0.05$. M: microscopy; C: culture; G1: infected untreated control group; G2: infected and treated with 10 mg/kg itraconazole once daily by oral gavage; G3: AzA-TEs gel- treated group (5 mg/kg); G4: AzA gel, and G5: plain-gel-treated groups topically twice a day.

Most treated animals were culture negative, but some animals remained microscopy positive on day 14 PT (Table 5). This could be due to the non-viable conidia and hyphae that are detected using microscopy and would not grow on culture [35,66]. The mycological cure rate in *M. canis* infected and treated animals after 14 days from onset of treatment was 83%

but, in the *T. mentagrophytes* model, the cure rate was 83% in AzA-TEs gel-treated group and 66.76% in itraconazole and AzA groups. Similarly, cure rates after treatment with antifungal agents ranged from 80–100% were reported in other studies [40,67]. However, the failure of mycological cure was observed in the *T. mentagrophytes* infected animals [35,68].

The superiority in the anti-fungal activity of the AzA-TEs gel formulation over other formulations (Figure 5) may be attributed to the high flexibility of the TEs, helping its penetration through the fungal cell wall and preventing ergosterol synthesis led to fungal cell membrane lysis and cell death [69]. Moreover, the lipid nanoparticles have small size that could enhance the presence of the nanoparticles to be in direct contact with the SC and confirms the entry of encapsulated drugs into the skin [70]. In addition, the extra potential of ethanol could kill organisms by denaturing their proteins and dissolving their lipids, apart from skin fluidization and penetration [71].

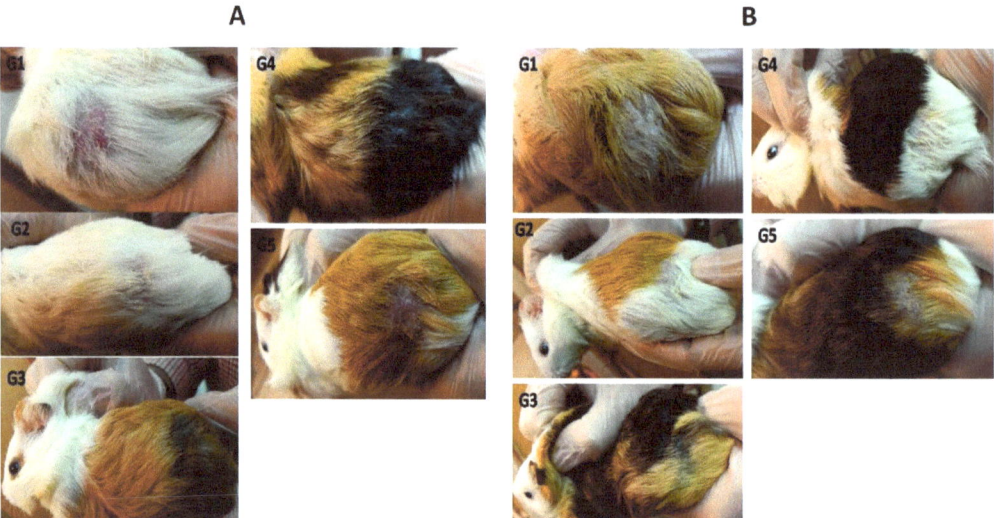

Figure 5. *M. canis* (**A**) and *T. mentagrophytes* (**B**) infected guinea pig models at day 14 post-treatment. G1: infected untreated control group; G2: infected and treated with 10 mg/kg itraconazole once daily through oral gavage; G3: AzA-TEs gel-treated group (5 mg/kg); G4: AzA gel, and G5: plain-gel-treated groups topically twice a day.

4. Conclusions

The TEs formulations proved efficacious in different skin conditions, skin cancer and cosmetics. They ensure better skin penetration and hence improved both local skin retention and transdermal action. Despite these advantages, the optimization of TEs composition is quite challenging. Several factors affect the formulation such as the nature of the drug and formulation variables. In the current study, AzA-TEs were successfully prepared using the thin film hydration method. The formulation variables for AzA-TEs were optimized and the optimized formulation showed a small size, high ZP and EE%, a prolonged release, and successful skin penetration. The obtained results from in vitro testing and in vivo models essentially imply that the therapeutic effects of AzA-TEs in dermatophytosis are directly mediated by their antidermatophyte activity. The TEs are promising carriers for enhancing the antidermatophyte activity of AzA by deep penetration through skin layers. In future, further studies related to human activity, stability, and toxicity should be performed. In addition, scaling up to an industrial scale should be studied and optimized. These results provide an important perspective on developing a safe and efficient antifungal drug for treating dermatophytoses.

Author Contributions: Conceptualization, A.M.N., N.M.B. and S.A.S.; methodology, A.M.N., N.M.B., S.A.S., Y.H.T. and N.M.S.; software, A.M.N., N.M.B., S.A.S. and Y.H.T.; validation, A.M.N., N.M.B. and S.A.S.; formal analysis, A.M.N., N.M.B., S.A.S. and Y.H.T.; investigation, A.M.N., N.M.B. and S.A.S.; resources, A.M.N., N.M.B., S.A.S., Y.H.T. and N.M.S.; data curation, A.M.N., N.M.B., S.A.S. and Y.H.T.; writing—original draft preparation, A.M.N., N.M.B., S.A.S., Y.H.T. and N.M.S.; writing—review and editing, A.M.N., N.M.B., S.A.S. and Y.H.T.; visualization, A.M.N., N.M.B. and S.A.S.; supervision, A.M.N., N.M.B. and S.A.S. All authors have read and agreed to the published version of the manuscript.

Funding: This research received no external funding.

Institutional Review Board Statement: The protocol of this study was approved by the ethical committee of the Faculty of Pharmacy, Port-Said University (REC-PHARM.PSU.22-6).

Data Availability Statement: The datasets generated or analyzed during the current study are available from the corresponding author upon reasonable request.

Conflicts of Interest: The authors declare no conflict of interest.

References

1. Bongomin, F.; Gago, S.; Oladele, R.O.; Denning, D.W. Global and multi-national prevalence of fungal diseases-estimate precision. *J. Fungi* **2017**, *3*, 57. [CrossRef]
2. White, T.; Findley, K.; Dawson, T.; Scheynius, A.; Boekhout, T.; Cuomo, C.; Xu, J.; Saunders, C.W. Fungi on the skin: Dermatophytes and Malassezia. *Cold Spring Harb. Perspect. Med.* **2014**, *4*, a019802. [CrossRef]
3. Havlickova, B.; Czaika, V.A.; Friedrich, M. Epidemiological trends in skin mycoses worldwide. *Mycoses* **2008**, *51*, 2–15. [CrossRef] [PubMed]
4. Dogra, S.; Kaul, S.; Yadav, S. Treatment of dermatophytosis in elderly, children, and pregnant women. *Indian Dermatol. Online J.* **2017**, *8*, 310–318. [CrossRef] [PubMed]
5. Aditya, K.G.; Jennifer, E.R.; Melody, C.; Elizabeth, A.C. Dermatophytosis: The management of fungal infections. *SKINmed: Dermatol. Clin.* **2005**, *4*, 305–310. [CrossRef]
6. Kim, J.-Y. Human fungal pathogens: Why should we learn? *J. Microbiol.* **2016**, *54*, 145–148. [CrossRef] [PubMed]
7. Kotla, N.G.; Chandrasekar, B.; Rooney, P.; Sivaraman, G.; Larrañaga, A.; Krishna, K.V.; Pandit, A.; Rochev, Y. Biomimetic lipid-based nanosystems for enhanced dermal delivery of drugs and bioactive agents. *ACS Biomater. Sci. Eng.* **2017**, *3*, 1262–1272. [CrossRef] [PubMed]
8. Malamatari, M.; Taylor, K.M.; Malamataris, S.; Douroumis, D.; Kachrimanis, K. Pharmaceutical nanocrystals: Production by wet milling and applications. *Drug Discov. Today* **2018**, *23*, 534–547. [CrossRef]
9. Jain, S.; Tiwary, A.K.; Sapra, B.; Jain, N.K. Formulation and evaluation of ethosomes for transdermal delivery of lamivudine. *AAPS PharmSciTech* **2007**, *8*, 249–257. [CrossRef]
10. El Maghraby, G.; Williams, A.; Barry, B.W. Skin delivery of 5-fluorouracil from ultradeformable and standard liposomes in-vitro. *J. Pharm. Pharmacol.* **2001**, *53*, 1069–1077. [CrossRef]
11. Song, C.K.; Balakrishnan, P.; Shim, C.K.; Chung, S.J.; Chong, S.; Kim, D.D. A novel vesicular carrier, transethosome, for enhanced skin delivery of voriconazole: Characterization and in vitro/in vivo evaluation. *Colloids Surf. B Biointerfaces* **2012**, *92*, 299–304. [CrossRef] [PubMed]
12. El-Menshawe, S.F.; Sayed, O.M.; Abou-Taleb, H.A.; El Tellawy, N. Skin permeation enhancement of nicotinamide through using fluidization and deformability of positively charged ethosomal vesicles: A new approach for treatment of atopic eczema. *J. Drug Deliv. Sci. Technol.* **2019**, *52*, 687–701. [CrossRef]
13. Mahmood, S.; Mandal, U.K.; Chatterjee, B. Transdermal delivery of raloxifene HCl via ethosomal system: Formulation, advanced characterizations and pharmacokinetic evaluation. *Int. J. Pharm.* **2018**, *542*, 36–46. [CrossRef]
14. Garg, V.; Singh, H.; Bhatia, A.; Raza, K.; Singh, S.; Singh, B.; Beg, S. Systematic development of transethosomal gel system of piroxicam: Formulation optimization, in vitro evaluation, and ex vivo assessment. *AAPS PharmSciTech* **2016**, *18*, 58–71. [CrossRef] [PubMed]
15. Islam, N.; Irfan, M.; Zahoor, A.F.; Iqbal, M.S.; Syed, H.K.; Khan, I.U.; Rasul, A.; Khan, S.-U.; Alqahtani, A.M.; Ikram, M.; et al. Improved bioavailability of ebastine through development of transfersomal oral films. *Pharmaceutics* **2021**, *13*, 1315. [CrossRef]
16. Kohli, A.; Alpar, H. Potential use of nanoparticles for transcutaneous vaccine delivery: Effect of particle size and charge. *Int. J. Pharm.* **2004**, *275*, 13–17. [CrossRef] [PubMed]
17. Tong, X.; Qi, X.; Mao, R.; Pan, W.; Zhang, M.; Wu, X.; Chen, G.; Shen, J.; Deng, H.; Hu, R. Construction of functional curdlan hydrogels with bio-inspired polydopamine for synergistic periodontal antibacterial therapeutics. *Carbohydr. Polym.* **2020**, *245*, 116585. [CrossRef]

18. Su, T.; Zhao, W.; Wu, L.; Dong, W.; Qi, X. Facile fabrication of functional hydrogels consisting of pullulan and polydopamine fibers for drug delivery. *Int. J. Biol. Macromol.* **2020**, *163*, 366–374. [CrossRef]
19. Zhang, M.; Huang, Y.; Pan, W.; Tong, X.; Zeng, Q.; Su, T.; Qi, X.; Shen, J. Polydopamine-incorporated dextran hydrogel drug carrier with tailorable structure for wound healing. *Carbohydr. Polym.* **2021**, *253*, 117213. [CrossRef] [PubMed]
20. Tomić, I.; Juretić, M.; Jug, M.; Pepić, I.; Čižmek, B.C.; Filipović-Grčić, J. Preparation of in situ hydrogels loaded with azelaic acid nanocrystals and their dermal application performance study. *Int. J. Pharm.* **2019**, *563*, 249–258. [CrossRef]
21. Moolakkadath, T.; Aqil, M.; Ahad, A.; Imam, S.S.; Iqbal, B.; Sultana, Y.; Mujeeb, M.; Iqbal, Z. Development of transethosomes formulation for dermal fisetin delivery: Box–Behnken design, optimization, in vitro skin penetration, vesicles–skin interaction and dermatokinetic studies. *Artif. Cells Nanomed. Biotechnol.* **2018**, *46* (Suppl. S2), 755–765. [CrossRef]
22. Salem, H.F.; Kharshoum, R.M.; Awad, S.M.; Mostafa, M.A.; Abou-Taleb, H.A. Tailoring of retinyl palmitate-based ethosomal hydrogel as a novel nanoplatform for acne vulgaris management: Fabrication, optimization, and clinical evaluation employing a split-face comparative study. *Int. J. Nanomed.* **2021**, *16*, 4251–4276. [CrossRef]
23. Kadam, T.; Darekar, A.; Gondkar, S.; Saudagar, R. Development and validation of spectrophotometric method for determination of azelaic acid. *Asian J. Res. Pharm. Sci.* **2015**, *5*, 83. [CrossRef]
24. Sudhakar, K.; Mishra, V.; Jain, S.; Rompicherla, N.C.; Malviya, N.; Tambuwala, M.M. Development and evaluation of the effect of ethanol and surfactant in vesicular carriers on Lamivudine permeation through the skin. *Int. J. Pharm.* **2021**, *610*, 121226. [CrossRef]
25. Albash, R.; Abdellatif, M.M.; Hassan, M.; Badawi, N.M. Tailoring Terpesomes and Leciplex for the Effective Ocular Conveyance of Moxifloxacin Hydrochloride (Comparative Assessment): In-vitro, Ex-vivo, and In-vivo Evaluation. *Int. J. Nanomed.* **2021**, *16*, 5247–5263. [CrossRef]
26. Nasr, A.M.; Elhady, S.S.; Swidan, S.A.; Badawi, N.M. Celecoxib Loaded In-Situ Provesicular Powder and Its In-Vitro Cytotoxic Effect for Cancer Therapy: Fabrication, Characterization, Optimization and Pharmacokinetic Evaluation. *Pharmaceutics* **2020**, *12*, 1157. [CrossRef]
27. Teaima, M.; Abdelmonem, R.; Adel, Y.A.; El-Nabarawi, M.A.; El-Nawawy, T.M. Transdermal Delivery of Telmisartan: Formulation, in vitro, ex vivo, Iontophoretic Permeation Enhancement and Comparative Pharmacokinetic Study in Rats. *Drug Des. Dev. Ther.* **2021**, *15*, 4603–4614. [CrossRef] [PubMed]
28. Hung, W.-H.; Chen, P.-K.; Fang, C.-W.; Lin, Y.-C.; Wu, P.-C. Preparation and evaluation of azelaic acid topical microemulsion formulation: In vitro and in vivo study. *Pharmaceutics* **2021**, *13*, 410. [CrossRef]
29. Teaima, M.H.; Badawi, N.M.; Attia, D.A.; El-Nabarawi, M.A.; Elmazar, M.M.; Mousa, S.A. Efficacy of pomegranate extract loaded solid lipid nanoparticles transdermal emulgel against Ehrlich ascites carcinoma. *Nanomed. Nanotechnol. Biol. Med.* **2022**, *39*, 102466. [CrossRef] [PubMed]
30. Albash, R.; Abdelbary, A.A.; Refai, H.; El-Nabarawi, M.A. Use of transethosomes for enhancing the transdermal delivery of olmesartan medoxomil: In vitro, ex vivo, and in vivo evaluation. *Int. J. Nanomed.* **2019**, *14*, 1953–1968. [CrossRef]
31. Malik, D.S.; Kaur, G. Nanostructured gel for topical delivery of azelaic acid: Designing, characterization, and in-vitro evaluation. *J. Drug Deliv. Sci. Technol.* **2018**, *47*, 123–136. [CrossRef]
32. de Hoog, G.S.; Guarro, J. *Atlas of Clinical Fungi*; Centraalbureau Voor Schimmelcultures: Baarn, The Netherlands, 1995.
33. Gozubuyuk, G.; Aktas, E.; Yigit, N. An ancient plant Lawsonia inermis (henna): Determination of in vitro antifungal activity against dermatophytes species. *J. Med. Mycol.* **2014**, *24*, 313–318. [CrossRef]
34. Taha, M.; Tartor, Y.H.; Abdul-Haq, S.I.M.; El-Maati, M.F.A. Characterization and Antidermatophyte Activity of Henna Extracts: A Promising Therapy for Humans and Animals Dermatophytoses. *Curr. Microbiol.* **2022**, *79*, 59. [CrossRef]
35. Brasch, J.; Christophers, E. Azelaic acid has antimycotic properties in vitro. *Dermatology* **1993**, *186*, 55–58. [CrossRef]
36. Silva, M.R.R.; Oliveira, J.G.; Fernandes, O.F.L.; Passos, X.S.; Costa, C.R.; Souza, L.K.H.; Lemos, J.A.; de Paula, J.R. Antifungal activity of Ocimum gratissimum towards dermatophytes. *Mycoses* **2005**, *48*, 172–175. [CrossRef] [PubMed]
37. CLSI. *M38–A2 Reference Method for Broth Dilution Antifungal Susceptibility Testing of Filamentous fungi*; CLSI: Berwyn, PA, USA, 2017. Available online: https://clsi.org/media/1894/m38ed3_sample.pdf (accessed on 20 February 2023).
38. Schwarz, S.; Silley, P.; Simjee, S.; Woodford, N.; Van Duijkeren, E.; Johnson, A.P.; Gaastra, W. Assessing the antimicrobial susceptibility of bacteria obtained from animals. *J. Antimicrob. Chemother.* **2010**, *65*, 601–604. [CrossRef] [PubMed]
39. Saunte, D.M.; Hasselby, J.P.; Brillowska-Dabrowska, A.; Frimodt-Møller, N.; Svejgaard, E.L.; Linnemann, D.; Nielsen, S.S.; Hædersdal, M.; Arendrup, M.C. Experimental guinea pig model of dermatophytosis: A simple and useful tool for the evaluation of new diagnostics and antifungals. *Med. Mycol.* **2008**, *46*, 303–313. [CrossRef] [PubMed]
40. Borgers, M.; Xhonneux, B.; Van Cutsem, J. Oral itraconazole versus topical bifonazole treatment in experimental dermatophytosis: Orale Itraconazol-vs topische Bifonazol-Behandlung bei experirnenteller Dermatophytose. *Mycoses* **1993**, *36*, 105–115. [CrossRef]
41. Soleimanian, Y.; Goli, S.A.H.; Varshosaz, J.; Sahafi, S.M. Formulation and characterization of novel nanostructured lipid carriers made from beeswax, propolis wax and pomegranate seed oil. *Food Chem.* **2018**, *244*, 83–92. [CrossRef] [PubMed]
42. Ahad, A.; Aqil, M.; Kohli, K.; Sultana, Y.; Mujeeb, M.; Ali, A. Formulation and optimization of nanotransfersomes using experimental design technique for accentuated transdermal delivery of valsartan. *Nanomed. Nanotechnol. Biol. Med.* **2012**, *8*, 237–249. [CrossRef] [PubMed]

43. Vasanth, S.; Dubey, A.; Ravi, G.S.; Lewis, S.A.; Ghate, V.M.; El-Zahaby, S.A.; Hebbar, S. Development and investigation of vitamin C-enriched adapalene-loaded transfersome gel: A collegial approach for the treatment of acne vulgaris. *AAPS PharmSciTech* **2020**, *21*, 61. [CrossRef] [PubMed]
44. Ahmed, T.A.; Alzahrani, M.M.; Sirwi, A.; Alhakamy, N.A. Study the antifungal and ocular permeation of ketoconazole from ophthalmic formulations containing trans-ethosomes nanoparticles. *Pharmaceutics* **2021**, *13*, 151. [CrossRef] [PubMed]
45. Limsuwan, T.; Amnuaikit, T. Development of ethosomes containing mycophenolic acid. *Procedia Chem.* **2012**, *4*, 328–335. [CrossRef]
46. Nasr, A.M.; Moftah, F.; Abourehab, M.A.S.; Gad, S. Design, Formulation, and Characterization of Valsartan Nanoethosomes for Improving Their Bioavailability. *Pharmaceutics* **2022**, *14*, 2268. [CrossRef]
47. Qushawy, M.; Nasr, A.; Abd-Alhaseeb, M.; Swidan, S.A. Design, optimization and characterization of a transfersomal gel using miconazole nitrate for the treatment of candida skin infections. *Pharmaceutics* **2018**, *10*, 26. [CrossRef] [PubMed]
48. Balata, G.F.; Faisal, M.M.; Elghamry, H.A.; Sabry, S.A. Preparation and characterization of ivabradine HCl transfersomes for enhanced transdermal delivery. *J. Drug Deliv. Sci. Technol.* **2020**, *60*, 101921. [CrossRef]
49. Ogiso, T.; Yamaguchi, T.; Iwaki, M.; Tanino, T.; Miyake, Y. Effect of positively and negatively charged liposomes on skin permeation of drugs. *J. Drug Target.* **2001**, *9*, 49–59. [CrossRef]
50. Jain, S.; Umamaheshwari, R.B.; Bhadra, D.; Jain, N.K. Ethosomes: A novel vesicular carrier for enhanced transdermal delivery of an antiHIV agent. *Indian J. Pharm. Sci.* **2004**, *66*, 72.
51. Salem, H.F.; Kharshoum, R.M.; Abou-Taleb, H.; Aboutaleb, H.A.; Abouelhassan, K.M. Progesterone-loaded nanosized transethosomes for vaginal permeation enhancement: Formulation, statistical optimization, and clinical evaluation in anovulatory polycystic ovary syndrome. *J. Liposome Res.* **2019**, *29*, 183–194. [CrossRef]
52. van den Bergh, B.A.; Wertz, P.W.; Junginger, H.E.; Bouwstra, J.A. Elasticity of vesicles assessed by electron spin resonance, electron microscopy and extrusion measurements. *Int. J. Pharm.* **2001**, *217*, 13–24. [CrossRef]
53. El Zaafarany, G.M.; Awad, G.A.S.; Holayel, S.M.; Mortada, N.D. Role of edge activators and surface charge in developing ultradeformable vesicles with enhanced skin delivery. *Int. J. Pharm.* **2010**, *397*, 164–172. [CrossRef]
54. Amnuaikit, T.; Limsuwan, T.; Khongkow, P.; Boonme, P. Vesicular carriers containing phenylethyl resorcinol for topical delivery system; liposomes, transfersomes and invasomes. *Asian J. Pharm. Sci.* **2018**, *13*, 472–484. [CrossRef] [PubMed]
55. Heidari, H.; Razmi, H. Multi-response optimization of magnetic solid phase extraction based on carbon coated Fe_3O_4 nanoparticles using desirability function approach for the determination of the organophosphorus pesticides in aquatic samples by HPLC–UV. *Talanta* **2012**, *99*, 13–21. [CrossRef] [PubMed]
56. Tarassoli, Z.; Najjar, R.; Amani, A. Formulation and optimization of lemon balm extract loaded azelaic acid-chitosan nanoparticles for antibacterial applications. *J. Drug Deliv. Sci. Technol.* **2021**, *65*, 102687. [CrossRef]
57. Eissa, M.A.; Hashim, Y.Z.H.-Y.; Nasir, M.H.M.; Nor, Y.A.; Salleh, H.M.; Isa, M.L.; Abd-Azziz, S.S.S.; Warif, N.M.A.; Ramadan, E.; Badawi, N.M. Fabrication and characterization of Agarwood extract-loaded nanocapsules and evaluation of their toxicity and anti-inflammatory activity on RAW 264.7 cells and in zebrafish embryos. *Drug Deliv.* **2021**, *28*, 2618–2633. [CrossRef]
58. Badawi, N.M.; Attia, Y.M.; El-Kersh, D.M.; Hammam, O.A.; Khalifa, M.K. Investigating the Impact of Optimized Trans-Cinnamic Acid-Loaded PLGA Nanoparticles on Epithelial to Mesenchymal Transition in Breast Cancer. *Int. J. Nanomed.* **2022**, *17*, 733–750. [CrossRef]
59. Bisht, A.; Hemrajani, C.; Upadhyay, N.; Nidhi, P.; Rolta, R.; Rathore, C.; Gupta, G.; Dua, K.; Chellappan, D.K.; Dev, K.; et al. Azelaic acid and Melaleuca alternifolia essential oil co-loaded vesicular carrier for combinational therapy of acne. *Ther. Deliv.* **2021**, *13*, 13–29. [CrossRef]
60. Chittasobhon, N.; Smith, J.M. The production of experimental dermatophyte lesions in guinea pigs. *J. Investig. Dermatol.* **1979**, *73*, 198–201. [CrossRef] [PubMed]
61. Van Cutsem, J. Animal models for dermatomycotic infections. *Curr. Top. Med. Mycol.* **1989**, *3*, 1–35.
62. Kumar, P.; Ramteke, P.; Pandey, A.C.; Pandey, H. Evaluation of antifungal activity of blended cinnamon oil and usnic acid nanoemulsion using candidiasis and dermatophytosis models. *Biocatal. Agric. Biotechnol.* **2019**, *18*, 101062. [CrossRef]
63. Treiber, A.; Pittermann, W.; Schuppe, H.-C. Efficacy testing of antimycotic prophylactics in an animal model. *Int. J. Hyg. Environ. Health* **2001**, *204*, 239–243. [CrossRef] [PubMed]
64. Ghannoum, M.A.; Hossain, M.A.; Long, L.; Mohamed, S.; Reyes, G.; Mukherjee, P.K. Evaluation of antifungal efficacy in an optimized animal model of *Trichophyton mentagrophytes*-dermatophytosis. *J. Chemother.* **2004**, *16*, 139–144. [CrossRef] [PubMed]
65. Sieber, M.; Hegel, J. Azelaic acid: Properties and mode of action. *Ski. Pharmacol. Physiol.* **2014**, *27* (Suppl. S1), 9–17.
66. Tartor, Y.H.; El-Neshwy, W.M.; Merwad, A.M.A.; El-Maati, M.F.A.; Mohamed, R.E.; Dahshan, H.M.; Mahmoud, H.I. Ringworm in calves: Risk factors, improved molecular diagnosis, and therapeutic efficacy of an Aloe vera gel extract. *BMC Vet. Res.* **2020**, *16*, 421. [CrossRef] [PubMed]
67. Van Cutsem, J. Oral and parenteral treatment with itraconazole in various superficial and systemic experimental fungal infections. Comparisons with other antifungals and combination therapy. *Br. J. Clin. Pract.* **1990**, *44* (Suppl. S71), 32–40.
68. Nagino, K.; Shimohira, H.; Ogawa, M.; Uchida, K.; Yamaguchi, H. Comparison of the therapeutic efficacy of oral doses of fluconazole and itraconazole in a guinea pig model of dermatophytosis. *J. Infect. Chemother.* **2000**, *6*, 41–44. [CrossRef]

69. Nayak, D.; Tawale, R.M.; Aranjani, J.M.; Tippavajhala, V.K. Formulation, optimization and evaluation of novel ultra-deformable vesicular drug delivery system for an anti-fungal drug. *AAPS PharmSciTech* **2020**, *21*, 140.
70. Lalvand, M.; Hashemi, S.J.; Bayat, M. Effect of fluconazole and terbinafine nanoparticles on the treatment of dermatophytosis induced by *Trichophyton mentagrophytes* in guinea pig. *Iran. J. Microbiol.* **2021**, *13*, 608. [CrossRef]
71. Maheshwari, R.G.S.; Tekade, R.K.; Sharma, P.A.; Darwhekar, G.; Tyagi, A.; Patel, R.P.; Jain, D.K. Ethosomes and ultradeformable liposomes for transdermal delivery of clotrimazole: A comparative assessment. *Saudi Pharm. J.* **2012**, *20*, 161–170. [CrossRef]

Disclaimer/Publisher's Note: The statements, opinions and data contained in all publications are solely those of the individual author(s) and contributor(s) and not of MDPI and/or the editor(s). MDPI and/or the editor(s) disclaim responsibility for any injury to people or property resulting from any ideas, methods, instructions or products referred to in the content.

MDPI AG
Grosspeteranlage 5
4052 Basel
Switzerland
Tel.: +41 61 683 77 34

Antibiotics Editorial Office
E-mail: antibiotics@mdpi.com
www.mdpi.com/journal/antibiotics

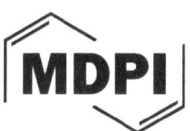

Disclaimer/Publisher's Note: The title and front matter of this reprint are at the discretion of the Guest Editor. The publisher is not responsible for their content or any associated concerns. The statements, opinions and data contained in all individual articles are solely those of the individual Editor and contributors and not of MDPI. MDPI disclaims responsibility for any injury to people or property resulting from any ideas, methods, instructions or products referred to in the content.

www.ingramcontent.com/pod-product-compliance
Lightning Source LLC
LaVergne TN
LVHW072354090526
838202LV00019B/2543